Emotional Intelligence:
Modern Outlook and Applications

Emotional Intelligence: Modern Outlook and Applications

Edited by **Charles Freeman**

FOSTER
ACADEMICS

New Jersey

Published by Foster Academics,
61 Van Reypen Street,
Jersey City, NJ 07306, USA
www.fosteracademics.com

Emotional Intelligence: Modern Outlook and Applications
Edited by Charles Freeman

International Standard Book Number: 978-1-63242-125-8 (Hardback)

Printed in the United States of America.

Contents

Preface

This book was inspired by the evolution of our times; to answer the curiosity of inquisitive minds. Many developments have occurred across the globe in the recent past which has transformed the progress in the field.

The modern outlooks as well as applications of emotional intelligence are described in this detailed book. Emotional intelligence is an evolving field for applied research and possible interventions, both in scholastic, academic, educational and organizational contexts, as well as at an individual level in terms of people's well-being and life satisfaction. This book displays an interest to give an international point of view, rich of stimuli and perspectives for research and intervention, in relation to a promising variable of current interest, such as emotional intelligence. This book aims to further contribute to affirmation of a particularly promising variable such as emotional intelligence which needs additional interest and concentration in both research and application domain.

This book was developed from a mere concept to drafts to chapters and finally compiled together as a complete text to benefit the readers across all nations. To ensure the quality of the content we instilled two significant steps in our procedure. The first was to appoint an editorial team that would verify the data and statistics provided in the book and also select the most appropriate and valuable contributions from the plentiful contributions we received from authors worldwide. The next step was to appoint an expert of the topic as the Editor-in-Chief, who would head the project and finally make the necessary amendments and modifications to make the text reader-friendly. I was then commissioned to examine all the material to present the topics in the most comprehensible and productive format.

I would like to take this opportunity to thank all the contributing authors who were supportive enough to contribute their time and knowledge to this project. I also wish to convey my regards to my family who have been extremely supportive during the entire project.

Editor

Part 1

Emotional Intelligence:
Theory, Research and Future Perspectives

Emotional Intelligence

Adrian Furnham
Research Department of Clinical, Educational and Health Psychology
University College London
UK

"Emotional intelligence is an organising framework for categorising abilities relating to understanding, managing and using feelings (P SALOVEY & J MAYER 1994)
"Emotional Intelligence: long neglected core component of mental ability or faddish and confused idea massively commercialised" (A. FURNHAM 2001)

1. Introduction

It has been suggested that there are now well over 10,000 scholarly books, chapters and papers on emotional intelligence. This is remarkable given that it has only been 21 years since the topic first appeared under that name in the psychological literature. If you Google Amazon you will find around 20 books with Emotional Intelligence in the title and three to five times that number dealing with the concept in one form or another.

The history of emotional intelligence is this: In 1920 the concept of "Social Intelligence" was first introduced; in 1990 the first published scientific paper on the topic using this term; in 1995 Goleman wrote the best seller "Emotional Intelligence"; in 1997 the first popular self-report questionnaire was developed; in 2003 the first ability measure devised. There is now a comprehensive Wikipaedia entry on the topic and various very serious handbooks and reviews.

A few authors are very well known. One very well known model is that of Bar-On (1988). According to the Bar-On model, *emotional intelligence consists of interrelated emotional and social competencies, skills and facilitators that determine how well we understand and express ourselves, understand others and relate with them, and cope with daily demands, challenges and pressures.* The emotional and social competencies, skills and facilitators included in this broad definition of the construct are based on the 5 meta-factors: intrapersonal EQ, interpersonal EQ, Stress management EQ, Adaptability EQ and General Mood EQ. Other models, notably that of Petrides and Furnham (2000 ab, 2003) is given below.

Since first coined by Thorndike (1920) and echoed later by Guilford (1967) psychologists have been interested in the "social intelligences". These are nearly always put in "inverted commas" because, strictly speaking, they are not intelligences but conceived of as social skills, even dispositions/traits that have both multiple causes and multiple consequences.

There are many explanations for the long standing interest in the "social intelligences". Cognitive ability/intelligence rarely explains more than a third to a half of the variance in any outcome measure, be it academic achievement, job performance or health. The question is, do the social intelligences account for incremental variance over IQ test results? A second reason is that it is difficult to improve or teach cognitive ability.Third, for over twenty years new advocates of "multiple intelligence" have been enormously successful in persuading people both of their existence and importance, despite the quality of their empirical evidence.

The question is what is social intelligence? Eysenck (1985) conceived of a useful model that differentiated three types of intelligence – biological, psychometric and social – and what factors influenced it. As we shall see there remains debate and discussion as to whether EI is a "real" intelligence or rather a social intelligence.

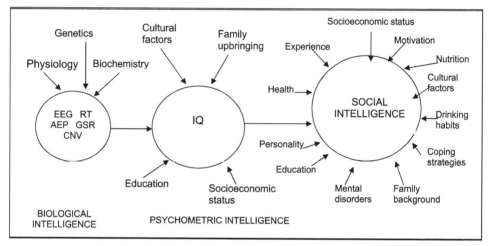

Fig. 1. Eysenck's representation of three different conceptions of "intelligence". In this model many things, like cognitive ability, predict social intelligence.

Mackintosh (1998) argued that social intelligence was social competence and success in social interaction that is adaptive and can be seen in other animal species. It allows individuals to understand others' hopes, fears, beliefs and wishes. He noted that it is not too difficult to define social intelligence (mainly in terms of social skills) nor devise tests to measure it. He doubted two things: first, if these many social and interpersonal skills actually load on a single dimension, and second whether they are uncorrelated with, and therefore related to, standard IQ measures of cognitive ability.

Various researchers have reviewed the concept of social intelligence including its discriminant validity, relationship to personality and classic cognitive ability, its role in "life tasks" and how it develops over time. They believe it is multifactional, relating to such issues as social sensitivity, social insight and social communication. In other words it is much more of a social or personality variable than a cognitive variable which is more about information processing and accumulation. Hence trait emotional intelligence (Petrides & Furnham, 2001, 2003, 2006). Others like Landy (2006) are much more circumspect about the concept. This is nicely described in the title of his chapter heading: "The long, frustrating and fruitless search for social intelligence".

2. Multiple intelligences

Over the past decade or so there has been an explosion in the number of "multiple intelligences" discovered. Hardly a year goes by before yet another is discovered. The following table shows 14 'different intelligences'.

	Multiple Intelligence	Author	Year
1.	Analytical	Sternberg	1997
2.	Bodily-kinesthetic	Gardner	1999
3.	Creative	Sternberg	1997
4.	Emotional	Salovey and Mayer	1990
5.	Interpersonal	Gardner	1999
6.	Intrapersonal	Gardner	1999
7.	Mathematical	Gardner	1999
8.	Musical	Gardner	1999
9.	Naturalistic	Gardner	1999
10.	Practical	Sternberg	1997
11.	Sexual	Conrad and Milburn	2001
12.	Spatial	Gardner	1999
13.	Spiritual	Emmons	2000
14.	Verbal	Gardner	1999

Table 1. The many identified multiple intelligences

Among academic researchers social intelligences are not usually considered part of cognitive ability and "intelligences" is always put in inverted commas. There are two reasons for this: *first*, there is very little good, empirical evidence supporting the idea that these are separate, distinguishable factors from each other; *second*, they seem unrelated to traditional measures of intelligence. More interesting, in a variety of studies, Furnham (2001) has shown lay people believe many of the multiple intelligences (i.e. musical, bodily-kinesthetic, emotions) are *not* linked to traditional ideas of intelligence.

The two figures most powerfully involved with the multiple intelligence world are Sternberg (1997) and Gardner (1983, 1999). Gardner (1983) defined intelligence as "the ability to solve problems or to create products that are valued within one or more cultural setting" (p.11) and specified seven intelligences. He argued that *linguistic/verbal* and *logical/mathematical intelligences* are those typically valued in educational settings. Linguistic intelligence involves sensitivity to the spoken and written language and the ability to learn languages. Logical-mathematical intelligence involves the capacity to analyse problems logically, solve maths problems and investigate issues scientifically. These two types of intelligence dominate intelligence tests.

Three other multiple intelligences are arts based: *musical intelligence* which refers to skill in the performance, composition and appreciation of musical patterns; *bodily kinaesthetic intelligence* which is based on the use of the whole or parts of the body to solve problems or to fashion products; and *spatial intelligence* which is the ability to recognise and manipulate patterns in space. There are also two personal intelligences: *interpersonal intelligence* which is the capacity to understand the intentions, motivations and desires of other people and to work effectively with them; and *intrapersonal intelligence* which is the capacity to understand oneself and to use this information effectively in regulating one's life. It is these latter two intelligence that *combined* make up emotional intelligences.

However, in his later book Gardner (1999) defines intelligence as a "biopsychological potential to process information that can be activated in a cultural setting to solve problems or create products that are of value in a culture" (p.33-34). In it, he introduces three possible new intelligences although he notes: "The strength of the evidence for these varies, and whether or not to declare a certain human capacity another type of intelligence is certainly a judgement call" (p.47). However, he only added one new intelligence, namely *naturalistic intelligence* which is "expertise in the recognition and classification of the numerous species – the flora and fauna – of his or her environment" (p.43). It is the capacity to taxonomise: to recognise members of a group, to distinguish among members of a species and to chart out the relations, formally or informally, among several species. The other two were spiritual and existential intelligences. *Spiritual intelligence* is the ability to master a set of diffuse and abstract concepts about being, but also mastering the craft of altering one's consciousness in attaining a certain state of being. This has recently become an issue of considerable debate (Emmons, 2000). *Existential intelligence* is yet more difficult to define: "the capacity to locate oneself with respect to the furthest reaches of the cosmos – the infinite and infinitesimal – and the related capacity to locate oneself with respect to such existential features of the human condition as the significance of life, the meaning of death, the ultimate fate of the physical and the psychological worlds and such profound experiences as love of another person or total immersion in a work of art" (p.61).

Despite its popularity in educational circles, Gardner's theory has been consistently attacked and criticised by those working empirically in the area (Allix, 2000; Klein, 1997; Morgan, 1996: White, 2005). Visser, Ashton and Vernon (2006) tested 200 participants giving them eight tests of the Gardner intelligences. Factor analysis reveal, against the Gardner theory, a large g factor. The highest loading tests on this g factor were Linguistic (Verbal), Logical/Mathematical, Spatial, Naturalistic and Interpersonal intelligences. The authors concluded: "Results support previous findings that highly diverse tests of purely cognitive abilities share strong loadings on a factor of general intelligence and that abilities involving sensory, motor or personality influences are less strongly g-loaded". (p.487). Later they conclude: " The substantial g-loadings of all purely cognitive tests in the current study contradict Gardner's assertion that there are at least eight independent intelligence domains. Although Gardner has acknowledged the existence of g and has conceded that the eight intelligences might not be entirely independent, his contention that positive correlations between various cognitive tasks are largely due to verbal demands was clearly not supported in this study, in which those verbal demands were minimized. Instead, measures of Linguistic, Spatial, Logical-Mathematical, Naturalistic, and Interpersonal intelligences showed a positive manifold of correlations, substantial loadings on a g factor, and substantial correlations with an outside measure of general intelligence. The common element that saturated the highly g loaded tests most strongly was their demand on reasoning abilities, not their specifically verbal content.

Sternberg (1997) has also developed a multi-dimensional model also known as the "triarchic" theory of "successful" intelligence. This posits that human intelligence comprises three aspects, that is, componential, experiential and contextual. The *componential* aspect refers to a person's ability to learn new things, to think analytically and to solve problems. This aspect of intelligence is manifested through better performance on standard intelligence tests, which require general knowledge and ability in areas such as arithmetic and vocabulary. The *experiential* aspect refers to a person's ability to combine different experiences in unique and creative ways. It concerns original thinking and creativity in both the arts and the sciences. Finally, the *contextual* aspect refers to a person's ability to deal with practical aspects of the environment and to adapt to new and changing contexts. This aspect of intelligence resembles what lay people sometimes refer to as "street smarts". Sternberg (1997) popularised these concepts and refers to them as analytic, creative and practical intelligence. However, practical intelligence theory has also attracted very serious criticism. Gottfredson (2003) in an extremely exhaustive review of all the work in the area disputes Sternberg's central claim that there exists a general factor of practical intelligence (made up of the three intelligences) that is distinct from academic intelligence as usually conceived.

Interest in emotional intelligence began at the same time as an interest in the multiple intelligences. Throughout this period there was disillusionment with orthodox intelligence (cognitive ability) testing. It was believed that IQ tests were devise and discriminatory and that most people knew of very clever people who were quite obviously not very successful at work. The concept of EI seemed to "arrive" just at the right time to become very popular.

3. Defining emotional intelligence

Despite its popularity, and the fact that most people claim to have heard of it, very few can accurately define emotional intelligence. Sceptics claim that "charm and influence" became "social and interpersonal skills" which has become "emotional intelligence". The new term and concept chimed with the zeitgeist and became very popular. It spawned a huge industry particularly with those interested in success at work. Many books make dramatic claims: for instance that cognitive ability or traditional academic intelligence contributes only about 20% to general life success (academic, personal and work) while the remaining 80% is directly attributable to EI.

Below is a simple 2x2 way of conceiving on EI: self vs other; emotional awareness vs management.

Goleman's (1995) book told a simple and interesting story about emotional intelligence that helped explain its appeal. Technical training in the essential job knowledge of any career is easy compared to teaching IQ skills. That is, as an adult it is comparatively more straight forward to teach a person the technical aspects of the job than the soft skills. The idea is that there is a critical period to acquire the basis of EI which is probably during early to late adolescence. The young person, often a male, may experience social anxiety, discomfort and rejection while attempting to interact with and influence others (specifically those they are attracted to, which is most often people of the opposite sex).

Hence they may over time find solace in computers and other activities with a high skills/low contact basis. Thus, in early adulthood, they appear to be technically competent in certain areas (IT, engineering) but still rather undeveloped in people skills and more specifically emotional awareness and regulation. They may even be 'phobic' about emotional issues and resistant to (social skills) training. It is also assumed that people are less able to pick up EI 'skills' as well as less willing to try. To acquire technical skills often requires considerable dedication so opportunities to acquire social skills (EQ) are, therefore, reduced. Then the low EQ person chooses technology rather than people for fun, comfort, a source of ideas because they do not understand emotions.

Emotional Competencies

Self Awareness • Emotional Self-Awareness • Self Confidence • Accurate Self-Assessment	_Social Awareness_ • Empathy • Organisational Awareness • Service Orientation
Self Management • Emotional Self-Control • Adaptability • Achievement Orientation • Optimism • Initiative • Transparency	_Relationship Management_ • Influence • Conflict Management • Ins. Leadership • Change Catalyst • Developing Others • Teamwork and Collaboration

Some adults often tend to be rigid, with poor self-control, poor social skills and are weak at building bonds. Understanding and using emotions/feelings are at the heart of business and indeed being human. Often business people prefer to talk about emotional competencies (rather than traits or abilities) which are essentially learned capabilities. Emotional competencies include: emotional self-awareness, emotional self-regulation, social-emotional awareness, regulating emotions in others: understanding emotions, etc. If one is to include older related concepts, like social skills or interpersonal competencies, it is possible to find a literature dating back thirty years showing these skills predict occupational effectiveness and success. Further, there is convincing empirical literature that suggests these skills can be improved and learnt.

4. Emotional intelligence as a management fads

The application of EI in the work place seems the virtual prototype of a fad. Furnham (2006) suggested that all management fads have a similar natural history which has seven separate identifiable phases: One question is whether EQ will follow this trajectory, and if so, where is it now?

a. *Academic Discovery:* Faddish ideas can often be traced to the world of academia. A modest discovery may result in a paper in a specialist journal. These papers show the causal link between two factors relevant to work situations. These papers are not only complicated and heavily statistical but they are cautious and preliminary. Academics often call for replications, more research, they are hesitant and underline the complexity of all the actual and possible factors involved. The early social and emotional intelligence papers are a little like this. However, it is difficult to trace the concept to one study or paper.

b.   *Description of the Study:*This process can last a long time, and usually involves a lot of elaboration and distortion in the process. Someone reads the paper and provides a summary. Others hear it and repeat it. But with every repetition, the findings become stronger and the complexity weaker. In this sense effect size estimates go up and criticisms about experimental technique go down. The crucial findings are recorded and embellished.

c.   *Popularisation in a Best Seller:* The next stage is a business writer/guru takes up the call, hears about the finding, gives them a catchy title and before you know what the fad is about to begin. That one single, simple idea/finding/process soon becomes a book. This is where the Goleman (1998) book plays such an important role. It is very widely reviewed in the media around the world. It is at this stage that the fad becomes a *buzzword*.

d.   *Consultant Hype and Universalisation:* It is not the academic or the author that really powers the fad but an army of management consultants trying to look as if they are at the cutting edge of management theory. Because the concepts are easy to understand and are said to have wide application, the consultants seek to apply them everywhere. What made the EQ phenomena different? Two things: first the web which now has a very big impact on the rapid and universal popularisation of ideas. The second was the rapid development of measures of EQ. The concept not only struck home but it could be (supposedly) efficiently and validly measured very easily. It was the measurement of EQ that really appealed to the management consultants.

e.   *Total Commitment by "the believers":*At this point, the evangelists move from the consultants to the managers. For a small number of companies, the technique *seems* to have brought quick, massive benefits. They become happy and willing product champions, which only serves to sell more books and fan the fires of faddishness. EQ champions are paraded at conferences. EQ awareness, courses and training improve performance and make people into better managers.

f.   *Doubt, Scepticism and Defection:* After pride comes the fall. After a few years of heavy product selling, the appetite for the fad becomes diminished. The market is saturated. Various 'new and improved'; or just as likely 'shorter and simpler'; versions of the fad are introduced. But it is apparent that the enthusiasm is gone. Managerial doubt follows academic scepticism, followed by journalistic cynicism, and finally consultant defection. It may be that the whole process starts with people pointing out the poor cost-benefit analysis of introducing the fad. Or it may occur because someone goes back to the original finding and shows that the gap has widened so much between what was initially demonstrated and what is now done, that the two are different species.

g.   *New Discoveries:* The end of one fad is an ideal time for trainers, writers and consultant to spot a gap in the market. They know there is an incurable thirst for a magic bullet, fix-all solutions, so the whole process starts again. The really clever people begin to sense when the previous fad is reaching its sell-by-date, so that they have just enough time to write their new best seller to get the market just right.

Is EI a management or educational fad? Has it passed through the above phases? And if so where is it now? Certainly the academics are only now beginning to respond with careful, considered research that attempts to unpick the concept. Suddenly the academic journals, particularly in differential psychology, are bursting with papers that take (hopefully) a disinterested scientific and measured look at EI (Austin, 2004; Chan, 2004; Roberts, Zeidner & Matthews, 2001). There has also appeared a serious, thoughtful and balanced review of work in the area (Matthews, Zeidner & Roberts, 2002). Academic researchers are not immune to fad and fashion. However the lag time is longer and thus what interests the two worlds of science and practice may easily be out-of-synchrony.

5. The components of EQ

There remains still no agreement about what features, factors, abilities or skills do or do not form part of EI. As more and more tests of, and books about EI appear on the market the situation gets worse rather than better. Most, but not all theories and systems include ideas about emotional awareness and regulation. Some distinguish between intra and interpersonal emotional skills. Some use the concept of ability, others of skills, and some of competencies.

Facets	High Scorers perceive themselves as being or having……
Adaptability	Flexible and willing to adapt to new conditions
Assertiveness	Forthright, frank and willing to stand up for their rights
Emotion expression	Capable of communicating their feelings to others
Emotion management (others)	Capable of influencing other people's feelings
Emotion perception (self-and others)	Clear about their own and other people's feelings
Emotion regulation	Capable of controlling their emotions
Impulsiveness (low)	Reflective and less likely to give into their urges
Relationship skills	Capable of having fulfilling personal relationships
Self-Esteem	Successful and self-confident
Self-Motivation	Driven and unlikely to give up in the face of adversity
Social competence	Accomplished networkers with excellent social skills
Stress management	Capable of withstanding pressure and regulating stress
Trait empathy	Capable to taking someone else's perspective
Trait happiness	Cheerful and satisfied with their lives
Trait optimism	Confident and likely to 'look on the bright side' of life.

Table 2. Common facets in salient models of EI

This lack of agreement is typical at the beginning of the academic exploration of a new concept. Indeed disagreement can continue for decades as big egos slog it out both conceptually and empirically to prove the validity and veridicality of their system. It does however make it particularly frustrating and confusing for the interested lay person.

A central unresolved question is what are the facets or components of EI. Thus early models distinguished between the perception, appraisal and expression of emotion in self and others; using emotion to facilitate thinking; the use of emotional knowledge to understand

and analyse emotions as well as the reflective regulation of emotions to promote growth. Some writers talk of *emotional literacy* (which involves the knowledge and understanding of one's own emotions and how they function), *emotional fitness* (which involves trustworthiness and emotional hardiness and flexibility), *emotional depth* (which involves emotional growth and intensity), and *emotional alchemy* (which involves using emotions to discover creative opportunities).

Others "divide up" EI into factors like self-awareness, self-regulation, self-motivation, empathy, and social skills. One more popular conception has 15 components (Petrides & Furnham, 2003)

These fifteen scales can be combined into four related, but independent, factors labelled well-being, self-control skills, emotional skills and social skills.

Another measure, less impressive psychometrically, but well marketed, has different scales and dimesions

Intrapersonal (self-awareness and self-expression)

- **Self-Regard**: To accurately perceive, understand and accept oneself
- **Emotional Self-Awareness**: To be aware of and understand one's emotions
- **Assertiveness**: To effectively and constructively express one's emotions and oneself
- **Independence**: To be self-reliant and free of emotional dependency on others
- **Self-Actualization**: To strive to achieve personal goals and actualize one's potential

Interpersonal (social awareness and interpersonal relationship)

- **Empathy**: To be aware of and understand how others feel
- **Social Responsibility**: To identify with one's social group and cooperate with others
- **Interpersonal Relationship**: To establish mutually satisfying relationships and relate well with others

Stress Management (emotional management and regulation)

- **Stress Tolerance**: To effectively and constructively manage emotions
- **Impulse Control**: To effectively and constructively control emotions

Adaptability (change management)

- **Reality-Testing**: To objectively validate one's feelings and thinking with external reality
- **Flexibility**: To adapt and adjust one's feelings and thinking to new situations
- **Problem-Solving**: To effectively solve problems of a personal and interpersonal nature

General Mood (self-motivation)

- **Optimism**: To be positive and look at the brighter side of life
- **Happiness**: To feel content with oneself, others and life in general

Other scales have yet different dimensions depending on how EI is defined and measured. This makes life rather complicated for the practitioner who is not always clear as to what measure to use and why.

6. Measurement

Dispute about what to measure when trying to ascertain a person's EI is paradoxically clearer but much more passionate when it comes to EI. Psychometricians make a basic distinction between measures of *maximum* performance (e.g. IQ tests – right or wrong answers) and measures of *typical* response (e.g. personality questionnaires, preference answers) which has far-reaching implications. Self-report measurement leads to the idea of EI as a personality trait ('trait EI' or 'emotional self-efficacy), whereas potential maximum-performance measurement would lead to ideas of EI as a cognitive ability ('ability EI' or 'cognitive-emotional ability).

Thus trait EI and ability EI are two *different constructs*. The primary basis for discriminating between trait EI and ability EI is found in the type of measurement approach one chooses to employ. Many dispute the more fundamental point that EI could ever be actually measured by cognitive ability tests. That is, EI concepts, like emotional regulation, can never be reliably and validly measured by an objective ability test because of the subjective nature of emotional experience.

A major difficulty with the measurement of ability EI is that emotional experiences are inherently subjective and, consequently lack the objectivity required to make them amenable to robust, valid and reliable maximum performance measurement. There is no simple way of applying truly veridical criteria in the objective scoring of items relating to the intrapersonal component of ability EI (e.g. "I am aware of my emotions as I experience them") simply because the application of such scoring procedures would require direct access to privileged information, such as inner feelings and private cognitions, that is available only to the individual who is being assessed.

This dispute has not prevented many people developing both types of tests. There currently exists well over a dozen trait EI type tests which look essentially like personality tests. On the other hand, there are those who see EI as a "real" intelligence or ability that needs to be measured as such. The most well established measure is called the MSCEIT. It measures four factors: perceiving and identifying emotions (the ability to recognise how you and those around you are feeling), using emotions to facilitate thought (the ability to generate emotion, and then reason with this emotion), understanding emotions (the ability to understand complex emotions and emotional 'chains', and how emotions evolve), and managing emotions (the ability to manage emotions in yourself and in others)

The eight task-level scores are reported for research and qualitative use only. The MSCEIT asks test takers to:

Identify the emotions expressed by a face or in designs.

Generate a mood and solve problems with that mood.

Define the causes of different emotions. Understand the progression of emotions.

Determine how to best include emotion in our thinking in situations that involve ourselves or other people.

The 'objective' scoring is based on two types of scoring systems. The first is called consensus scoring which is based on popular agreement. So, show a large group a photo and/or play music and ask them to identify the emotion of the person in the photo and the emotion engendered by the music. If 82% think the photo shows the person is angry then that becomes the correct answer for the question. Equally if 73% say the music makes one maudlin then that is the correct answer. The second way in which it is hoped to achieve objective scoring is through expert scoring. Here various researchers whose specialty is the emotions are asked to make judgements: i.e. do the test. Their scores are thought of as best. Both methods are used in conjunction to determine test scores.

Measure	Authors	Reliability α	Reliability test-retest	Predictive Validity	Incremental Validity	Convergent / Discriminant Validity	Factor Structure
EARS. Emotional Accuracy Research Scale	Mayer & Geher, 1996	Low (.24 for target scoring, and .53 for consensus scoring)	?	?	?	Small and unstable correlations with self-report empathy	Unclear (4 factors?)
EISC. Emotional Intelligence Scale for Children	Sullivan, 1999	Low to moderate	?	?	?	?	?
MEIS. Multifactor Emotional Intelligence Scale	Mayer, Caruso & Salovey, 1999	Good for global ability EI (.70-.85), but low (.35-.66) for branches 3 & 4 (better for consensus than for expert scoring)	?	Unclear	?	Small to moderate correlations with crystallized intelligence (Gc) Low correlations with the Big Five	Unclear (3 factors?)
MSCEIT. Mayer Salovey Caruso Emotional Intelligence Test	Mayer, Salovey, & Caruso, 2002	Better for version 2 than version 1 (.68-.71)	?	Well-being, verbal SAT scores.	Social deviance (over personality and verbal intelligence)	Convergence between general consensus and expert consensus scoring. Very low correlations (<.30) with trait EI measures	Unclear (4 factors?)
FNEIPT. Freudenthaler & Neubauer Emotional Intelligence Performance Test	Freudenthaler & Neubauer, 2003	Moderate: .69 for "managing own emotions," and .64 for "managing others' emotions"	?	?	?	"Managing own emotions" correlated with self-reported intrapersonal EI (.51) and, "managing others' emotions" correlated with self-report interpersonal EI (.25). Both subscales correlated with the Big Five (.18 to -.51)	Unclear (2 factors?)

Note: Information in this table is necessarily succinct and readers are encouraged to consult the original sources for specific details. Entries designated 'unclear' do not necessarily indicate conflicting evidence, as they may also refer to lack of adequate data. Question marks indicate that we have been unable to obtain data for the relevant entry.

Table 3. *Summary of Ability EI Measures*

There are thus two very different ways to measure EI. One looks like a personality test and indeed see EI as a type of personality trait. The other is more like an ability test. The former is much easier and cheaper to administer than the latter. But the real question is which is the more *accurate and reliable measure*. Studies have shown that scores from the two tests are modestly positively correlated. Researchers still argue which is the better measure, but at the very heart of the debate is whether EI is just another personality trait or conceptualised more accurately as a real part of intelligence.

Perez et al (2005) did an excellent comprehensive review of the extant measures in the area. No doubt more have appeared since then.

Three things are interesting about the attached tables. First, how very many tests exist which suggests many have been rather rushed.

Second, how very little data exists to demonstrate their validity which is the gold standard for psychometricians. Third, that there does not seem to be any attempt to look at the relationship between these measures in a systematic review.

Measure	Authors	Reliability α	Reliability test-retest	Predictive Validity	Incremental Validity	Convergent/ Discriminant Validity	Factor Structure
TMMS. Trait Meta Mood Scale	Salovey et al., 1995	.70-.85	?	Depression, mood recovery, goal orientation	?	Moderate correlations with the Big Five	3 factors, but no global score
EQ-i. Emotional Quotient Inventory	Bar-On, 1997	Generally good (about .85)	Good	Mental health, coping, work and marital satisfaction	?	Moderate to high correlations with the Big Five	Unclear
SEIS. Schutte Emotional Intelligence Scales	Schutte et al., 1998	.70-.85	?	Social support, life and marital satisfaction, depression, performance on cognitive tasks	Some evidence vis-a-vis the Big Five	Medium-to-high correlations with the Big Five	Unclear (3 or 4 factors), global score
EI-IPIP. Emotional Intelligence-based IPIP Scales	Barchard, 2001	.70-.85	?	?	?	?	?
ECI. Emotional Competence Inventory	Boyatzis, Goleman, & Hay/McBer, 1999	.70-.85 for global score >.85 for social skills	Adequate, but based on small samples	Moderate correlations with managerial styles and organizational climate. Low correlations with career success	?	Unclear (small samples); uncorrelated with critical thinking and with analytical reasoning	Unclear (4 factors?)

Measure	Authors	Reliability α	Reliability test-retest	Predictive Validity	Incremental Validity	Convergent/ Discriminant Validity	Factor Structure
EISRS. Emotional Intelligence Self-Regulation Scale	Martinez-Pons, 2000	.75-.94	?	Depression, life satisfaction, positive affect	?	Unclear	Unclear (1 factor?)
DHEIQ. Dulewicz & Higgs Emotional Intelligence Questionnaire	Dulewicz & Higgs, 2001	Low to moderate (.54-.71)	?	Organizational level advancement	?	Unclear	Unclear
TEIQue. Trait Emotional Intelligence Questionnaire	E.g., Petrides, 2001; Petrides, Pérez, & Furnham, 2003	Generally good (about .85)	Good (.50 to .82; global score .78; 12-month period)	Mental health (depression, personality disorders, dysfunctional attitudes), adaptative coping styles, job stress, job performance, organizational commitment, deviant behaviour at school, sensitivity to mood induction	Good vis-a-vis Giant Three, Big Five, and positive and negative affect	The TEIQue can be isolated in Giant Three and Big Five factor space	4 factors, global score
SPTB. Sjöberg Personality Test Battery (EI Scale)	Sjöberg, 2001	.70-.85	?	Anti-authoritarian attitudes, emotion identification skills, social orientation	?	Moderate correlations with extraversion (.37) and neuroticism (-.50)	?
TEII. Tapia Emotional Intelligence Inventory	Tapia, 2001	.70-.85	Good (.60 to .70)	?	?	?	4 factors, global score
SUEIT. Swinburne University Emotional Intelligence Test	Palmer & Stough, 2002	Generally good (about .85)	Good (.82 to .94; 1-month period)	Well-being, occupational stress	?	Moderate correlations with neuroticism (-.41), extraversion (.44), openness (.27)	?
WEIP-3. Workgroup Emotional Intelligence Profile (version 3)	Jordan et al., 2002	.70-.85	?	Self-monitoring, empathy	?	Small to moderate correlations with TMMS	Unclear (7 factors?)

Measure	Authors	Reliability α	Reliability test-retest	Predictive Validity	Incremental Validity	Convergent / Discriminant Validity	Factor Structure
EIS. Emotional Intelligence Scales	Van der Zee et al., 2002	Adequate for 'other-ratings' (.70-.85). Low for self-ratings (<.60).	?	Academic performance, social success	Some evidence vis-a-vis the Big Five	Low correlations with IQ. Moderate to high correlations with the Big Five	Unclear (3 factors?)
WLEIS. Wong & Law Emotional Intelligence Scales	Wong & Law, 2002	.70-.85	?	Job performance and satisfaction. Organizational commitment, turnover intention	?	Small negative correlations with IQ	4 factors, global score
LEIQ. Lioussine Emotional Intelligence Questionnaire	Lioussine, 2003	.70-.85	?	?	?	Moderate correlations with the Big Five	Unclear (7 factors?)

Note: Information in this table is necessarily succinct and readers are urged to consult the original sources for specific details. Entries designated 'unclear' do not necessarily indicate conflicting evidence, as they may also refer to lack of adequate data. Question marks indicate that we have been unable to obtain data for the relevant entry.

Table 4. *Summary of Trait EI Measures*

7. Emotional intelligence at work

It was no doubt Goleman's book that electrified the public and popularised the term. He has retried to capture attention more recently with *Social Intelligence* (Goleman, 2006). In his *second* book he extended his ideas to the workplace. Now he has over 25 facets subsumed under five domains. Any one inspecting this system (see below) would be astounded by the conceptual muddle at both levels. Thus personality traits, like Conscientiousness, are subsumed under the domain of self-regulation. Equally unrelated psychological concepts like initiative and optimism, are classified under motivation. It seems difficult, in fact to determine, what is not a facet of EQ. That is: does it have any divergent validity?

But the book seems to have an over inclusive view of what EQ is. There are lists of facets and features, some derivative of each other, some quite unrelated to anything about emotion (see Table 5). It does echo themes in the zeitgeist; hence its popularity. The book is also easy to dip into; with many summaries and précis. Hence, there were, and indeed still are, a rash of magazine and newspaper articles that popularised the book and the concept. This is not "trickle down" economics, rather a waterfall of publicity. The sheer amount of positive publicity given to the book must be one of the factors involved in its success and the popularity of the concept at the heart of it.

Personal Competence
Self-Awareness: *Knowing one's internal states, preferences, resources and intuitions*
- **Emotional Awareness**: recognising emotions and their effects
- **Accurate self-assessment**: knowing own strengths and limits
- **Self-confidence**: strong sense of self-worth and capabilities

Self-Regulation: *managing one's internal states, impulses and resources*
- **Self Control**: keeping disruptive emotions and impulses in check
- **Trustworthiness**: maintaining standards of honesty and integrity
- **Conscientiousness**: taking responsibility for personal performance
- **Adaptability**: flexibility in handling change
- **Innovation**: being comfortable with novel ideas, approaches and new information

Motivation: *Emotional tendencies that guide or facilitate reaching goals*
- **Achievement drive**: striving to improve or meet a standard of excellence
- **Commitment**: aligning with the goals of the group or organisation
- **Initiative**: readiness to act on opportunities
- **Optimism:** persistence in pursuing goals despite obstacles or setbacks

Personal Competence
Empathy: *Awareness of others' feelings, needs and concerns*
- **Understanding others**: sensing others' feelings and perspectives and taking an active interest in their concerns.
- **Developing others**: sensing others' development needs and bolstering their abilities
- **Service orientation**: anticipating, recognising and meeting customer needs
- **Leveraging diversity**: cultivating opportunities through different kinds of people
- **Political awareness**: reading a group's emotional currents and power relationships

Social Skills: *Adeptness at inducing desirable responses in others*
- **Influence**: wielding effective tactics for persuasion
- **Communication**: listening openly and sending convincing messages
- **Conflict management**: negotiating and resolving disagreements
- **Leadership:** inspiring and guiding individuals and groups
- **Change catalyst:** initiating or managing change
- **Building bonds:** nurturing instrumental relationships
- **Collaboration and co-operation:** working with others toward shared goals
- **Team capabilities:** creating group synergy in pursuing collective goals.

Table 5. The Emotional Intelligences at work

In his 1995 book, Goleman claimed that cognitive ability (i.e. intelligence) contributed around 20% toward life success but the remaining 80% is directly attributable to emotional intelligence. In a later book, Goleman (1998) lists 25 social competencies from conflict management to self-control all of which make-up social competencies that lead success at work.

Equally in their book entitled "Executive EQ", Cooper and Sawaf (1997) put forth the four cornerstones of emotional intelligence at the executive level: *emotional literacy* (involves the knowledge and understanding of one's own emotions and how they function), *emotional fitness* (involves trustworthiness and emotional hardiness and flexibility), *emotional depth* (involves emotional growth and intensity), and *emotional alchemy* (involves using emotions to discover creative opportunities).

But how to explain how EQ works: the process to explain why EQ is correlated with or essential for business success. Consider some of the explanations for how EQ operates in the workplace and why people with higher EI are supposed to be more successful. First, high EQ people are better at communicating their ideas, intentions and goals. They are more articulate, assertive and sensitive. Second, EQ is closely associated with team-work social skills which are very important at work. Next, business leaders, high in EQ, build supportive climates which increase organisational commitment which in turn leads to success. Fourth, high EQ leaders are perceptive and know their own and their teams' strengths and weaknesses which enable them to leverage the former and compensate for the latter. Fifth, EQ is related to effective and efficient copying skills which enable people to deal with demands, pressure and stress better. Sixth, high EQ leaders can accurately identify what followers feel and need, as well as, being more inspiring and supportive. They generate more excitement, enthusiasm and optimism. Seventh, high EQ managers, unlike their low EQ companions, are less prone to negative, defensive and destructive coping and decision-making styles.

There is no doubt that social skills and emotional sensitivity of managers at work is very important. Emotional perceptiveness, sensitivity and management is more important is some jobs than others. More than 20 years ago after a study of airline steward staff, Hochschild (1983) wrote a book, The *Managed Heart: Commercialisation of Human Feeling*. In it she argued for a new concept: *emotional labour*. She said many jobs require physical and mental labour but some, uniquely, require emotional labour.

The idea is that service staff are required to express emotions they do not necessarily feel. They are required to smile, be positive and appear to be relaxed regardless what they are actually experiencing. Hochschild called this *surface acting*. However, in some jobs you are almost required to feel these emotions. This is called *deep acting*. The idea is that (canny) customers can spot the false display of emotion, so you have to learn the "inside-out smile".

Service staff have to learn to become method actors. Karl Marx said workers were alienated from the products of their labour. Equally, Hochschild believed service workers, whose emotions are "managed and controlled" by their employers, become alienated from their real feelings. Hochschild argued that this cost too much, in that it caused psychological damage in the long term. Yet there remains controversy, not so much about the concept but whether it is essentially damaging in the way it alienates workers from their true feelings (Seymore, 2000).

Since the start of the Millennium there have been a stream of empirical papers on EQ (Lopes et al., 2003; Petrides & Furnham, 2000ab, 2001, 2003). Some have focused very specifically on *EQ at work*. Thus Jordan et al (2002) developed a workgroup EQ scale to test hypotheses about the relationship between EQ, team process effectiveness and team goal focus. They did indeed find some evidence that low EQ teams did perform at lower levels than high EQ teams. Critics however would probably simply want to relabel EQ as social skills or emotional awareness.

Quebbeman and Rozell (2002) defined emotional intelligence in terms of self-awareness, self-regulation, motivation, empathy and social skills. They tested a model that suggested that work experiences trigger responses that are mediated by EQ and Neuroticism to produce affective outcomes, and thence behavioural outcomes. Similarly, Petrides and Furnham (2006) looked at the relationship between EQ, job stress, control and satisfaction as well as organisational commitment. EQ predicted perceived job control which predicted job satisfaction and thence commitment. However, they found significant sex differences in the whole process.

Many have subsequently discussed and tested the idea that emotional intelligence is related to work success. Some papers have been theoretical, others empirical. Thus, Quebberman and Rozell (2002) propose a model that posits how emotional intelligence is related to workplace aggression. Dulewicz and Higgs (2001) developed, and part tested, a model that puts EQ at the centre of the predictors of job performance. Thus, they believe that cognitive ability and specified management competencies contribute to a person's EQ (self-awareness, interpersonal sensitivity, etc). EQ is modified by other factors called drivers (decisiveness) and constrainers (lack of emotional resilience), but directly predicts performance. They argue that they have evidence to suggest that EQ is directly related to leadership through specific leadership competencies like creating the case for change, engaging others, as well as implementing and sustaining change.

Jordan et al (2002) looked at the work related performance of low vs high EQ work groups. They found high emotional intelligence teams operated at high levels of performance throughout the study period while low emotional intelligence teams, initially performed at a low level, but equalled the performance of the high emotional intelligence teams by the end of the study period. This suggests the power of EQ is rather limited.

Petrides and Furnham (2006) found in a study of British working adults that emotional intelligence was related to perceived job control, which predicted job satisfaction. They found, however, evidence of sex differences such that in males EQ was negatively predictive of perceived job stress while there was no significant relationship in females.

Zeidner, Matthews and Roberts (2004) provided a useful *critical overview of the role of EQ in the workplace*. As they note, often business people prefer to talk about emotional competencies (rather than traits or abilities), which are essentially learned capabilities. In this sense, EQ is "the potential to become skilled at learning certain emotional responses" (p.377). It, therefore, does not ensure that individuals will (as opposed to can) manifest competent behaviours at work. Thus, EQ is an index of potential. However, emotional competence does, it is argued, assist in learning (soft) interpersonal skills. They tried to specify these emotional competencies. They include: emotional self-awareness, emotional self-regulation, social-emotional awareness, regulating emotions in others, understanding emotions, etc. If one is to include older related concepts like social skills or interpersonal competencies then it is possible to find a literature dating back thirty years showing these skills predict occupational effectiveness and success. Further, there is convincing empirical literature that suggests these skills can be improved and learnt.

However Zeidner et al (2004) are quite rightly eager to squash the IQ vs EQ myth. They note (my italics) "*several unsubstantiated claims* have appeared in the popular literature and the media about the significance of EI in the workplace. Thus, EI has been claimed to validly predict a variety of successful behaviours at work, at a level exceeding that of intelligence... Of note, however, Goleman is unable to cite empirical data supporting any causal link between EI and any of its supposed, positive effects" (p.380).

The authors point out that EQ measures must demonstrate criterion, discriminant, incremental and predictive validity to be cost effective in business and scientifically sound. We know that general ability (IQ) predicts around 20 – 30 % of the variance in (higher) job performance across all jobs, all criteria, but more for complex jobs.

They review studies which provide positive, mixed and negative results. Quite rightly they offer critiques of the studies which purport to show EQ linked to work success. Typical problems include: The psychometric properties of the EQ measure; Not controlling for intelligence (cognitive ability) or personality factors; not having very robust measures of work-related behaviour; Not being able to disentangle the direction of causality through using longitudinal studies; and having too many impressionistic, anecdotal studies, too few of which are published in peer review journals.

The authors are also interested in the explanation for the process. Thus *if* EQ does predict satisfaction, productivity, team work etc. the question is what is the *process* or *mechanism* that accounts for this? It seems in the literature, there are various speculations to account for this:

- High EQ people are better at communicating their ideas, intentions and goals. They are more articulate, assertive and sensitive.
- EQ is closely associated with team-work social skills, that are very important at work.
- Business leaders, high in EQ, build supportive climates which increase organisational commitment, which in turn leads to success.
- High EQ leaders are perceptive and know their own and their teams' strengths and weaknesses, which enables them to leverage the former and compensate for the latter.
- EQ is related to effective and efficient coping skills, which enable people to deal with demands, pressure and stress better.
- High EQ leaders can accurately identify what followers feel and need, as well as, be more inspiring and supportive. They generate more excitement, enthusiasm and optimism.
- High EQ managers, unlike their low EQ companions, are less prone to negative, defensive and destructive coping and decision-making styles.

Zeidner et al (2004) end with an evaluative summary and guidelines to do good research in the area: "Overall, this section of our review suggests that the current excitement surrounding the potential benefits from the use of EI in the workplace may be premature or even misplaced. Whereas EI appears related to performance and affective outcomes, the evidence for performance is very limited and often contradictory. Much of the predictive validity of questionnaire measures of EI may be a product of their overlap with standard personality factors. Furthermore, the literature is replete with unsubstantiated generalisations, with much of the existing evidence bearing on the role of EI in occupational success either anecdotal or impressionistic and/or based on unpublished or in-house research. Thus, a number of basic questions still loom large: Do emotionally intelligent employees produce greater profits for the organisation? Does EI enhance well-being at the workplace? Are the affects of training in EI likely to result in increases in job performance and/or work satisfaction?" (p.380).

In order to provide both good theory and evidence to support the use of EQ in organisational settings, Zeidner et al (2004) recommend the following:

- The measure of EQ used needs to have reliability and validity and be clearly differentiated from related constructs. "A science of EI requires specifying the definition, number, type and range of primary emotional abilities within a formal psychometric model" (p.390).
- Researchers need to match the test to the job and specify precisely the context and process by which it works. They recommend an emotional task analysis to understand how EQ works in different jobs.
- Researchers need good measures of the criterion job behaviour; they need to look at facets or components of EQ and they need to measure other variables like IQ or personality traits. In short, despite some rather fantastic claims to the contrary, the guiding principle appears presently as "caveat emptor"." (p.393).

A special issue of the *Journal of Organisational Behaviour* (Vol 26) in 2005 was dedicated to EI in the workplace. This included a review of measures (Conte, 2005), but also a conceptual critique by Locke (2005) who concluded robustly that: "EI's extension into the field of leadership is even more unfortunate. By asserting that leadership is an emotional process, Goleman denigrates the very critical role played by rational thinking and actual intelligence in the leadership process. Given all the add-ons to the concept proposed by Goleman et al. (2002), any associations between leadership effectives and an EI scale that included these add-ons would be meaningless.

However, Ashkansy and Daus (2005) argue the concept and its measurement is sound and worthy of attention. They assert four things: Emotional intelligence is distinct from, but positively related to, other intelligences. It is an individual difference, where some people are more endowed, and others are less so. It develops over a person's life span and can be enhanced through training. It involves, at least in part, a person's abilities to identify and to perceive emotion (in self and others), as well as possession of the skills to understand and to manage those emotions successfully.

Daus and Ashkansy (2005) also identified and refuted three claims by their critics namely: Emotional intelligence is dominated by opportunistic "academics-turned-consultants" who have amassed much fame and fortune based on a concept that is shabby science at best. The measurement of emotional intelligence is grounded in unstable, psychometrically flawed instruments, which have not demonstrated appropriate discriminant and predictive validity to warrant/justify their use. There is weak empirical evidence that emotional intelligence is related to anything of importance in organisations.

The area is thus alive and well with vigorous debate about concepts, measurement and usefulness. From an academic perspective it seems very important to establish the independence of either trait or ability emotional intelligence from related concepts and provide robust measures of it. More importantly there remains a great deal of work to be done on demonstrating how, when and why emotional intelligence impacts work related behaviour. If the area has done nothing else, it has succeeded in making emotions at work a topic worth of investigation.

8. Conclusion

If you "google" emotional intelligence you will notice that there are over 7 million hits. This is true testament to the popularity of the concept that has come of age. The academics are now catching up and there are now reviews and meta-analyses which show the predictive power of EI. Thus, for instance, Martins, Ramalho and Morin (2010) in a comprehensive meta-analysis showed EI was clearly, strongly and explicably linked to mental and physical health. Mavroveli & Sanchez-Ruiz (2011) showed EI related to academic behaviour and school achievement. In a masterly review one of the most important researchers in the area Petrides (2011) noted how the applications of EI have been to organizational, clinical, health, educational and social psychology.

However it should not be thought that the area has escaped criticism and debate. Still some wonder if EI adds anything beyond traditional personality and cognitive ability variables (Bastian, Burns & Nettelbeck, 2005). There is accumulating evidence that EI does indeed add incremental evidence over classic personality and ability measures to predict career-making decision difficulties (Di Fabio & Palazzeschi, 2009a) and scholastic success (Di Fabio & Palazzeschi, 2009b).

Another issue of great interest and importance is whether EI can be trained: that is whether EI is in some sense a trainable skill. Recent evidence by Di Fabio and Kenny (2011) suggests that specific training can have significant beneficial success. However we need to know more what type of training is most successful and why.

There also remains a bitter war between those who hold an ability vs a trait conception of EI. (Petrides, 2010). Yet the field has come a long way in 20 years. Academics are still trying to test the claims of the early enthusiasts and beginning to understand where EI "fits in" with what we know about individual differences. It remains an exciting time for all those working in this area.

9. Acknowledgements

Many sections of this chapter are based on previous papers that I have written. I remain, as always, constantly in debt to my good friend and colleague Dr Dino Petrides for allowing me to access his amazing knowledge of the whole story of emotional intelligence, particularly on how it is measured

10. References

Allix, N. (2000). The theory of multiple intelligences: A case of missing cognitive matter. *Australian Journal of Education, 44*, 272 – 293.

Ashkanasy, N., & Daus, C. (2005). Rumours of the death of emotional intelligence is organisational behaviour are vastly exaggerated. *Journal of Organisational Behaviour, 26*, 441 – 452.

Austin, E. (2004). An investigation of the relationship between trait emotional intelligence and emotional task performance. *Personality and Individual Differences, 36*, 1855 – 1864.

Austin, E. J., Saklofske, D. H., Huang, S. H. S., & McKenney, D. (2004). Measurement of trait emotional intelligence: Testing and cross-validating a modified version of Schutte et al.'s (1998) measure. *Personality and Individual Differences, 36*, 555 – 562.

Barchard, K.A.(2001) Seven components potentially related to emotional intelligence. http://ipip.ori.org

Bar-On, R. (1988) *The development of a concept of psychological well-being.* Unpublished Doctoral Dissertation: Rhodes University, South Africa

Bar-On, R. (1997). *BarOn Emotional Quotient Inventory (EQ-i): Technical manual.* Toronto, Canada: Multi-health Systems.

Bastian, V., Burns, N., & Nettelbeck, T. (2005) Emotional intelligence predicts life skills, but not as well as personality and cognitive abilities. *Personality and Individual Differences, 39*, 1135-1145.

Boyatzis, R.E.,Goleman, DF.,& Hay/McBer, (1999) Emotional competence inventory. Boston: HayGroup

Brackett, M. A., & Mayer, J. D. (2003). Convergent, discriminant and incremental validity of competing measures of emotional intelligence. *Personality and Social Psychology Bulletin, 29*, 1147 – 1158.

Brody, N. (2005). What cognitive intelligence is and what emotional intelligence is not. *Psychological Inquiry, 15*, 234 – 238.

Chamorro-Premuzic, T., & Furnham, A. (2005). *Intellectual Competence.* London: Lawrence Erlbaum.

Chan, D. (2004). Perceived emotional intelligence and self-efficacy among Chinese secondary school teachers in Hong Kong. *Personality and Individual Differences, 36*, 1781 – 1795.

Ciarrochi, J., Chan, A. Y. C., & Caputi, P. (2000). A critical evaluation of the emotional intelligence construct. *Personality and Individual Differences, 28*, 539 – 561.

Conrad, S., & Milburn, M. (2001). *Sexual Intelligence.* Crown Publishers, New York.

Conte, J. (2005). A review and critique of emotional measures. *Journal of Organisational Behaviour, 26*, 433 – 440.

Cooper, R. K., & Sawaf, A. (1997). *Executive EQ: Emotional intelligence in leadership and organisations.* New York: Grosset, Putnam.

Daus, C., & Ashkanasy, N. (2005). The case for the ability-based model of emotional intelligence in organisational behaviour. *Journal of Organisational Behaviour, 26*, 453 – 466.

Di Fabio, A., & Kenny, M. (2011) Promoting emotional intelligence and career decision making among Italian high school students. *Journal of Career Assessment. 19*, 21-34.

Di Fabio, A., & Palazzeschi, L. (2009a) Emotional intelligence, personality traits and career decision difficulties. *International Journal for Educational and Vocational Guidance, 9*, 135-146.

Di Fabio, A., & Palazzeschi, L. (2009b) An indepth look at scholastic success: Fluid intelligence, personality traits or emotional intelligence? *Personality and Individual Differences, 46*, 581-585.

Dulewicz, S. V., & Higgs, M. J. (2001). *EI general and general 360 user guide.* Windsor, UK.

Emmons, R. (2000). 'Is spirituality an intelligence?' *International Journal for the Psychology of Religion, 10*, 3-26.

Eysenck, H. (1998). *Intelligence: A New Look.* New Brunswick, NJ. Transaction Publishers.

Eysenck, H. (Ed). (1985). *A model for intelligence.* Berlus: Springer-Verlag.

Freudenthaler, H. H., & Neubauer, A. C. (2003, July). *The localisation of emotional intelligence within human abilities and personality.* Poster presented at the 11th Biennial Meeting of the International Society for the Study of the Individual Differences (ISSID), Graz, Austria.

Furnham, A. (2001). Self-estimates of intelligence: Culture and gender differences in self and other estimates of both general (g) and multiple intelligences. *Personality and Individual Differences, 31,* 1381 – 1405.

Furnham, A. (2004). 'Arc lay people lumpers or splitters'. *Learning and Individual Differences, 14,* 153 – 168.

Furnham, A. (2005). Gender and personality difference in self and other ratings of business intelligence. *British Journal of Management, 16,* 91 – 103.

Furnham, A. (2006). Explaining the popularity of emotional intelligence. In K. Murphy (Ed). *A Critique of Emotional Intelligence.* New York: LEA, p.141 – 159.

Furnham, A., & Bunclark, K. (2006). Sex differences in parents' estimations of their own and their children's intelligences. *Intelligences, 39,* 1-14.

Furnham, A., & Petrides, K. V. (2004). Parental estimates of five types of intelligence. *Australian Journal of Psychology, 56,* 10 – 17.

Furnham, A.,& Petrides, K. V. (2003). Trait emotional intelligence and happiness. *Social Behaviour and Personality, 31, 815 – 823.*

Gardner, J. (1983). *Frames of mind: The theory of multiple intelligences.* New York: Basic Books.

Gardner, J. (1999). *Intelligence reframed: Multiple intelligence for the 21st century.* New York: Basic Books.

Goleman, D. (1995). *Emotional Intelligence: Why it can matter more than IQ.* New York: Bantam Books.

Goleman, D. (1998). *Working with emotional intelligence.* New York: Bantam Books.

Goleman, D. (2006). *Social Intelligence: The New Science of Human Relationships.* New York: Bntum Books.

Gottfredson, L. (2003). Dissecting practical intelligence theory. *Intelligence, 31,* 343 – 397.

Greenspan, S. I. (1989). Emotional intelligence. In K. Field, B. J Cohler, & G. Wood (Eds). *Learning and education: psychoanalytical perspectives* (pp. 209 – 243). Madison, CT: International Universities Press.

Guilford, J. (1967). *The Nature of Human Intelligence.* New York: McGraw-Hill.

Harvey, M., Novicevic, M., and Kiessling, T. (2002). Development of multiple IQ maps for the use in the selection of impatriate managers: a practical theory'. *International Journal of Intercultural Relations, 26,* 493 – 524.

Higgs, M. J., & Dulewicz, S. V. (1999). *Making sense of emotional intelligence.* Windsor, UK: Nfer-Nelson.

Hochschild, A. (1983). *The Managed Heart: Commercialisation of Human Feeling.* Berkeley: University of California Press.

Jensen, A. (1998). *The g Factor: The Science of Mental Ability.* Praeger, New York.

Jordan, P. J., Ashkanasy, N. M., hartel, C. E. J., & Hooper, G. S. (2002). Workgroup emotional intelligence scale development and relationship to team process effectiveness and goal focus. *Human Resource Management Review, 12,* 195 – 214.

Klein, P. (1997). 'Multiplying the problems of intelligence by eight: A critique of Gardner's Theory'. *Canadian Journal of Education, 22,* 377 – 394.

Landy, F. (2006). The long, frustrating and fruitless search for social intelligence: A cautionary late. In K. Murphy (Ed) *A Critique of Emotional Intelligence*. Maliwah NJ: Erlbaum, pp.81-123

Leuner, B. (1966). Emotionale Intelligenz und Emanzipation (Emotional Intelligence and Emancipation). *Praxis der Kinderpsychologie und Kinderpsychiatry, 15,* 196 – 203.

Lioussine, D. V. (2003, July). *Gender differences in emotional intelligence.* Poster presented at the 11th Biennial Meeting of the International Society for the Study of the Individual Differences (ISSID), Graz, Austria.

Locke, E. (2005). Why emotional intelligence is an invalid concept. *Journal of Organisational Behaviour, 26,* 425 – 431.

Lopes, P., Salovey, P., & Straus, R. (2003). Emotional intelligence, personality and the perceived quality of social relationships. *Personality and Individual Differences, 35,* 641 – 658.

MacCann, C., Matthews, G., Zeidner, M., & Roberts, R. D. (2004). The assessment of emotional intelligence: On frameworks, fissures and the future. In G. Geher (Ed.). *Measuring emotional intelligence: common ground and controversy* (pp.21 – 52. Hauppauge, NY: Nova Science.

Mackintosh, N. (1998). *IQ and human intelligence.* Oxford: Oxford University Press.

Martinez-Pons, M. (2000). Emotional intelligence as a self-regulatory process: A social cognitive view. *Imagination, Cognition and Personality, 19,* 331 – 350.

Martins, A., Ramalho, N., & Morin, E. (2010) A comprehensive meta-analysis of the relationship between emotional intelligence and health. *Personality and Individual Differences, 49,* 554-564.

Matthews, G., Zeidner, M., & Roberts, R. D. (2002). *Emotional intelligence: Science and myth.* Cambridge, MA: MIT Press.

Matthews, G., Zeidner, M., & Roberts, R. D. (2008). Measuring emotional intelligence: promises, pitfalls, solutions? In A. D. Ong, & M van Dulmen (Eds.), *Handbook of methods in positive psychology.* Oxford, UK: Oxford University Press.

Mavroveli, S., Sanchez-Ruiz, M.J. (2011) Trait emotional intelligence influences on academic achievement and school behaviour. *British Journal of Educational Psychology, 81,* 112-134.

Mayer, J. D., & Geheer, G. (1996). Emotional intelligence and the identification of emotion. *Intelligence, 22,* 89 – 113.

Mayer, J. D., & Salovey, P. (1997). What is emotional intelligence? In P. Salovey & D J. Sluyter (Eds.), *Emotional development and emotional intelligence:* Educational implications (pp.3 – 31). New York: Basic Books.

Mayer, J. D., DiPaolo, M., & Salovey, P. (1990). Perceiving affective content in ambiguous visual stimuli: A component of emotional intelligence. *Journal of Personality Assessment, 54,* 772 – 781.

Mayer, J. D., Salovey, P., & Caruso, D. R. (2000). Models of emotional intelligence. In R. J. Sternberg (Ed.). *The Handbook of Intelligence* (pp. 396 – 420). New York: Cambridge University press.

Mayer, J. D., Salovey, P., & Caruso, D. R. (2002). *The Mayer-Salovey-Caruso Emotional Intelligence Test (MSCEIT): user's manual.* Toronto, Canada: Multi-Health Systems.

Mayer,J.D. Caruso,D.R.,& Salovey,P. (1999). Emotional intelligence meets traditional standards for an intelligence. Intelligence, 27, 267-298.

Morgan, H. (1996). An analysis of Gardners theory of multiple intelligence. *Roeper Review,* *18,* 263 – 269.

Nardi, D. (2001). *Multiple intelligences and personality type.* New York, Telog.

Neisser, U. (1976). General academic and artificial intelligence. In L. Resnick (Ed.). *The Nature of Intelligence.* Erlbaum: Hillsdale, NJ.

O'Connor, R. M., & Little, I. S. (2003). Revisiting the predictive validity of emotional intelligence: Self-report versus ability-based measures. *Personality and Individual Differences, 35,* 1893 – 1902.

Palmer, B. R., & Stough, C. (2002). *Swinburne University Emotional Intelligence Test (Workplace SUEIT). Interim technical manual (Version 2).* Victoria, Australis: Swinburne University of Technology.

Palmer, B. R., Manocha, R., Gignac, G., & Stough, C. (2003). Examining the factor structure of the Bar-On Emotional Quotient Inventory with an Australian general population sample. *Personality and Individual Differences, 35,* 1191 – 1210.

Perez, J., Petrides, K. V., & Furnham, A. (2005). Measuring trait emotional intelligence. In R. Schulze & R. Roberts (Eds). *Emotional Intelligence: An International handbook.* Gottingen: Hogrefe, pp. 181 – 201.

Petrides, K. V. (2001). *A psychometric investigation into the construct of emotional intelligence.* University College London: Doctoral dissertation.

Petrides, K. V., & Furnham, A. (2000a). Gender differences in measured and self-estimated trait emotional intelligence. *Sex Roles, 42,* 449 – 461.

Petrides, K. V., & Furnham, A. (2000b). On the dimensional structure of emotional intelligence. *Personality and Individual Differences, 29,* 313 – 320.

Petrides, K. V., & Furnham, A. (2001). Trait emotional intelligence: psychometric investigation with reference to established trait taxonomies. *European Journal of Personality, 15,* 425 – 448.

Petrides, K. V., & Furnham, A. (2003). Trait emotional intelligence: behavioural validation in two studies of emotion recognition and reactivity to mood induction. *European Journal of Personality, 17,* 39 – 57.

Petrides, K. V., & Furnham, A. (2006). The role of trait emotional intelligence in a gender-specific model of organisational variables. *Journal of Applied Social Psychology, 36,* 552-569..

Petrides, K. V., Frederickson, N., & Furnham, A. (2004). The role of trait emotional intelligence in academic performance and deviant behaviour at school. *Personality and Individual Differences, 36,* 277 – 293.

Petrides, K. V., Furnham, A., & Frederickson, N. (2004). Emotional intelligence. *The Psychologist, 17,* 574 – 577.

Petrides, K. V., Furnham, A., & Mavroveti, S. (2006). *Trait emotional intelligence: Moving forward in the field of EI.* In G. Matthews, M. Zeidner, & R. Roberts (Eds) *Emotional Intelligence: Known and Unknowns.* Oxford: OUP.

Petrides, K., V., Perez, J. C., & Furnham, A. (2006). On the criterion and incremental validity of Trait Emotional Intelligence, *Emotion and Cognition.*

Petrides, K.V. (2010). Trait emotional intelligence theory. *Industrial and Organizational Psychology, 3,* 136-139.

Petrides, K.V. (2011) Ability and trait emotional intelligence.In T.Chamorro-Premuzic, S. Von Stumm & A Furnham. (Eds). *The Wiley-Blackwell Handbook of Individual Differences.*Oxford: Blackwell.

Quebbeman, A., & Rozell, E. (2002). Emotional intelligence and dispositional affectivity and moderators of workplace aggression. *Human Resource Management Review, 12,* 125 – 143.

Riggio, R., Murphy, S., & Pirozzolo, F. (2002). *Multiple Intelligences and Leadership.* Lawrence Erlbaum, London.

Roberts, R., Zeidner, M. R., & Matthews, G. (2001). Does emotional intelligence meet traditional standards for an intelligence. Some new data and conclusions. *Emotion, 1,* 243 – 248.

Saklofske, D. H., Austin, E. J., & Minski, P. S. (2003). Factor structure and validity of a trait emotional intelligence measure. *Personality and Individual Differences, 34,* 707 – 721.

Sala, F. (2002). Emotional Competence Inventory: Technical manual. Boston: Hay/McBer Group.

Salovey, P., & Mayer, J. D. (1990). Emotional intelligence. *Imagination, Cognition and Personality, 9,* 185 – 211.

Salovey, P., & Mayer, J.D. (1994). Some final thoughts about personality and intelligence. In R.J. Sternberg & P. Ruzgis (Eds) *Personality and Intelligence.* Cambridge; CUP, pp 303-318.

Salovey, P., Mayer, J. D., Goldman, S., Turvey, C., & Paflai, T. (1995). Emotional attention, clarity and repair: Exploring emotional intelligence using the Trait Meta-Mood Scale. In J. W. Pennebaker (Ed.), *Emotion, disclosure, and health* (pp. 125 – 154). Washington, DC: American Psychological Association.

Salovey, P., Woolery, A., & Mayer, J. D. (2001). Emotional intelligence: Conceptualisation and measurement. In G. Fletcher & M. Clark (Eds.), *The Blackwell Handbook of Social Psychology* (pp.279 – 307). London: Blackwell.

Schutte, N. S., Malouff, J. M. Hall, L. E., Haggerty, D. J., Cooper, J. T., Golden, C. J., et al. (1998). Development and validation of a measure of emotional intelligence. *Personality and Individual Differences, 25,* 167 – 177.

Schutte, N. S., malouff, J. M., Bobik, C., Coston, T. D., Greeson, C., Jedlicka, C., et al. (2001). Emotional intelligence and interpersonal relations. *Journal of Social Psychology, 141,* 523 – 536.

Seymore, D. (2000). Emotional labour. *Hospitality Management, 19,* 159 – 171.

Sjoberg, L. (2001). Emotional intelligence: A psychometric analysis. *European Psychologist, 6,* 79 – 95.

Spain, J. S., Eaton, L. G., & Funder, D. C. (2000). Perspectives on personality: The relative accuracy of self versus others for the prediction of emotion and behaviour. *Journal of Personality, 68,* 837 – 867.

Sternberg, R. (1985). *Beyond IQ: A Triarchic Theory of Human Intelligence.* Cambridge University Press, New York.

Sternberg, R. (1997). *Successful Intelligence.* Plume, New York.

Sullivan, A. K. (1999). The emotional intelligence scale for children. *Dissertation Abstracts International, 60,* 68.

Tapia, M. (2001). Measuring emotional intelligence. *Psychological Reports, 88,* 353 – 364.

Thorndike, E. L. (1920). Intelligence and its use. *Harper's Magazine, 140,* 227 – 235.

Van der Zee, K., Schakel, L., & Thijs, M. (2002). The relationship of emotional intelligence with academic intelligence and the big five. *European Journal of Personality, 16,* 103 – 125.

Visser, B., Ashton, M., & Vernon, P. (2006) Beyond g: Putting multiple intelligence theory to the test. *Intelligence, 34,* 487-502.

Warwick, J., & Nettelbeck, T. (2004). Emotional intelligence is…..? *Personality and Differences, 37,* 1091 – 1100.

Watson, D. (2000). *Mood and temperament.* New York: Guilford.

Weisinger, H. (1998). *Emotional intelligence at work: The untapped edge for success.* San Fransisco: Jossey-Bass.

White, J. (2005). Howard Gardner: The myth of multiple intelligences. *Viewpoint, 16,* 1 – 11,

Wong, C-S., & Law, K. S. (2002). *The effects of leader and follower emotional intelligence.*

Zeidner, M., Matthews, G., & Roberts, R. (2004). Emotional intelligence in the workplace: A critical review. *Applied Psychology, 33,* 371 – 399.

2

Emotional Intelligence:
A New Variable in Career Decision-Making

Annamaria Di Fabio

Department of Psychology, University of Florence
Italy

1. Introduction

This chapter introduces emotional intelligence as an innovative variable in career decision-making processes. It also discusses recent empirical studies and outlines new research and intervention perspectives. In recent years, interest has grown in the significance of individual differences in career decision-making (Gati et al., 2010; Savickas, 2004). Awareness has also gradually increased that career decision-making is complex and multidimensional and that individual characteristics have to be taken into account in order to understand the way in which individuals deal with their career decisions (Gati et al., 2010). From this perspective, emotional intelligence appears to be a particularly promising variable in career decision-making processes (Di Fabio & Kenny, 2011).

The chapter will deal first with the principal decisional variables in the career field (career indecision and indecisiveness, career decision-making difficulties, decisional styles) and then describe the evolution of the emotional intelligence construct. Next, it will consider the role of emotional intelligence as a new variable in the career decision-making process (Caruso & Wolfe, 2001; Di Fabio & Blustein, 2010; Di Fabio & Kenny, 2011; Di Fabio & Palazzeschi, 2008b, 2009; Emmerling & Cherniss, 2003; Kenny & Di Fabio, 2009; Kidd, 1998; Young, 2010; Young & Valach, 1996) and also discuss various empirical studies on emotional intelligence.

2. Decisional variables

2.1 Career indecision and indecisiveness

The career indecision construct is used in the literature to underline the problems that can arise during career decision-making (Gati et al., 1996). The construct is designed to explain why some individuals experience uncertainty about their educational and vocational future while others are more involved and confident in making their own choices (Wanberg & Muchinsky, 1992).

From a theoretical point of view, different approaches can be used to examine different aspects of indecision (Kelly & Lee, 2002). The vocational interests approach, supported by Holland and Holland (1977), holds that indecision results from difficulties in personal and vocational identity and from insufficient crystallization of interests. Holland's (1959) theory categorizes individuals into six personality types that correspond to specific professional areas (RIASEC). Accordingly, individuals who belong simultaneously to two or more types could be more undecided about which career path to take. Individuals with low scores in all personality types could also have interests that are not sufficiently defined to lead to a clear career choice. Another possibility is that individuals with high scores in all personality types could have so many interests that they cannot come to a clear decision. Finally, individuals with a wide range of skills could have difficulties in choosing among the various alternatives (Holland, 1959).

According to Super's approach (1953), indecision can correspond to a normal stage of career development. Osipow (1999) supports the thesis, developed earlier by Super (1953), that indecision should not necessarily be considered a persistent problem but rather a normal stage that all people go through during their lifetime. It is possible to distinguish between evolutive indecision (indecision), which corresponds to a normal stage in life in terms of development, and chronic or generalized indecision, known as indecisiveness, which is a personality characteristic that manifests itself in the difficulty that certain individuals have in taking decisions in any contexts of their lives. More recently, Savickas (2004) distinguished between undecided individuals (characterized by a momentary inability to choose but having the potential to make decisions based on their development level, the availability of information, and their decisional training and social support), and indecisive individuals (characterized by chronic anxiety and lack of problem-solving abilities).

3. Career decision-making difficulties

The theoretical and applicative relevance of the career indecision construct is underlined and contextualized by Gati et al. (1996) who state that the increasing rate of change in the world of work increases the number of individual transitions from one job to another during the lifetime of a person. A primary purpose of career counseling is to facilitate the construction of the career decision-making process, particularly with regard to overcoming the difficulties encountered during the process.

The research on career decision-making has devoted considerable attention to the categorization of the various facets of career indecision. Tinsley (1992) argues that, historically, two lines of research have been established: one purely theoretical and one empirical, that is characterized by attempts to devise measures to detect career indecision. However, the two lines of research were developed independently of each other, and, in an attempt to integrate them, Gati et al. (1996) proposed and empirically tested a taxonomy of difficulties individuals may experience. The career decision-making process can be subdivided into different components each of which involves different types of difficulties (Gati et al., 1996). Thus, the various difficulties that individuals may encounter during the career decision-making process can be classified into different categories, and difficulties with the same characteristics can be allocated to the same categories (Campbell & Cellini, 1981). According to Gati et al. (1996), a 'tree' can be used to list the difficulties: the two main groups of difficulties can be distinguished temporally – those that may be encountered before (lack of readiness) and those that may be encountered after the start of the decision-making process (lack of information, inconsistent information). The three main categories of difficulties (lack of readiness, lack of information, inconsistent information) each have a number of subcategories, giving a total of ten subcategories.

Regarding lack of readiness, three specific subcategories of difficulties can be identified: lack of motivation (low willingness to make a decision), indecisiveness (general difficulty in making a decision) and dysfunctional beliefs (distorted perception of careers and the decision-making process, irrational expectations and dysfunctional thoughts about the process).

Regarding lack of information, four specific subcategories of difficulties can be identified: lack of information about the decision-making process (lack of knowledge on how to make a decision appropriately and, particularly, on the steps in the career decision-making process); lack of information about the self (where individuals feel they do not have enough information about themselves, for example about their career preferences, their abilities, and so on); lack of information about occupations (lack of information on career options, for example what alternatives exist and the characteristics of these alternatives); lack of information about ways of obtaining information and getting help with career decision-making.

Regarding inconsistent information, three specific subcategories of difficulties can be identified: unreliable information (where individuals feel they are getting contradictory information about themselves and possible occupations); internal conflicts (an internal state of confusion that arises from the difficulty in reaching compromises on incompatible factors that individuals consider important); external conflicts (the gap between individual preferences and those of significant others, or the differing opinions of significant others).

3.1 Decisional styles

In recent decades, a gradual shift has occurred from economic and probabilistic decision-making models to decision maker characteristics (Arroba, 1977; Harren, 1979; Mann et al., 1997; Scott & Bruce, 1995). The early normative models that characterized the study of decision-making processes (Edwards, 1954; Luce & Raiffa, 1957; Von Winterfeldt & Edwards, 1986; Von Neumann & Morgenstern, 1947) have gradually been replaced by research on how the problem and the situation influence decision-making (Kleindorfer et al., 1993; Payne, Bettman, & Jhonson, 1993), and also by research on the influence of personal factors in choice modalities (Brew et al., 2001), suggesting therefore the existence of different types of decisional styles (Arroba, 1977; Harren, 1979; Janis & Mann, 1977; Jepsen, 1974; Mann et al., 1997; Scott & Bruce, 1995).

In the debate on decisional styles, attention swung from task and decisional situation variables (Driver et al., 1990; Scott & Bruce, 1995) to more cognitive, individual variables (Andersen, 2000; Hunt et al., 1989; Keegan, 1984; Mckenny & Keen, 1974; Mitroff, 1983) until a more timely and integrated decisional style definition could be formulated (Thunholm, 2004).

In the literature, the concept of decisional style was first used to indicate the primary mode employed by individuals to resolve decisional conflict (Janis & Mann, 1977; Mann et al., 1997; Radford et al., 1993). Decisional style was subsequently defined as individuals' habitual pattern of making decisions (Driver, 1979) or as the typical way of perceiving and responding to individual decision-making tasks (Harren, 1979).

The term decisional style was also often used synonymously with cognitive style (Andersen, 2000; Hunt et al., 1989; Keegan, 1984; Mckenny & Keen, 1974; Mitroff, 1983), a term which, in the career decision-making field, refers to the procedures for selecting and processing information that are central to understanding the decision-making process (Hunt et al., 1989). Driver et al. (1990), however, refer to decisional style as learned habit and state that the key difference between styles is the amount of information considered during the decision-making process as well as the number of alternatives identified in the decision-making: in this case, the task and context clearly influence individual differences on how meaning is attributed to the collected data.

Scott and Bruce (1995, p. 820) further defined decisional style as "the learned habitual response pattern exhibited by an individual when confronted with a decision situation. It is not a personality trait, but a habit-based propensity to react in a certain way in a specific decision context". The role of habit and situational factors as predictors of decisional behaviour is thus highlighted.

More recently, Thunholm (2004, p. 941) formulated a more integrated definition of decisional style as a "pattern of response given by an individual in a decisional situation. This pattern of response is determined by the decisional situation, by the decisional task and by the same decider". The deciders demonstrate individual differences in habits as well as in basic cognitive abilities such as information processing, self-evaluation and self-control, which impact consistently on the pattern of response in different tasks and situations.

Interest in different types of decisional styles also gradually developed (Arroba, 1977; Harren, 1979; Janis & Mann, 1977; Jepsen, 1974; Mann et al., 1997; Mann et al., 1989; Scott & Bruce, 1995). The model by Scott and Bruce (1995) identifies five decisional styles in behavioural terms: the rational style, characterized by extensive information research and a systematic evaluation of identified alternatives; the intuitive style, characterized by confidence in one's own intuition and feelings; the dependent style, characterized by seeking the advice and opinions of others before deciding; the avoidant style, characterized by an attempt to avoid decision-making as far as possible; the spontaneous style, characterized by immediate intuition and the desire to reach a decision as quickly as possible.

Mann et al.'s (1997) taxonomy identifies four decisional styles: avoidance, which refers to the tendency to avoid conflict by giving others the responsibility for making a decision; vigilance, which refers to the careful and involved clarification of the goal to be reached through the decision-making process and the thorough evaluation of each option prior to deciding; procrastination, which refers to the tendency to postpone confronting a decisional problem; hypervigilance, which refers to the tendency to attempt, frenetically, to resolve a conflict that arises from having to make choices.

4. Evolution of the emotional intelligence construct

Emotional intelligence is considered a relatively new and growing research area, which has attracted interest at various levels (Zeidner et al., 2004). Emotional intelligence as a construct was first defined by Thorndike in 1920 as the ability to perceive one's own and others' emotions, motives and behaviours, and to use them to act optimally. In 1966, Leuner coined the term emotional intelligence, and, in 1988, Bar-On came up with the term Emotional Quotient (EQ). The emotional intelligence construct has elicited increasing interest since the nineties, especially from psychologists and researchers who have developed different models and definitions.

An early proposition of emotional intelligence was articulated by Mayer et al. (2000) who distinguished between mental ability models and mixed models: the first defined emotional intelligence in terms of individual cognitive abilities in processing emotional information, and the second conceptualized emotional intelligence as a construct that included a mix of cognitive abilities with other characteristics such as aspects of personality.

A second proposition of emotional intelligence called into question the different measures of emotional intelligence arguing that the type of measurement rather than the theory itself determines the nature of the different EI models (Petrides & Furnham, 2000, 2001). In line with this view, Petrides and Furnham (2000, 2001) distinguish between the trait EI (or the trait emotional self-efficacy) and the ability EI (formally defined as information-processing EI). This distinction is not linked to the ability model and the mixed model discussed earlier: Petrides and Furnham's proposition is indeed based on the method of measuring the construct (self-report *vs* maximum performance), and it sees the assessed construct as qualitatively different. Trait EI represents a constellation of emotion-related self-perceptions located at the lower levels of personality. Information-processing emotional intelligence, on the other hand, concerns emotional abilities (e.g. the ability to identify, express and label emotions). Trait EI is thus assessed through self-reported measures while information-processing emotional intelligence refers to objective maximum performance measures (Petrides & Furnham, 2000).

Finally, a further distinction regarding emotional intelligence should be considered, namely that the various models in the literature are distinguished according to whether they are focused on specific abilities or on the overall integration of these abilities (Mayer et al., 2008). Mayer et al. differentiate between specific-ability approaches that concentrate on a particular ability or abilities that can be considered fundamental to emotional intelligence; integrative-model approaches that consider emotional intelligence an overall ability; and the mixed-model approaches that include a wide range of non-cognitive factors.

The empirical studies that will be discussed later in this chapter deal in particular with Bar-On's (1997, 2002) theoretical model of emotional intelligence and also with the model by Salovey and Mayer (1990, Mayer & Salovey, 1997).

In Bar-On's (1997, 2002) model, emotional intelligence is conceptualized as a multifactorial construct where emotional, personal and social competencies converge and determine the modalities through which individuals relate with themselves and with others and that support them in coping effectively with environmental demands and pressures. Emotional intelligence develops over time, it changes in an individual's life and it can be improved through training programmes. Bar-On's (1997) model is hierarchical and includes a global dimension of emotional intelligence, five principal dimensions and fifteen subdimensions. The principal dimensions and their fifteen subdimensions are the following: 1) intrapersonal emotional Intelligence, which refers to awareness of one's own emotions and ability to express one's own feelings and communicate own's one needs. It concerns: self-regard, emotional self-awareness, assertiveness, independence and self-actualization; 2) interpersonal emotional intelligence, which refers to the ability both to establish cooperative, constructive and satisfactory relationships and to understand the feelings of others. It concerns: empathy, social responsibility and interpersonal relationships; 3) stress management, which refers to the ability to control and regulate emotions. It concerns: stress tolerance and impulse control; 4) adaptability, which refers to the ability of use emotions to implement effective strategies for problem-solving. It concerns: reality testing, flexibility and problem-solving; 5) general mood, which refers to the ability to be optimistic, to feel and express positive feelings and to draw pleasure from the presence of others. It includes: optimism and happiness. Based on the Bar-On model, the Emotional Quotient Inventory (EQ-i, Bar-On, 1997) was developed as a self-report questionnaire for detecting perceived emotional intelligence. There is also a short version (Bar-On, 2002).

The first model of Salovey and Mayer (1990) includes three categories of adaptive abilities: appraisal and expression of emotion, regulation of emotion and utilization of emotions in solving problems. The first category includes the dimension of appraisal and expression of emotion in the self and appraisal of emotion in others. The component of appraisal and expression of emotion in the self is further subdivided into verbal and non-verbal subcomponents while the appraisal of emotion in others component consists of the non-verbal perception and empathy subcomponents. The second category, regulation of emotion, consists of regulation of emotion in the self component and the regulation of emotion in others components. The third category, utilization of emotions, includes the flexible planning, creative thinking, redirected attention and motivation components. Mayer and Salovey (1997) later revised their EI model by focusing more on the cognitive aspects of the construct. The revised model includes four components that develop over time ranging from basic psychological processes to higher and more integrated processes on a psychological level: 1) perceiving emotions; 2) facilitating thought; 3) understanding emotions; 4) managing emotions. According to this model, the first and the second components are part of the experiential emotional intelligence area while the third and the fourth components flow into the strategic emotional intelligence area. Based on this proposition, the Mayer-Salovey-Caruso Emotional Intelligence Test (MSCEIT, Mayer et al., 2002) was developed for detecting ability-based emotional intelligence.

5. Emotional intelligence: An innovative variable in career decision-making

Emotions seemingly play an important role in career decision-making processes, but often this influence is not fully understood and recognized (Emmerling & Cherniss, 2003; Young, 2010). The literature on career development has increasingly focused on the role of emotions in career decision-making. Kidd (1998) maintains that emotion, in addition to cognition, is a key determining factor in career choice and career behaviour. Caruso and Wolfe (2001) argue that emotions play a crucial role in career development and selection.

According to Young et al. (1996), the role of emotion in career construction is understandable in the light of the action theory approach, which holds that career is built through the everyday actions. The authors argue that emotions are linked to the purposes, projects and needs of every individual. They accordingly advance three reasons in support of the importance of emotions in career construction: emotions motivate action, they regulate it, and they permit access to and the development of narratives about chosen career paths (Young et al., 1996). Young and Valach (1996) argue that career development is closely connected to emotions and that, therefore, the awareness of one's emotions is essential to building one's career path. In support of the importance of emotions in career decision-making, Cooper (1997) argues that those who trust their feelings and allow themselves to be guided by them have more successful career paths. In studying the role of emotions in the career choice process, emotional intelligence is introduced as a critical variable for career success (Brown et al., 2003; Di Fabio & Blustein, 2010; Di Fabio & Kenny, 2011; Di Fabio & Palazzeschi, 2008a, 2008b, 2009; Emmerling & Cherniss, 2003). People with high emotional intelligence generally have greater awareness of their emotions and have a greater capacity to integrate emotional experience with their thoughts and actions (Emmerling & Cherniss, 2003). Emmerling and Cherniss (2003) consequently stress the key role that emotional intelligence plays in the processes of career exploration and career decision-making. Brown et al. (2003) state that individuals with greater emotional intelligence will probably place more trust in their own capacity to confront tasks related to career decision-making. Emmerling and Cherniss (2003) argue that people with high emotional intelligence are more aware of their own interests and professional values and that they can communicate these interests and values more efficiently during career counseling. The authors similarly believe that such people are better able to manage their own emotional response to career decision-making. Emmerling and Cherniss (2003) conclude that people who are better able to understand and manage their own emotions will probably also be better able to predict the emotional consequences of a potential career choice and avoid jobs that imply unpleasant responsibilities and tasks for them. Instead, they will choose career options that will bring them greater job and life satisfaction. Emotional intelligence is therefore a particularly promising variable for better understanding career decision-making processes. The link between emotional intelligence and different decisional variables (career decision-making difficulties, decisional styles, indecisiveness) has been empirically analyzed (Di Fabio & Blustein, 2010; Di Fabio & Kenny, in press; Di Fabio & Palazzeschi, 2007, 2008a, 2009, Di Fabio et al., submitted).

On the basis of the relationship between career decision-making difficulties, defined according to the model by Gati et al. (1996), and the EI construct according to the model by Bar-On (1997), based on the results of a study conducted on a sample of Italian interns (Di Fabio & Palazzeschi, 2008a), it appears that less emotional intelligence is associated with a greater lack of readiness regarding the difficulties that the individual may encounter before starting the decisional process; a greater lack of information in respect of the decisional process, the self, occupations (and the way to obtain such information); a greater inconsistency of information in respect of not only the lack of consistent information but also in respect of internal and external conflicts. The study also reveals that the intrapersonal dimension of emotional intelligence explains more of each of the three dimensions on the Career Decision-making Difficulties Questionnaire (CDDQ, Gati et al., 1996) and stresses the importance of one's own emotions in the construction of one's own career. Furthermore, a study on a sample of Italian interns (Di Fabio & Palazzeschi, 2009) – still using the career decision-making difficulties model by Gati et al. (1996), the Big Five personality model accessed through the Big Five Questionnaire (BFQ, Caprara et al., 1993) and the EI model by Bar-On (1997, 2002) – showed that the dimensions of emotional intelligence add a percentage of incremental variance compared to the variance explained by personality traits in respect of each of three subdimensions of the CDDQ. The results reveal the role of personality traits as well as emotional intelligence in career decision difficulties thus demonstrating the interesting contribution that emotional intelligence can make in career decision-making. This is because personality traits are seen as stable in the literature (Costa & McCrae, 1992) whereas emotional intelligence is considered a characteristic that can be improved through specific training (Di Fabio & Kenny, 2011). Furthermore, the EI dimension that best explains each of the three dimensions of the CDDQ is the intrapersonal dimension again highlighting the importance of awareness of one's own emotions.

A study on university students (Di Fabio & Palazzeschi, 2008b) using the General Decision Making Style questionnaire (GDMS, Scott & Bruce, 1995) to evaluate decisional styles and the Bar-On Emotional Quotient Inventory: Short (Bar-On EQ-i:S, Bar-On, 2002) to evaluate emotional intelligence, showed 1) that the Adaptability dimension of emotional intelligence impacts positively on the Rational decisional style thus highlighting the role of the ability to use emotions in resolving problems and making use of an adaptive decisional style characterized by an attentive and rational way of proceeding; 2) that the Interpersonal dimension of emotional intelligence impacts positively on the Intuitive style suggesting that the ability to comprehend the feelings of others is central in the use of a style characterized by trusting one's own intuitions and feelings; 3) that the Intrapersonal dimension of emotional intelligence impacts inversely on the Dependent decisional style thus indicating that a limited awareness of one's own emotions is linked to a decisional style characterized by the need to entrust one's self to others for decision-making; 4) that the Intrapersonal dimension impacts inversely on the Avoidant decisional style suggesting that limited awareness of one's own emotions plays a role in the use of a decisional style characterized by the avoidance of decision-making; 5) that the Adaptability dimension of emotional intelligence impacts inversely on the Spontaneous decisional style indicating that limited competence in using emotions for problem-solving is linked to the use of a decisional style characterized by the wish to make decisions immediately and as fast as possible.

A later study (Di Fabio & Blustein, 2010) on high school students using the Melbourne Decision Making Questionnaire (MDMQ, Mann et al., 1997) and the Bar-On Emotional Quotient Inventory: Short (Bar-On EQ-i:S, Bar-On, 2002), revealed that the Intrapersonal dimension is linked inversely to disadaptive decisional styles indicating that a lack of awareness of one's own emotions may be related to the use of inadequate decisional styles. The Adaptability dimension is strongly related to the Vigilance adaptive style highlighting the importance of the ability to use emotions to realize effective strategies in problem solving. Another study (Di Fabio & Palazzeschi, 2007) conducted on a sample of interns using the MDMQ (Mann et al., 1997), the Big Five Questionnaire (BFQ, Caprara et al., 1993) and the Bar-On EQ-i: S (Bar-On, 2002), revealed that the emotional intelligence dimensions add a percentage of incremental variance with respect to personality traits in relation to adaptive as well as disadaptive decisional styles. In particular, for the Vigilance adaptive style, the percentage of incremental variance explained by emotional intelligence is greater than the percentage of incremental variance explained by personality traits. Furthermore, in this study, the Adaptability dimension had a greater inverse influence on the Vigilance adaptive style, and the Intrapersonal dimension had a greater inverse influence on the Disadaptive decisional styles.

Concerning decisional styles, a further investigation was conducted using, simultaneously, self-reported emotional intelligence as well as ability-based emotional intelligence. The study by Di Fabio and Kenny (in press) on Italian high school students using the GDMS by Scott and Bruce (1995) to evaluate decisional styles, the Bar-On Emotional Quotient Inventory (Bar-On EQ-i, 1997) to evaluate self-reported emotional intelligence and the Mayer Salovey Caruso Emotional Intelligence Test (MSCEIT, Mayer et al., 2002) to evaluate ability-based emotional intelligence, revealed that self-reported emotional intelligence with respect to ability-based emotional intelligence largely explained decisional styles thus underlining the principal role of self-assessment of one's emotional skills and personal qualities.

Another study investigated the different roles that emotional intelligence could play in career indecision and indecisiveness. Research by Di Fabio et al. (submitted) on Italian university students looked at the relationship between career indecision and personality traits, career decision-making self-efficacy, perceived social support and self-reported emotional intelligence according to the Bar-On model (1997). The results showed that emotional intelligence explained a percentage of the incremental variance with respect to both personality traits and career decision-making self-efficacy and perceived social support in relation to both career indecision and indecisiveness. While career indecision was better explained by emotional intelligence, indecisiveness was better explained by personality. The study could thus investigate in depth the two constructs and highlight their convergences as well as their divergences.

The above studies showed the possible emergence of an attractive operating scenario at various levels in educational/vocational guidance and career counseling. What makes emotional intelligence an interesting, innovative variable in the research and intervention field is that, whereas personality characteristics are considered substantially stable, there is broad consensus in the literature that emotional intelligence is an improvable characteristic (Bar-On, 1997; Di Fabio & Kenny, 2011; Mayer et al., 2002). Psychologists have also been encouraged to develop intervention programmes that promote emotional and social growth as well as academic success and career development (Walsh et al., 2002). Training programmes on emotional intelligence (Di Fabio & Kenny, 2011; Kotsou et al., 2011; Nelis et al., 2009) would be particularly relevant given the links found with the decision variables (Di Fabio & Blustein, 2010; Di Fabio & Kenny, 2011, in press; Di Fabio & Palazzeschi, 2007, 2008a, 2008b, 2009; Di Fabio et al., submitted).

An emotional intelligence training programme specifically developed according to the model by Mayer and Salovey (1997) for Italian high school students (Di Fabio, 2010) not only increased the emotional intelligence (both ability-based and self-reported) but also reduced the career decision-making difficulties and indecisiveness of the students (Di Fabio & Kenny, 2011).

During the preliminary intervention phase, four classes (91 participants) were randomly chosen from the final high school year in a school system in the Province of Florence. The two classes that showed no significant differences between the mean scores of the studied variables were selected to take part in the research, which contained an experimental group and a control group for the administration of the instruments at T1 and T2. The following instruments were admistered collectively in the classroom: the MSCEIT (Mayer et al., 2002); the Emotional Intelligence Scale (EIS, Schutte et al., 1998); the Indecisiveness Scale (IS, Frost & Shows, 1993); and the Career Decision-Making Difficulties Questionnaire (CDDQ, Gati et al., 1996). Di Fabio and Kenny's (2011) study showed that the intervention was effective not only in improving emotional intelligence, both ability-based and self-reported, but also in reducing indecisiveness and career indecision with effects that remained a month after the intervention (Di Fabio & Kenny, 2011). This further underlined the link between emotional intelligence and decisional variables.

6. Conclusions

The literature review earlier in the chapter, which focused on the links between emotional intelligence and career decisional variables, identified promising innovations in the field of research and intervention. Current prevention models recognize the need to reduce risks and increase resources and strengths (Kenny & Hage, 2009; Kenny et al., 2009). Here, it is particularly important to identify variables that may represent strengths for the individual and that can be used in specific interventions. In this regard, emotional intelligence is seen as a particularly promising variable in the literature (Bar-on, 1997; Kotsou et al., 2011; Mayer et al., 2002; Nelis et al., 2009). The importance of developing interventions that support career development and career decision-making is underlined by research that documents the links between career decision-making difficulties, psychological distress, low levels of psychological well-being and school problems (American College Health Association, 2004; Fouad et al., 2006; Multon et al., 2001).

Recent research suggests that interventions that strengthen emotional intelligence could well promote progress in professional development (Ellis & Ryan, 2005). The importance of emotional awareness and abilities in managing emotions is receiving increasing recognition in the literature on career development (Brown et al., 2003; Emmerling & Cherniss, 2003; Kidd, 1998; Young, 2010). The studies cited in this chapter also highlight the relationship between the emotional intelligence construct and career decision-making difficulties (Di Fabio & Palazzeschi, 2008a, 2009, Di Fabio et al., submitted), decisional styles (Di Fabio & Blustein, 2010; Di Fabio & Kenny, in press; Di Fabio & Palazzeschi, 2007, 2009) and indecisiveness (Di Fabio et al., submitted). It could be argued that interventions to improve emotional intelligence could also reduce career indecision and indecisiveness (Di Fabio & Kenny, 2011).

It should, however, be noted that the studies discussed in this chapter cannot summarily be generalized as the results were obtained from non-representative samples of participants. Future research should therefore use more representative samples of the Italian population and also verify the results in other national contexts. A further limitation in most of the reviewed studies was the exclusive use of self-report measures for assessing emotional intelligence. As suggested (Di Fabio & Kenny, in press) with regard to decisional styles defined according to the GDMS model by Scott and Bruce (1995), it might be interesting to use instruments that can detect both ability-based emotional intelligence and self-reported measures. This would help clarify aspects of overlap and the specificity of the ability-based emotional intelligence model and the self-reported emotional intelligence model regarding different decisional variables.

Despite these limitations, emotional intelligence seems to be a particularly promising variable in respect of decisional issues in the career field (Di Fabio & Blustein, 2010; Di Fabio & Kenny, 2011, in press; Di Fabio & Palazzeschi, 2007, 2008a, 2008b, 2009; Di Fabio et al., submitted). In their interventions, practitioners could determine clients' emotional intelligence abilities and use specific ways to increase these abilities. The enhancement of emotional intelligence could be a new component of interventions to promote career development and of programmes aimed at the development of young people (Di Fabio & Kenny, 2011). Recognition of the role of emotional intelligence in different career decisional situations could also help define operational scenarios for different levels of prevention: a level of intervention for psycho-emotional enhancement (primary prevention) (Di Fabio & Blustein, 2010; Hage et al., 2007; Kenny & Di Fabio, 2009); screening interventions (secondary prevention) for early specific training in emotional intelligence (Di Fabio & Kenny, 2011; Dulewicz & Higgs, 2004; Emmerling & Cherniss, 2003); career counseling intervention (tertiary prevention) for the identification of specific paths for clients who could benefit from programmes on specific aspects of emotional intelligence. Guidance and career counseling could be enriched by identifing clients with difficulties in perceiving and working with emotions in order to calibrate specific types of intervention. Preventive services and interventions in support of career development could help prevent dysfunctions and minimize social costs related to career indecision and psychological stress (Fouad et al., 2006). The costs associated with providing preventive interventions could reduce future demands for more expensive health and social services (Swisher et al., 2004). Increasing attention is being given to the role of individual variables in career decision-making in an attempt to develop more effective and individualized interventions (Bernaud, 2008). From this perspective, emotional intelligence appears to be a very promising variable in terms of research and intervention. Here it should be remembered that many counselors believe that emotions play a significant role in career decision-making (Young, 2010). The importance of reintroducing the study of emotions and doing more research on their role in career decision-making processes has rightfully been emphasized as a new challenge in the field of guidance and career counseling (Young, 2010).

7. References

American College Health Association. (2004). *Healthy Campus 2010*. Retrieved from http://www.acha.org/info_resources/hc2010.cfm

Andersen, J. A. (2000). Intuition in managers: Are intuitive managers more effective? *Journal of Managerial Psychology*, Vol. 15, No. 1, (2000), pp. 46-67, ISSN 0268-3946

Arroba, T. (1977). Styles of decision making and their use: An empirical study. *British Journal of Guidance and Counselling*, Vol. 5, No. 2, (July 1977), pp. 149-158, ISSN 0306-9885

Bar-On, R. (1988). *The development of a concept of psychological well-being*. Unpublished Doctoral Dissertation, Rhodes University, South Africa.

Bar-On, R. (1997). *The Emotional Intelligence Inventory (EQ-I): Technical manual*, Multi-Health Systems, Toronto, Canada.

Bar-On, R. (2002). *Bar-On Emotional Quotient Inventory: Short. Technical manual*, Multi-Health Systems, Toronto, Canada

Bernaud, J.-L. (2008). International seminar *Counseling and guidance in employment services*, Medici-Riccardi Palace, Florence, Italy (December, 2008)

Brew, F. P., Hesketh, B., & Taylor, A. (2001). Individualist-collectivist differences in adolescent decision making and decision styles with Chinese and Anglos. *International Journal of Intercultural Relations*, Vol. 25, No. 1, (January 2001), pp. 1-19, ISSN 0147-1767

Brown, C., George-Curran, R., & Smith, M. L. (2003). The role of emotional intelligence in the career commitment and decision-making process. *Journal of Career Assessment*, Vol. 11, No. 4, (November 2003), pp. 379-392, ISSN 1069-0727

Campbell, R. E., & Cellini, J. V. (1981). A diagnostic taxonomy of adult career problems. *Journal of Vocational Behavior*, Vol. 19, No. 2, (October 1981), pp. 175-190, ISSN 0001-8791

Caprara, G. V., Barbaranelli, C., & Borgogni, L. (1993). *BFQ: Big Five Questionnaire. Manual* (2nd ed.), Giunti O.S., Florence, Italy

Caruso, D. R., & Wolfe, C. J. (2001). Emotional intelligence in the workplace. In: *Emotional intelligence in everyday life: A scientific inquiry*, J. Ciarrocchi, J. P. Forgas, & J. Mayer (Eds.), 150-167, Taylor & Francis, ISBN 1-84169-028-7, Philadelphia

Cooper, R. K. (1997). Applying emotional intelligence in the work place. *Training & Development*, Vol. 51, No. 12, (December 1997), pp. 31-38, ISSN 1055-9760

Costa, P. T., & McCrae, R. R. (1992). *NEO PI-R professional manual*, Psychological Assessment Resources, ISBN 978-9997924452, Odessa, FL

Di Fabio, A. (2010). *Potenziare l'intelligenza emotiva in classe. Linee Guida per il training* [Enhancing emotional intelligence at school: Guidelines for training], Giunti O.S., ISBN 978-88-09-74892-7, Florence, Italy

Di Fabio, A., & Blustein, D. L. (2010). Emotional intelligence and decisional conflict styles: Some empirical evidence among Italian high school students. *Journal of Career Assessment*, Vol. 18, No. 1, (February 2010), pp. 71-81, ISSN 1069-0727

Di Fabio, A., & Kenny, M. E. (2011). Promoting emotional intelligence and career decision making among Italian high school students. *Journal of Career Assessment*, Vol. 19, No. 1, (February 2011), pp. 21-34, ISSN 1069-0727

Di Fabio, A., & Palazzeschi, L. (2007). Intelligenza emotiva, tratti di personalità e stili decisionali: Alcune evidenze empiriche in un campione italiano di apprendisti [Emotional intelligence, personality traits and decisional styles: Some empirical evidence in an Italian sample of apprentices]. *Risorsa Uomo. Rivista di Psicologia del Lavoro e dell'Organizzazione*, Vol. 13, No. 4, (2007), pp. 469-486, ISSN 1128-0689

Di Fabio, A., & Palazzeschi, L. (2008a). Indécision vocationnelle et intelligence émotionnelle: Quelques données empiriques sur un échantillon d'apprentis italiens [Career decision difficulties and emotional intelligence: Some empirical evidence in an Italian sample of wage-earning apprentices]. *Pratiques Psychologiques*, Vol. 14, No. 4, (June 2008), pp. 213-222, ISSN 1269-1763

Di Fabio, A., & Palazzeschi, L. (2008b). Intelligenza emotiva: Nuove prospettive nel career decision-making [Emotional intelligence: New perspectives in career decision-making]. *Risorsa Uomo. Rivista di Psicologia del Lavoro e dell'Organizzazione*, Vol. 14, No. 4, (2008), pp. 459-471, ISSN 1128-0689

Di Fabio, A., & Palazzeschi, L. (2009). Emotional intelligence, personality traits and career decision difficulties. *International Journal for Educational and Vocational Guidance*, Vol. 9, No. 2, (July, 2009), pp. 135-146, ISSN 0251-2513

Di Fabio, A., Palazzeschi, L., Asulin-Peretz, L, & Gati, I. (submitted). Career indecision versus indecisiveness: associations with personality traits, career decision-making self-efficacy, perceived social support, and emotional intelligence. *Journal of Career Assessment*, ISSN 1069-0727

Driver, M. J. (1979). Individual decision making and creativity. In: *Organizational behaviour*, S. Kerr (Ed.), 59-94, Grid Publishing, Columbus, OH

Driver, M. J., Brousseau, K. E., & Hunsaker, P. L. (1990). *The dynamic decision maker*, Harper & Row, ISBN 978-1-55542-593-7, New York.

Dulewicz, V., & Higgs, M. (2004). Can emotional intelligence be developed? *International Journal of Human Resource Management*, Vol. 15, No. 1, (February 2004), pp. 95-111, ISSN 0958-5192

Edwards, W. (1954). Probability preferences among bets with differing expected values. *American Journal of Psychology*, Vol. 67, No. 1, (March 1954), pp. 56-67, ISSN 0002-9556

Ellis, R., & Ryan, J. A. (2005). Emotional intelligence and positive psychology: Therapist tools for training/coaching clients to move beyond emotional relief. *Annals of the American Psychotherapy Association*, Vol. 8, No. 3, (September 2005), pp. 42-43, ISSN 1535-4075

Emmerling, R. J., & Cherniss, C. (2003). Emotional intelligence and career choice process. *Journal of Career Assessment*, Vol. 11, No. 2, (May 2003), pp. 153-167, ISSN 1069-0727

Fouad, N. A., Guillen, A., Harris-Hodge, E., Henry, C., Novakovic, A., Terry, S., & Kantamneni, N. (2006). Need, awareness, and use of career services for college students. *Journal of Career Assessment*, Vol. 14, No. 4, (November 2006), pp. 407-420, ISSN 1069-0727

Gardner, H. (1983). *Frames of mind: The theory of multiple intelligences*, Basic Books, ISBN 978-0-465-02433-9, New York

Gati, I., Krausz, M., & Osipow, S. H. (1996). A taxonomy of difficulties in career decision-making. *Journal of Counseling Psychology*,Vol. 43, No. 4, (October 1996), pp. 510-526, ISSN 0022-0167

Gati, I., Landman, S., Davidovitch, S., Asulin-Peretz, L., & Gadassi, R. (2010). From career decision-making styles to career decision-making profiles: A multidimensional approach. *Journal of Vocational Behavior*, Vol. 76, No. 2, (April 2010), pp. 277-291, ISSN 0001-8791

Guilford, J. P. (1956). The structure of intellect. *Psychological Bulletin*, Vol. 53, No. 4, (July 1956), pp. 267-293, ISSN 0033-2909

Hage, S., Romano, J., Conyne, R., Kenny, M., Mathews, C., Schwartz, J. P., & Waldo, M. (2007). Best practice guidelines on prevention in practice, research, training, and social advocacy for psychologists. *The Counseling Psychologist*, Vol. 35, No. 4, (July 2007), pp. 493-566, ISSN 0011-0000

Harren, V. A. (1979). A model of career decision making for college students. *Journal of Vocational Behavior*, Vol. 14, No. 2, (April 1979), pp. 119-133, ISSN 0001-8791

Holland, J. L. (1959). A theory of vocational choice. *Journal of Counseling Psychology*, Vol. 6, No. 1, (1959), pp. 35-44, ISSN 0022-0167

Holland, J. L., & Holland, J. E. (1977). Vocational indecision: More evidence and speculation. *Journal of Counseling Psychology*, Vol. 24, No. 5, (September 1977), pp. 404-414, ISSN 0022-0167

Hunt, R. G., Krzystofiak, F. J., Meindl, J. R., & Yousry, A. M. (1989). Cognitive style and decision making. *Organizational Behavior and Human Decision Processes*, Vol. 44, No. 3, (December 1989), pp. 436-453, ISSN 0749-5978

Janis, I. L., & Mann, L. (1977). *Decision making: A psychological analysis of conflict, choice, and commitment*, Free Press, ISBN 978-0-02-916190-6, New York

Jepsen, D. A. (1974). Vocational decision-making strategy-types: An exploratory study. *Vocational Guidance Quarterly*, Vol. 23, No. 1, (September 1974), pp. 17-23, ISSN 0042-7764

Keegan, W. J. (1984). *Judgements, choices and decisions*, Wiley, ISBN 978-0-471-86834-7, New York

Kelly, K. R., & Lee, W. C. (2002). Mapping the domain of career decision problems. *Journal of Vocational Behavior*, Vol. 61, No. 2, (October 2002), pp. 302-326, ISSN 0001-8791

Kenny, M. E., & Di Fabio, A. (2009). Prevention and career development. *Risorsa Uomo. Rivista di Psicologia del Lavoro e dell'Organizzazione*, Vol. 15, No. 4, (2009), pp. 361-374, ISSN 1128-0689

Kenny, M. E., & Hage, S. M. (2009). The next frontier: Prevention as an instrument of social justice. *Journal of Primary Prevention*, Vol. 30, No. 1, (January 2009), pp. 1-10, ISSN 0278-095X

Kenny, M. E., Horne, A. M., Orpinas, P., & Reese, L. E. (2009). Social justice and the challenge of preventive interventions: An Introduction. In: *Realizing social justice: The challenge of preventive interventions*, M. E. Kenny, A. M. Horne, P. Orpinas, & L. E. Reese (Eds.), 3-14, American Psychological Association, ISBN 978-1-4338-0411-3, Washington, DC

Kidd, J. M. (1998). Emotion: An absent presence in career theory. *Journal of Vocational Behavior*, Vol. 52, No. 3, (June 1998), pp. 275-288, ISSN 0001-8791

Kleindorfer, P. R., Kunreuther, H. C., & Schoemaker, P. J. H. (1993). *Decision sciences: An integrative perspective*, University Press, ISBN 978-0-521-32867-8, Cambridge, NY

Kotsou, I., Nelis, D., Grégoire, J., & Mikolajczak, M. (2011). Emotional Plasticity: Conditions and Effects of Improving Emotional Competence in Adulthood. *Journal of Applied Psychology*, Vol. 96, No. 4, (July 2011), pp. 827-839, ISSN 0021-9010

Leuner, B. (1966). Emotional intelligence and emancipation. *Praxis der Kinderpsychologie und Kinderpsychiatrie*, Vol. 15, No. 6, (September 1966), pp. 196-203, ISSN 0032-7034

Luce, R. D., & Raiffa, H. (1957). *Games and decisions*, Wiley, New York

Mann, L., Burnett, P., Radford, M., & Ford, S. (1997). The Melbourne Decision Making Questionnaire: An instrument for measuring patterns for coping with decisional conflict. *Journal of Behavioral Decision Making*, Vol. 10, No. 1, (March, 1997), pp. 1-19, ISSN 0894-3257

Mann, L., Harmoni, R., & Power, C. (1989). Adolescent decision making: The development of competence. *Journal of Adolescence*, Vol. 12, No. 3, (September 1989), pp. 265-278, ISSN 0140-1971

Mayer, J. D., Roberts, R. C., & Barsade, S. G. (2008). Human abilities: Emotional intelligence. *Annual Review of Psychology*, Vol. 59, (January 2008), pp. 507-536, ISSN 0066-4308

Mayer, J. D., & Salovey, P. (1997). What is emotional intelligence? In: *Emotional development and emotional intelligence: Educational implications*, P. Salovey & D. Sluyter (Eds.), 3-31, Basic Books, ISBN 978-0-465-09587-2, New York

Mayer, J. D., Salovey, P., & Caruso, D. R. (2000). Selecting a measure of emotional intelligence: The case of ability scales. In: *The handbook of emotional intelligence*, R. Bar-On & J. D. Parker (Eds.), 320-342, Jossey Bass, ISBN 978-0-7879-4984-6, San Francisco

Mayer, J. D., Salovey, P., & Caruso, D. R. (2002). *Mayer-Salovey-Caruso Emotional Intelligence Test (MSCEIT): User's manual*, Multi-Health Systems, ISBN 978-0-72952-630-2 Toronto, Canada

Mckenny, J., & Keen, P. (1974). How managers' mind work. *Harvard Business Review*, Vol. 52, (May-June 1974), pp. 79-90, ISSN 0017-8012

Mitroff, I. I. (1983). *Stakeholders of the organizational mind*, Jossey-Bass, ISBN 978-0-87589-580-2, San Francisco

Multon, K. D., Heppner, M. J., Gysbers, N. C., Zook, C., & Ellis-Kalton, C. A. (2001). Client psychological distress: An important factor in career counselling. *Career Development Quarterly*, Vol. 49, No. 4, (June 2001), pp. 324-335, ISSN 0889-4019

Nelis, D., Quoidbach, J., Mikolajczak, M., & Hansenne M. (2009). Increasing emotional intelligence: (How) is it possible? *Personality and Individual Differences*, Vol. 47, No. 1, (July 2009), pp. 36-41, ISSN 0191-8869

Osipow, S. H. (1999). Assessing Career Indecision. *Journal of Vocational Behavior*, Vol. 55, No. 1, (August 1999), pp. 147-154, ISSN 0001-8791

Payne, J. W., Bettman, J. R., & Johnson, E. J. (1993). *The adaptive decision maker*, University Press, ISBN 978-0-521-42526-1, Cambridge, NY

Petrides, K. V., & Furnham, A. (2000). On the dimensional structure of emotional intelligence. *Personality and Individual Differences*, Vol. 29, No. 2, (August 2000), pp. 313-320, ISSN 0191-8869

Petrides, K. V., & Furnham, A. (2001). Trait emotional intelligence: Psychometric investigation with reference to established trait taxonomies. *European Journal of Personality*, Vol. 15, No. 6, (December 2001), pp. 425-428, ISSN 0890-2070

Radford, M. H. B., Mann, L., Otha, Y., & Nakane, Y. (1993). Differences between Australian and Japanese students in decisional self-esteem, decisional stress and coping styles. *Journal of Cross Cultural Psychology*, Vol. 24 4, No. 3, (September 1993), pp. 284-297, ISSN 0022-0221

Salovey, P., & Mayer, J. D. (1990). Emotional intelligence. *Imagination, Cognition and Personality*, Vol. 9, No. 3, (1990), pp. 185-211, ISSN 0276-2366

Savickas, M. (2004). Vocational psychology. In: *Encyclopedia of Applied Psychology*, C. Spielberger (Ed.), 655-667, Elsevier, ISBN 978-0-12-657410-4, Amsterdam, Netherlands

Schutte, N. S., Malouff, J. M., Hall, L. E., Haggerty, D. J., Cooper, J. T., Golden, C. J., & Dornheim, L. (1998). Development and validation of a measure of emotional intelligence. *Personality and Individual Differences*, Vol. 25, No. 2, (August, 1998), pp. 167-177, ISSN 0191-8869

Scott, S. G., & Bruce, R. A. (1995). Decision-making style: The development and assessment of a new measure. *Educational and Psychological Measurement*, Vol. 55, No. 5, (October 1995), pp. 818-831, ISSN 0013-1644

Super, D. E. (1953). A theory of vocational development. *American Psychologist*, Vol. 8, No. 5, (May, 1953), pp. 185-190, ISSN 0003-066X

Swisher, J. D., Scherer, J., & Yin, R. K. (2004). Cost-benefit estimates in prevention research. *The Journal of Primary Prevention*, Vol. 25, No. 2, (October 2004), pp. 137-148, ISSN 0278-095X

Thorndike, R. K. (1920). Intelligence and its uses. *Harper's Magazine*, Vol. 140, (January 1920), pp. 227-235, ISSN 0017-789X

Thunholm, P. (2004). Decision-making style: Habit, style or both? *Personality and Individual Differences*, Vol. 36, No. 4, (March 2004), pp. 931-944, ISSN 0191-8869

Tinsley, H. E. A. (1992). Career decision making and career indecision. *Journal of Vocational Behavior*, Vol. 41, No. 3, (December 1992), pp. 209-211, ISSN 0001-8791

Von Neumann, J., & Morgenstern, O. (1947). *Theory games and economic behaviour*, Princeton University Press, ISBN 978-0-691-13061-3, Princeton, NJ

Von Winterfeldt, D., & W. Edwards (1986). *Decision analysis and behavioral research*, Cambridge University Press, ISBN 978-0-521-27304-6, New York

Walsh, M. E., Galassi, J. P., Murphy, J. A., & Park-Taylor, J. (2002). A conceptual frame work for counseling psychologists in schools. *The Counseling Psychologist*, Vol. 30, No. 5, (September 2002), pp. 682-704, ISSN 0011-0000

Wanberg, C. R., & Muchinsky, P. M. (1992). A typology of career decision status: Validity extension of the vocational decision status model. *Journal of Counseling Psychology*, Vol. 39, No. 1, (January 1992), pp. 71-80, ISSN 0022-0167

Young, R. A. (2010, July). *Counselling Psychology: The ways forward*. Paper presented at 27th International Congress of Applied Psychology, Melbourne, Australia.

Young, R. A., & Valach, L. (1996). Interpretation and action in career counseling. In: *Handbook of career counseling theory and practice*, M. L. Savickas & W. B. Walsh (Eds.), 361-375, Davies-Black, ISBN 978-0-89106-080-2, Palo Alto, CA

Young, R. A., Valach, L., & Collin, A. (1996). A contextual explanation of career. In: *Career choice and development*, D. Brown & L. Brooks (Eds.), (3rd ed.), 477-512, Jossey-Bass, ISBN 978-0-7879-0204-9, San Francisco

Zeidner, M., Matthews, G., & Roberts, R. D. (2004). Emotional intelligence in the workplace: A critical review. *Applied Psychology: An International Review*, Vol. 53, No. 3, (July 2004), pp. 371-399, ISSN 0269-994X

3

The Impact of Emotional Intelligence on Health and Wellbeing

Reuven Bar-On
University of Texas Medical Branch
USA

1. Introduction

The purpose of this chapter is to examine the impact of emotional intelligence on health and wellbeing. Following a brief introduction to emotional intelligence and the way this construct is conceptualised and measured, the author summarises a number of studies that shed light on the relationship between emotional intelligence, health and wellbeing. This process narrows the focus on what are thought to be the key predictors of health and wellbeing. Potential limitations of the studies reviewed are discussed, recommendations for future research are made, and implications for applying the findings to enhance health and wellbeing are pondered. The author stresses the importance of their application in parenting, education and healthcare in particular.

2. A brief introduction to emotional intelligence

Emotional intelligence has become a major topic of interest in scientific circles as well as in the lay public since the publication of a book by the same name in 1995 [1]. Despite the heightened level of interest in this 'new idea' since the publication of Daniel Goleman's bestseller, scholars have been studying various aspects of this construct for much of the 20th century; and the historical roots of emotional and social intelligence can be traced back to the 19th century [2]. At this point of the discussion, it is important to draw the reader's attention to the fact that a variety of different terms have been used to describe emotional intelligence over the years; and the various terms that have been used to describe it are italicised below to provide the reader with a sense of how these terms have changed over time.

The first known work in this scholarly field was published by Charles Darwin as early as 1872 and focused on the importance of *emotional expression* for survival and adaptation [2].

Publications began appearing in the 20th century with the work of Edward Thorndike on *social intelligence* in 1920 [3]. Many of these early studies focused on describing, defining and attempting to assess socially competent behaviour [3-7]. Edgar Doll published the first instrument designed to measure *socially intelligent behaviour* in young children [6]. Possibly influenced by Thorndike and Doll, David Wechsler included two subscales ("Comprehension" and "Picture Arrangement") in his well-known test of cognitive intelligence that appear to have been designed to measure social intelligence [8]. A year after the first publication of this test in 1939, Wechsler described the influence of *non-intellective factors* on intelligent behaviour which was yet another reference to this construct [9]. In the first of a number of publications following this early description moreover, he argued that our models of human intelligence would not be complete until we can adequately describe these factors [10].

Scholars began to shift their attention from describing and assessing social intelligence to understanding the purpose of interpersonal behaviour and the role it plays in effective adaptability [11], which was essentially how Darwin described this behaviour with respect to survival and adaptation. This line of research helped define human effectiveness from the social perspective as well as strengthened one very important aspect of Wechsler's definition of general intelligence: "The capacity of the individual to act purposefully" [12, p. 7]. Additionally, this helped position social intelligence as part of general intelligence.

Scholarly activity in the area of social intelligence continued uninterruptedly from the early 1920s to the present and included scientific studies conducted by many prominent psychologists in the field [3, 4, 10, 13-16]. The early definitions of social intelligence influenced the way *emotional intelligence* was later conceptualised. Contemporary theorists like Peter Salovey and John Mayer originally viewed emotional intelligence as part of social intelligence [17, p. 189], which suggests that both concepts are related and may, in fact, represent interrelated components of the same construct.

In the late 1940s, scientific inquiry began to centre around *alexithymia* [18, 19], which is the essence of emotional intelligence at the pathological end of the continuum in that it focuses on the ability, or rather the inability, to recognise, understand and describe emotions [20]. Based on a recent computerised search, it is interesting to note that more than 1,000 articles, chapters and books have been published that are related to alexithymia and how it affects physical and psychological health; and the vast majority of these publications appeared long before the publication of Daniel Goleman's 1995 bestseller popularising the topic [1].

Two new directions that paralleled and possibly evolved from alexithymia were *psychological mindedness* [21] and *emotional awareness* [22].

From the 1970s, many mental healthcare practitioners began evaluating the *psychological mindedness* of patients to assess their suitability for psychotherapy and ability to benefit from it.

Research exploring the neural circuitry that governs emotional awareness [23], as well as additional emotional and social aspects of this concept [23-31], has begun to provide tangible evidence of the anatomical foundations of this construct which some have prematurely and inaccurately described as 'an intangible myth' [32-34].

The literature reveals various attempts to combine the emotional and social components of this wider construct. For example, Howard Gardner [35] explains that his conceptualisation of *personal intelligences* is based on *intrapersonal intelligence* and *interpersonal intelligence*. Additionally, Carolyn Saarni [36] describes *emotional competence* as including eight interrelated emotional and social skills. And Reuven Bar-On has shown that *emotional-social intelligence* is composed of a number of intrapersonal and interpersonal competencies and skills that combine to determine effective human behaviour [37-39].

Based on the above, it is more accurate to refer to this construct as "emotional-social intelligence" rather than "emotional intelligence" or "social intelligence" as Bar-On has suggested for a number of years [39]. Throughout this chapter, this wider construct is interchangeably referred to as "emotional-social intelligence" and, at times, "emotional and social intelligence" or simply "emotional intelligence" (EI).

Since the time of Thorndike [3], a number of different conceptualisations of emotional intelligence have appeared creating an interesting mixture of confusion, controversy and opportunity regarding how best to define and measure this construct. In an effort to help clarify matters, the *Encyclopedia of Applied Psychology* [40] suggested that there are three basic conceptual and psychometric models: (a) the Salovey-Mayer model [41] which defines this construct as the ability to perceive, understand, manage and use emotions to facilitate thinking, measured by an ability-based measure [42]; (b) the Goleman model [43] which views this construct as a wide range of competencies and skills that drive human performance, measured by multi-rater assessment [44]; and (c) the Bar-On model [37-39] which describes an array of interrelated emotional and social competencies and skills that impact intelligent behaviour, measured by self-report [38, 45], multi-rater assessment and structured interview [46-48].

For a detailed historical overview of subjective wellbeing and its relationship with emotional intelligence, the reader is referred to Bar-On's seminal article on the topic [49].

3. The conceptual and psychometric model of emotional intelligence used in this chapter

From Darwin to the present, most conceptual and psychometric models of emotional-social intelligence have included one or more of the following factorial components: (a) the ability to recognise, understand, express and utilise emotions and feelings; (b) the ability to understand how others feel and use this information to relate with them; (c) the ability to manage and control emotions so they work for us and not against us; (d) the ability to use input from emotions and feelings to manage change, adapt and solve problems of a personal and interpersonal nature; and (e) the ability to be optimistic, positive and self-motivated to navigate through life and cope with challenges as they arise. The Bar-On conceptual and psychometric model of emotional intelligence captures all these components and is described below, in light of the fact that the present chapter relies primarily on this particular model to study and understand the relationship between this construct, health and wellbeing.

According to the Bar-On model, *emotional-social intelligence is an array of interrelated emotional and social competencies, skills and behaviours that determine how effectively we understand and express ourselves, understand others and relate with them, and cope with daily demands, problems and pressure* [38, 39, 50]. The emotional and social competencies, skills and behaviours referred to in this conceptualisation include the 15 factors that are described in Appendix A.

The Emotional Quotient Inventory (EQ-i) was developed, over a period of 17 years, to assess the 15 factorial components of the Bar-On model [37-39, 50, 51]. The EQ-i is a self-report measure of emotionally and socially intelligent behaviour that provides an estimate of one's emotional-social intelligence. A detailed description of how this instrument was developed, normed and validated, together with its psychometric properties, are found elsewhere in the literature [e.g., 37-39, 50-55]. In brief, the EQ-i comprises 133 items in the form of short sentences and employs a 5-point response scale. A list of the inventory's items is found in the instrument's technical manual [38]. The EQ-i is suitable for individuals 17 years of age and older and takes approximately 20 to 30 minutes to complete online. The individual's responses render a Total EQ score and scores on the following 15 scales described in Appendix A: Self Regard, Emotional Self-Awareness, Assertiveness, Independence, Self-Actualization, Empathy, Social Responsibility, Interpersonal Relationship, Stress Tolerance, Impulse Control, Reality Testing, Flexibility, Problem Solving, Optimism, and Happiness. Average to above average scores on the EQ-i indicate that the respondent is effective in emotional and social functioning. The higher the scores, the more positive the prediction for effective functioning in meeting daily demands and challenges. On the other hand, low scores suggest an inability to be effective and the possible existence of emotional, social and/or behavioural problems. The EQ-i has a built-in correction factor that automatically adjusts the scale scores based on scores obtained from the instrument's validity indices; and this is a very important feature for self-report measures in that it reduces the potentially distorting effects of response bias thereby increasing the accuracy of the results.

The EQ-i was originally constructed as an experimental instrument designed to examine the conceptual model of *emotional and social functioning* that the author began developing in the early 1980s during his doctoral studies [37]. At that time, he hypothesised that effective emotional and social functioning should eventually lead to a sense of psychological wellbeing. It was reasoned that the results gained from applying such an instrument on large and diverse population samples would reveal more about emotionally and socially intelligent behaviour and about the underlying construct of emotional-social intelligence. Based on findings obtained from applying the EQ-i in a wide range of studies from the early 1980s to the present day, the author has moulded his conceptualisation of this construct over time. In 2011, a mildly revised version of the EQ-i -- referred to as the "EQ-i 2.0" -- was renormed [www.mhs.com]. Although some of the items were reworded and others added, the 15 factorial structure of the Bar-On model was confirmed, for the most part, in spite of the cosmetic changes that were introduced.

4. Examining the relationship between emotional intelligence, health and wellbeing

The remainder of this chapter is devoted entirely to examining and summarising the nature of the relationship between emotional intelligence, health and wellbeing. In order to do this, the following three areas need to be explored empirically:

- The nature of the relationship between emotional intelligence and physical health
- The nature of relationship between emotional intelligence and subjective wellbeing
- The nature of the relationship between health and subjective wellbeing

5. The nature of the relationship between emotional intelligence and physical health

To explore and understand the nature of the relationship between emotional intelligence (EI) and physical health, the findings of five studies are presented below. These findings address the question of whether emotionally intelligent people are healthier than those who are less emotionally intelligent, and *vice versa*. In presenting these studies, the specific EI factors involved will be summarised and discussed at the end of this section.

The 1st study. The first study reviewed here was based on the North American normative sample upon which the EQ-i was originally piloted and standardised for use in the United States and Canada [45]. This study was first described in 2004 [51] and has been cited by others in more than 90 publications since then.

When the 152-item beta version on the EQ-i was piloted in 1996 and 1997, the following item was eventually excluded from the final 133-item version of this instrument because it was thought to be associated more with self-perceived health (SPH) than with emotional intelligence (EI): "I feel good about my health in general." In spite of its limitations as an EI item, it was useful in providing a self-perceived evaluation of the respondents' physical health to help examine the EQ-i's validity as it relates to predicting health. It is important to note that a growing body of research findings indicate that self-perceived health is significantly correlated with clinically assessed health [56-61] which justified its use here as a valid measure of health.

Within the EQ-i's normative sample of 3,831 adults [38], 1,867 males and 1,945 females with an average age of 34.2 years responded to the above-mentioned SPH item. As the first step in studying the relationship between emotional intelligence and health, the degree of difference in SPH was examined between respondents with lower and higher levels of EI (i.e., those with Total EQ scores less than 1 SD below the mean and those with scores greater than 1 SD above the mean respectively). Because of the multivariate nature of the data and the methods used to collect that data, a one-way ANOVA was applied to examine the differences in their SPH; and the results are presented in Table 1 below.

	Low EI (n=528)	High EI (n=547)	F score	p level
SPH	3.49 ± 1.05	4.64 ± 0.67	463.58	<.001

Table 1. Differences in self-perceived physical health (SPH) between individuals with lower and higher levels of emotional intelligence (EI) based on a one-way ANOVA.

The results in Table 1 indicate that people who are more emotionally intelligent feel healthier than those who are less emotionally intelligent. To confirm these findings, it was important to evaluate whether individuals who perceive themselves as healthy are more emotionally intelligent that those who feel they are less healthy. Using the above-mentioned normative sample [38], the degree of difference in EI was examined between those respondents with lower and higher levels of SPH (i.e., those with SPH scores less than 1 SD below the mean and those with SPH scores greater than 1 SD above the mean respectively). A one-way ANOVA was once again applied to examine the differences in EI, and the results appear in Table 2.

	Low SPH (n=202)	High SPH (n=1,304)	F score	p level
Overall EI	416.4 ± 57.6	487.5 ± 45.3	398.25	<.001

Table 2. Differences in overall emotional intelligence (EI), based on EQ-i raw scores for the Total EQ scale, between individuals with lower and higher levels of self-perceived health (SPH).

The results in Table 2 suggest that individuals who are healthier are more emotionally intelligent than those who are less healthy. As such, this confirms the results in Table 1.

To better understand the overall impact of emotional intelligence (EI) on physical health as well as the specific constellation of EI factors that predict and differentiate between lower and higher levels of self-perceived health (SPH), a Multiple Regression Analysis was applied to the EQ-i normative data to examine the ability of the instrument's 15 subscales to predict SPH which was assessed with the previously mentioned item ("I feel good about my health in general"). This resulted in a Regression R of .49 demonstrating a moderate to high correlation between EI and SPH; and based on an R² of .24, nearly 25% of self-perceived physical health appears to be influenced by one's level of emotional intelligence. The strongest EI predictors of physical health that emerge from the regression model appear in Table 3 in the order of their predictive ability.

EQ-i subscales	β score	t value	p level
Self Regard	.403	15.52	<.001
Stress Tolerance	.097	4.07	<.001
Self-Actualization	.054	2.24	.025
Impulse Control	.039	2.09	.037

Table 3. The significant EI predictors of self-perceived health generated by Multiple Regression Analysis (n=3,812).

The results in Table 3 suggest that self regard (one's ability to understand and accept oneself) is the strongest predictor of health. To understand the specific EI factors measured by the EQ-i subscales appearing in Table 3, and elsewhere throughout this chapter, the reader is referred to Appendix A which describes what each of the subscales measure.

In order to more closely study those EI factors that are capable of distinguishing between less healthy and healthier individuals, a one-way ANOVA was applied to the EQ-i normative data. Raw scores for the instrument's 15 subscales were entered as the dependent variables, and low and high SPH levels (1 SD below and above the mean value respectively) were entered as the independent (grouping) variable. The statistically significant results are revealed in Table 4 in the order of their ability to distinguish between lower and higher levels of self-perceived health.

EI factors assessed by EQ-i subscales	Low SPH (n=202)	High SPH (n=1,304)	F score	p level
Self Regard	28.8 ± 7.2	37.0 ± 5.6	412.13	<.001
Happiness	32.7 ± 6.3	38.3 ± 4.7	266.32	<.001
Optimism	29.0 ± 5.6	33.7 ± 4.1	231.48	<.001
Stress Tolerance	29.1 ± 6.0	34.5 ± 5.3	204.38	<.001
Self-Actualization	33.8 ± 6.3	38.4 ± 4.7	185.15	<.001

Table 4. The ability of EI factors to distinguish between lower and higher levels of self-perceived health (SPH) based on a one-way ANOVA.

By observing the results of this study, that are presented in Tables 3 and 4, it can be seen that strongest EI predictors of physical health are self regard (in particular), self-actualisation, stress tolerance, optimism and happiness. Based on the way these EI factors are defined in Appendix A, the findings suggest that individuals who have good self-awareness and understand their weaknesses as well as their strengths, pursue activities that actualise their potential, manage emotions well and who are typically optimistic, positive and content are healthier individuals.

The 2nd study. The second study re-examined here more directly and objectively examined the impact of emotional intelligence on physical health. This study was based on a sub-sample of the Israeli normative sample, upon which the EQ-i was standardized for use in that country. It was first described in 2006 [50] and has been cited in more than 240 other publications since then. This particular sample included 941 male conscripts into the Israeli Defence Forces (IDF), with an average age of 18 years at the time this study was conducted in 2001. Upon mandatory conscription into the IDF, each conscript is thoroughly examined by medical staff at the Office of Mobilisation and receives a 5-digit medical profile or profiles based on their existing state of health. The first 4 digits of this profile reveal the specific nature of their medical condition/s, while the 5th digit indicates the severity of the condition/s. Severity ranges from 1 to 7. Typically a severity of 1 and 2 does not restrict the nature of the conscripts' 3-year tour of mandatory military service. The higher the severity level from 3 to 5, however, the more they are limited regarding where they can serve and what they can do. While level 7 automatically rejects conscripts from military service because of the specific nature and severity of their medical condition, level 6 requires that they be re-evaluated after a period of one year at which time they are either rejected from military service (i.e., 6 is raised to 7) or they begin to serve with a lower level of severity (i.e., level 6 is reduced to anywhere from 1 to 5 depending upon their medical condition when they are re-evaluated).

The above-mentioned system of receiving well-documented medical profiles represents an objective and accurate assessment of these individuals' state of health. At the time of their initial medical evaluation at Office of Mobilisation, 941 IDF conscripts were randomly identified with medical profiles ranging from 1 to 5. This group completed the EQ-i at the time of their initial medical examinations. Conscripts with psychiatric profiles were excluded from this sample, in order to limit the focus of the study to physical health. As was originally described [50], Multiple Regression Analysis was applied and rendered an overall correlation of .37 indicating a low moderate yet significant relationship between emotional intelligence and physical health for the sample studied. Based on re-examining the specific impact of emotional intelligence on three different grouped levels of severity (587 with level 1, 188 with level 2 and 166 with levels 3 through 5), four EI factors emerged as the strongest predictors of physical health; and they are listed in Table 5 in the order of their predictive ability.

EQ-i subscales	β score	t value	p level
Self-Actualization	.154	3.26	.001
Stress Tolerance	.127	2.16	.031
Optimism	.127	2.14	.032
Problem Solving	.104	2.22	.027

Table 5. The statistically significant EI predictors of clinically assessed health in IDF conscripts (n=941) based on Multiple Regression Analysis.

In addition to examining the impact of EI on health by conducting a regression analysis of the data, an analysis of variance was also applied to examine the ability of EI factors to differentiate between lower and higher levels of clinically-assessed health in this sample (i.e., 587 individuals with a severity level of 1 and 354 with severity levels from 2 to 5). A one-way ANOVA was used to examine the ability of EI to differentiate these two different levels of health, and the results are described below. The 5 EI factors, assessed by the EQ-i, which were able to significantly differentiate between lower and higher levels of physical health appear in Table 6 in the order of their ability to differentiate between less healthy and healthier individuals.

EQ-i Scales (EI Factors)	Less Healthy (n=354)	More Healthy (n=587)	F score	p level
Flexibility	27.8 ± 5.0	29.1 ± 4.4	16.91	<.001
Stress Tolerance	34.0 ± 5.9	35.3 ± 5.2	13.02	<.001
Optimism	31.4 ± 4.6	32.4 ± 4.4	9.81	.002
Interpersonal Relationship	44.3 ± 6.0	45.3 ± 5.7	5.87	.016
Happiness	38.6 ± 5.1	39.3 ± 4.5	4.13	.042

Table 6. Differences in emotional intelligence, based on EQ-i raw scores, between individuals with lower and higher levels of self-perceived health.

The results from the second study appearing in Tables 5 and 6 indicate that one's ability (a) to manage emotions and cope with stress, (b) be flexible and adaptable, (c) solve personal and interpersonal problems, (d) achieve personal goals designed to actualise their potential as well as the ability to be (e) optimistic and (f) content with themselves, others and life in general significantly differentiate between less healthy and healthier individuals.

The 3rd study. The third study presented in this section directly and objectively examines the impact of emotional intelligence on health in a clinical sample [62]. This study was conducted in the Department of Dermatology and Skin Science at the University of British Columbia in Vancouver and examined the relationship between emotional intelligence (EI) and alopecia areata (AA), which is an autoimmune disease characterised by hair loss. In this study, which was recently submitted for review, the EI of 42 AA patients were compared with a non-clinical sample of 77 individuals. The non-clinical control group was created by randomly selecting the EQ-i scores of 77 individuals from the North American normative sample upon which this psychometric instrument was originally normed in North America [38]. In the experimental group, each participant completed the EQ-i. The primary aim was to investigate EI differences between AA patients and the non-clinical control group. The clinical sample included 13 males and 29 females who were randomly selected from the Department of Dermatology and Skin Science; and the non-clinical control group included a matched proportion of males and females in the same age range of 19 to 68 with an average age of 40.7 years. A one-way ANOVA was employed to determine the extent of differences in EI between AA patients and the non-clinical control group. The results are shown in Table 7 below.

It can be seen, from the results in Table 7, that the AA patients experience more difficulty in managing their emotions and coping with stress (Stress Tolerance), are more pessimistic (Optimism) and unhappy (Happiness), have poor self-awareness and self-acceptance (Self

Regard) and are less motivated to pursue their interests and actualise personal goals (Self-Actualization) when compared with the non-clinical sample. Their ability to manage emotions and cope with stress is by far the most severe EI deficiency when compared with healthy individuals.

EQ-i scales	AA patient scores (n=42)	Non-clinical scores (n=77)	F score	p level
Stress Tolerance	91.4 ± 21.8	99.5 ± 9.1	8.11	.005
Happiness	95.5 ± 18.7	101.2 ± 8.4	5.33	.023
Optimism	95.4 ± 20.5	101.4 ± 8.7	4.96	.028
Self Regard	95.5 ± 18.6	100.9 ± 9.4	4.40	.038
Self-Actualization	96.6 ± 17.0	101.5 ± 9.0	4.29	.041

Table 7. A one-way ANOVA examination of differences in emotional intelligence, assessed with standardized EQ-i scores, between alopecia areata (AA) patients and a non-clinical sample.

The 4th study. The fourth study re-evaluated here examines the impact of emotional intelligence (EI) on health in a sample of coronary heart disease patients who suffered myocardial infarction (MI). This study was conducted by a graduate student in South Africa in 1996 [63], and the source in which it was described [38] was cited 380 times in other publications. The graduate student administered the EQ-i to 58 MI patients within 10 days of being hospitalised after suffering a heart attack; and their scores were compared with the EQ-i scores of 58 individuals who were randomly selected from the normative sample upon which this instrument was normed in South Africa. She applied a t-test to examine the difference in EI between the two groups, and the results are listed in Table 8 below.

EQ-i scales	MI patient Scores	Non-clinical Scores	t value	p level
Stress Tolerance	84.0	99.8	8.70	<.001
Flexibility	85.3	100.6	8.08	<.001
Self-Actualization	84.7	98.2	7.68	<.001
Happiness	86.1	98.6	7.46	<.001
Problem Solving	90.3	100.9	5.04	<.001

Table 8. Significant differences in emotional intelligence, assessed with standardized EQ-i scores, between the MI patients (n=58) and a non-clinical sample (n=58).

The results in Table 8 indicate that the MI patients exhibited significant deficiencies in their ability to manage emotions (Stress Tolerance), to solve problems of a personal and interpersonal nature (Problem Solving), to change and adapt (Flexibility) and appeared less motivated to pursue their personal goals (Self-Actualization) and less content with their lives (Happiness) when compared with the control group.

The 5th study. The fifth study discussed in this section examined differences in emotional intelligence between 35 cancer survivors and a matched non-clinical sample [64]. This study, which was cited in 12 other peer-reviewed publications, was conducted in the Paediatric Oncology Department at Rambam Hospital in Israel. A group of 35 late adolescents and young adults, who were considered to be "cancer survivors" (i.e., symptom free for at least five years), were randomly selected from hospital files. The individuals in this group were initially diagnosed with various types of cancer when they were children or young adolescents. In one of their follow-up examinations, they were asked to complete the EQ-i. Their scores were compared with the EQ-i scores of 35 randomly selected individuals from the local normative population sample matched for gender and age. The only EQ-i scale that was able to significantly distinguish the cancer survivors from the non-clinical control group was Optimism as can be seen in Table 9.

EQ-i scales	CA survivors Scores	Non-clinical Scores	F score	p level
Optimism	32.3 ± 5.1	29.6 ± 3.7	6.34	.014

Table 9. Significant differences in emotional intelligence between the adolescent cancer survivors (n=35) and a non-clinical sample (n=35).

As is observed in Table 9, the cancer survivors' level of optimism is significantly higher than the non-clinical subjects. This is an interesting finding, in light of the fact that optimism is considered a key facilitator of emotionally and socially intelligent behaviour [39]. Additionally, Barbara Fredrickson's research has demonstrated that positive emotions, such as optimism, joy and contentment, strategically broaden the "thought-action repertoire" that plays an important role in survival [65]. Based on her findings and those of others, such emotions create the desire to contemplate current life situations, to be flexible [66], open and integrate relevant information [67, 68] into new perceptions of the self and world enhancing one's ability to survive and creatively adapt [69]. This serves to broaden one's "cognitive organization" for the purpose of integrating a wide range of diverse information [70, p. 87]; and when individuals expand their focus of attention, problem-solving is more flexible, creative and effective than when they are in a negative or neutral mood state [65].

Summary: The results generated by the five studies reviewed in this section indicate that emotional intelligence has a significant impact on health as well as on the ability to cope with and possibly survive life-threatening medical conditions. Table 10 summarises the key findings from these studies that have examined the relationship between emotional intelligence on health.

EI factors assessed by the EQ-i	Study No. 1	Study No. 2	Study No. 3	Study No. 4	Study No. 5
Self Regard	√		√		
Stress Tolerance	√	√	√	√	
Flexibility		√		√	
Problem Solving		√		√	
Self-Actualization	√	√	√	√	
Optimism	√	√	√		√
Happiness	√	√	√	√	

Table 10. The 7 EI factors that appeared most often in Tables 1 through 9 that are significantly associated with physical health.

Table 10 shows that the four most important EI competencies, skills and behaviours that impact health appear to be (1) the ability to adequately manage emotions and cope with stress, (2) the ability to set personal goals and the drive to achieve them in order to actualise one's potential, (3) optimism as well as (4) the ability to feel content with oneself, others and life in general. Additionally, but to a lesser extent, (5) being aware of one's limitations and weaknesses as well as one's strengths, (6) flexibility and adaptability as well as (7) the ability to solve personal and interpersonal problems also appear to be important in attaining and maintaining good physical health.

6. The nature of the relationship between emotional intelligence and subjective wellbeing

Does emotional intelligence impact overall subjective wellbeing (SWB)? To address this question, it is helpful to re-examine an earlier study that empirically studied this relationship in 2005 [49] which was cited in 20 other publications. In that study, wellbeing was defined as a subjective state that emerges from a feeling of satisfaction with (a) one's physical health and oneself in general, (b) one's close interpersonal relationships and (c) one's occupation and financial situation. This comprehensive definition of subjective wellbeing comprises the key reoccurring themes used to describe this construct in the literature. Ryff [71], Helliwell and Putnam [72] consider all three of these particular aspects of SWB to be the essential features of this construct, while Oswald [73], Clark [74] and others have emphasised the occupational and financial component. It is important to note that the above three-factor conceptualisation also reflects very closely the most current description of this construct on the web (www.merriam-webster.com/dictionary/well-being -- September 1, 2011), which defines subjective wellbeing as the state of being happy, healthy and prosperous which is similar to the old adage of being "healthy, wealthy and wise."

In the 2005 study [49], a measure of SWB was used which captures the above definition of this construct. This measure was based on the item and factor analysis of 16 items that were originally designed to tap the physical, personal, interpersonal, occupational and financial aspects of subjective wellbeing in the 152-item beta version of the EQ-i [38]. In the initial stage, item analysis eliminated the 7 weakest items. Then, a varimax rotation of the 9 remaining items was applied and rendered three clearly identifiable factors. Three interpersonal satisfaction items loaded on the first factor (33.8% of the variance). One occupational and two financial satisfaction items loaded on the second factor (14.1% of the variance). And one personal and two physical health satisfaction items loaded on the third factor (11.2% of the variance). The specific items that load on these three factors appear in Appendix B. These nine items were excluded from the final version of the EQ-i together with additional items, which were originally designed to tap various aspects of quality of life and overall wellbeing as was previously mentioned.

Because of the limited number of items (3) in each of the final factorial components of this instrument, a 9-item composite scale of overall SWB was created by summing all of the items. The instrument is based on a self-report assessment modality, which remains the method of choice for measuring SWB [75, 76] irrespective of the criticism that is typically levelled against this type of assessment for other purposes. Additionally, Helliwell and Putnam [72] strongly support a near exclusive use of self-reports to measure this construct as do most of the other current researchers in this area. Moreover, a growing body of research findings demonstrate that responses on self-report measures reflect real differences across individuals corresponding with external reports of observed behaviour [77-79].

Using this 9-item SWB measure, the relationship between emotional intelligence and subjective wellbeing was then examined using Multiple Regression Analysis on the original North American normative sample for the EQ-i (n=3,385/3,831). The results indicated that the two constructs are highly correlated (R=.77 – F=380.41, p<.001). The three most significant EI predictors of SWB that emerge from the regression model are listed in Table 11.

EI Competencies assessed by the EQ-i	β score	t value	p level
Self Regard	.402	20.13	<.001
Happiness	.231	11.61	<.001
Self-Actualization	.165	9.08	<.001

Table 11. A multiple regression analysis of the impact of EI on general SWB (n=3,385), rendering a correlation of .77 and the following 3-factor predictive model.

Table 11 reveals a well defined 3-factor EI model that impacts subjective wellbeing and accounts for 60% of the variance (R²=.60). According to this model and based on the way these EI factors are defined in Appendix A, individuals who (a) understand and accept themselves, (b) strive to achieve personal goals and actualise their potential and who (c) are content with themselves, others and life, in general, typically experience a sense of wellbeing. It can be seen that the three factors in the regression model fairly closely parallel the factorial model of the SWB instrument for the most part.

Examining the contribution of emotional intelligence to wellbeing addresses a reoccurring theme in the literature regarding the need to empirically study those factors that impact SWB and to develop models that predict it [80]. The implications of the above-mentioned findings are that it is indeed possible to create models capable of predicting SWB as some scholars have envisaged [80].

7. The nature of the relationship between health and subjective wellbeing

Is one's level of self-perceived health significantly correlated with subjective wellbeing, and can subjective wellbeing, in turn, impact self-perceived health? To address the first part of this question, it is necessary to examine the degree of correlation between the previously-mentioned indicator of SPH ("I feel good about my health") and the above-mentioned SWB measure. Before doing that, however, the above item that is used as the SPH indicator was removed from 9-item SWB measure (Appendix B); otherwise, its inclusion would artificially increase the degree of correlation between SPH and SWB. Based on the North American sample upon which the EQ-i was originally normed (n=3,831), the resulting bivariate correlation that emerged is .56 accounting for 31% of the variance (R²=.31) This is a moderately high correlation suggesting that one's level of self-perceived health does indeed have a significant impact on one's overall sense of subjective wellbeing.

To address the second part of the above question (i.e., whether subjective wellbeing impacts self-perceived health), a Multiple Regression Analysis was applied to examine the extent to which SWB impacts SPH on the same population sample. The resulting correlation coefficient was once again .56 (R²=.31, F=343.16, p<.001) as expected, and the predictive regression model that emerged appears in Table 12 below.

Subjective Wellbeing	β score	t value	p level
I feel good about my physical fitness.	.435	30.34	<.001
Looking at both my good points and bad points, I feel good about myself.	.144	9.29	<.001
I feel good about my family life.	.089	5.71	<.001
I am happy with my intimate relations with others.	.054	3.50	.001
I'm happy with my work.	.043	3.04	.002

Table 12. A multiple regression analysis of the impact of SWB on SPH (n=3,753), which rendered a correlation of .56 and the following 5-factor predictive model.

The results presented here suggest that 31% of the variance (R²=.31) of self-perceived health is explained by subjective wellbeing. Additionally, the specific findings in Table 12 appear to indicate that satisfaction with (a) one's physical fitness and self-acceptance as wells as with (b) one's interpersonal relationships and with (c) work have a strong impact on one's health. Although physical health is typically considered to be a cause rather than an effect of SWB [72], the findings presented here suggest that there most likely is a reciprocal relationship between physical health and subjective SWB [65]. The chain of events are perhaps as follows: (a) EI factors contribute to health and overall SWB, and (b) SWB, in turn, contributes to physical health.

The above findings compare favourably with those previously obtained by Brackett and Mayer [81], who carried out one of the only other studies that directly examine the overall relationship between EI and SWB followed by Bar-On [49]. On a homogeneous sample of 207 university students, they examined the correlation between SWB (evaluated with Carol Ryff's measure of this construct [71]) and EI (assessed with both the MSCEIT [42] and the EQ-i [45]). The results revealed a correlation of .28 rendered by the MSCEIT and .54 rendered by the EQ-i. It is important to point out that Brackett and Mayer [81] did not describe the specific EI predictors of SWB in their article.

8. Discussion

This chapter presented findings from seven studies that empirically demonstrate that emotional intelligence (EI) significantly impacts physical health and overall subjective wellbeing. Those EI factors that have the strongest impact on health and wellbeing are the following:

1. Self regard (the ability to accurately perceive, understand and accept oneself)
2. Self-actualisation (the ability to pursue personal goals and actualise one's potential)
3. Stress tolerance (the ability to effectively and constructively manage emotions)
4. Optimism (the ability to be positive, hopeful and look at the brighter side of life)
5. Happiness (the ability to feel content with oneself, others and life in general)

Based on the way these EI factors are defined by the Bar-On model, it appears that people who (1) are accurately aware of and accept themselves, (2) pursue constructive personal goals, (3) are capable of effectively managing their emotions, (4) are optimistic and (5) content with themselves, their significant others and life in general tend to experience good health and wellbeing. It is interesting to note that stress tolerance and self-actualisation are also two of the most powerful EI contributors to mental health as well [50].

Although physical health was based on both self-report as well as objective medical evaluation in clinical and non-clinical samples, the primary limitation of the studies reviewed in this chapter is that the data were generated by one particular measure of emotional intelligence and one particular measure of wellbeing. These specific models of emotional intelligence and wellbeing, no matter how valid and reliable they might be, cannot logically provide an exhaustive and complete assessment of these constructs. Future studies in this area of scholarly inquiry should, therefore, use a wider variety of psychometric instruments to assess both emotional-social intelligence and subjective wellbeing. Additionally, the relationship between emotional intelligence, health and subjective wellbeing should also be studied on more diverse clinical and non-clinical samples. Not only should the cross-cultural element be taken into consideration in selecting the non-clinical samples in future studies, but the relationship between emotional intelligence, health and wellbeing should be re-examined in a wider variety of clinical samples. In light of the fact that all of the studies presented here were cross-sectional moreover, future studies should also attempt to longitudinally re-examine this relationship in order to better predict the ability to attain and maintain health as well as to survive and recover from life-threatening medical conditions.

The impact of additional (potential) predictors of health and wellbeing should also be empirically explored in future studies. For example, this could include personality factors, resilience and spiritual development. Two large studies, in which the author will be involved, are presently being designed and will shed more light on the psycho-social nature of physical health, recovery from illness and subjective wellbeing. One will look at the emotional, social and spiritual predictors of health as well as the effects of targeted intervention to enhance these specific predictors and, hopefully, health in a non-clinical sample. The other study will examine the impact of emotional intelligence, resilience and spirituality on breast cancer survivorship.

After demonstrating, in the present chapter, that emotional intelligence significantly impacts both physical health and subjective wellbeing, it is logical to ask whether emotionally and socially intelligent behaviour can be enhanced in order to improve health and wellbeing. In responding to this very important question, it is necessary to point out that numerous studies are described in the literature showing that emotionally and socially intelligent behaviour can indeed be enhanced at home [82-84], school [85-90], work [91-100] as well as in the clinical setting [63, 101, 102]. The findings indicate that EI factors are both teachable and learnable, and that these competencies, skills and behaviours, unlike personality traits, can be enhanced by relatively simple didactic methods over a relatively short period of time [103]. Not only do these studies show that such EI-oriented programmes can make a significant difference, they also support the notion that EI measures can effectively be used to monitor and measure progress achieved as a result of these programmes. What also needs to be done in future projects of this nature is to more extensively examine a variety of pre-

and post-intervention behavioural parameters to help evaluate the extent to which positive changes have been made as well as maintained overtime.

Since the mid 1960s, growing numbers of children around the world have been introduced to EI-enriching curricula such as those developed and promoted by Self-Science [85, 88], the Collaborative for Academic, Social, and Emotional Learning [82, 89] and the National School Climate Center [86]. Some of these programmes have targeted not only individual schools but cities [87], entire school districts [104] and even larger geographic areas [105].

Hopefully, the results presented here, together with future findings, will eventually make their way into parenting, education and healthcare. Parents and educators could benefit from these efforts by learning how best to raise and educate children to be more emotionally and socially intelligent, effective and healthy; and based on the findings presented in this chapter, it is reasonable to assume that such efforts in parenting and education will have a positive and, hopefully, lasting effect on overall subjective wellbeing. This could also add an important and valuable component to preventive medicine. Healthcare personnel could eventually benefit from assessing their patients' level of EI, overall wellbeing and other closely-associated predictive factors (e.g., personality traits, resilience and spiritual development). The results of this type of diagnostic screening could indicate the need to refer patients for remedial counselling designed to strengthen specific EI deficiencies needed to help improve physical health and wellbeing.

In closing, it is the hope of this author that research continues to expand in this very important area of scholarly inquiry and that the findings will be applied in order to help improve health and wellbeing for an ever increasing number of people worldwide.

9. Appendices

EQ-i scales	The EI competencies and skills assessed by each scale
Self Regard	*To accurately perceive, understand and accept oneself.*
Emotional Self-Awareness	*To be aware of and understand one's emotions.*
Assertiveness	*To effectively and constructively express one's emotions and oneself.*
Independence	*To be self-reliant and free of emotional dependency on others.*
Self-Actualization	*To strive to achieve personal goals and actualise one's potential.*
Empathy	*To be aware of and understand how others feel.*
Social Responsibility	*To identify with one's social group and cooperate with others.*
Interpersonal Relationship	*To establish mutually satisfying relationships and relate well with others.*
Stress Tolerance	*To effectively and constructively manage emotions.*
Impulse Control	*To effectively and constructively control emotions.*
Reality Testing	*To objectively validate one's feelings and thinking with external reality.*
Flexibility	*To adapt and adjust one's feelings and thinking to new situations.*
Problem Solving	*To effectively solve problems of a personal and interpersonal nature.*
Optimism	*To be positive, hopeful and look at the brighter side of life.*
Happiness	*To feel content with oneself, others and life in general.*

Appendix A. The EQ-i Scales and What They Assess

SWB Scale Components	The Items Included in Each SWB Component:
Physical & Personal SWB:	1. I feel good about my health in general.
	6. I feel good about my physical fitness.
	2. Looking at both my good points and bad points, I feel good about myself.
Interpersonal SWB:	3. I'm happy with the people I live with.
	7. I'm happy with my intimate relations with others.
	9. I feel good about my family life.
Occupational & Financial SWB:	4. I'm happy with my work.
	8. I'm happy with my financial situation.
	5. I'm satisfied with the money I have to live on.

Appendix B. The Experimental Scale Used to Examine SWB in the Present Study

10. References

[1] Goleman, D. (1995). *Emotional intelligence*. New York: Bantam Books.

[2] Darwin, C. (1872/1965). *The expression of the emotions in man and animals*. Chicago: University of Chicago Press.

[3] Thorndike, E. L. (1920). Intelligence and its uses. *Harper's Magazine, 1(40)*, 227-235.

[4] Moss, F. A., & Hunt, T. (1927). Are you socially intelligent? *Scientific American, 137*, 108-110.

[5] Moss, F. A., Hunt, T., Omwake, K. T., & Ronning, M. M. (1927). *Social intelligence test*. Washington, DC: Center for Psychological Servie.

[6] Doll, E. A. (1935). A generic scale of social maturity. *American Journal of Orthopsychiatry, 5*, 180-188.

[7] Chapin, F. S. (1942). Preliminary standardization of a social impact scale. *American Sociological Review, 7*, 214-225.

[8] Wechsler, D. (1955). *Manual for the Wechsler Adult Intelligence Scale*. New York, NY: The Psychological Corporation.

[9] Wechsler, D. (1940). Nonintellective factors in general intelligence. *Psychological Bulletin, 37*, 444-445.

[10] Wechsler, D. (1943). Nonintellective factors in general intelligence. *Journal of Abnormal Social Psychology, 38*, 100-104.

[11] Zirkel, S. (2000). Social intelligence: The development and maintenance of purposive behavior. In R. Bar-On and J. D. A. Parker (Eds.), *Handbook of emotional intelligence*. San Francisco: Jossey-Bass, pp. 3-27.

[12] Wechsler, D. (1958). *The measurement and appraisal of adult intelligence (4th ed.)*. Baltimore, MD: The Williams & Wilkins Company.

[13] Kelly, G. A. (1955). *A theory of personality: The psychology of personal constructs*. New York: Norton.

[14] Rogers, C. R. (1961). *On becoming a person (2nd ed.)*. Boston: Houghton Mifflin.

[15] Rotter, J. B. (1966). Generalized expectancies for internal versus external control of reinforcement. *Psychological Monographs, 80*, 1-28.

[16] Cantor, N., & Kihlstrom, J. (1987). *Personality and social intelligence*. Englewood Cliffs, NJ: Erlbaum.

[17] Salovey, P., & Mayer, J. D. (1990). Emotional intelligence. *Imagination, Cognition, and Personality, 9*, 185-211.

[18] Ruesch, J. (1948). The infantile personality. *Psychosomatic Medicine, 10*, 134-144.

[19] MacLean, P. D. (1949). Psychosomatic disease and the visceral brain: Recent developments bearing on the Papez theory of emotion. *Psychosomatic Medicine, II*, 338-353.

[20] Sifneos, P. E. (1967). Clinical observations on some patients suffering from a variety of psychosomatic diseases. *Acta Medicina Psychosomatica, 21*, 133-136.

[21] Appelbaum, S. A. (1973). Psychological mindedness: Word, concept, and essence. *International Journal of Psycho-Analysis, 54*, 35-46.

[22] Lane, R. D., & Schwartz, G. E. (1987). Levels of emotional awareness: A cognitive-developmental theory and its application to psychopathology. *American Journal of Psychiatry, 144*, 133-143.

[23] Lane, R. D. (2000). Levels of emotional awareness: Neurological, psychological and social perspectives. In R. Bar-On and J. D. A. Parker (Eds.), *Handbook of emotional intelligence*. San Francisco: Jossey-Bass, pp. 171-191.

[24] Damasio, A. R. (1994). *Descartes' error: Emotion, reason, and the human brain*. New York: Grosset/Putnam.

[25] LeDoux, J. (1996). *The emotional brain: The mysterious underpinnings of emotional life*. New York: Simon and Schuster.

[26] Bechara, A., Tranel, D., & Damasio, R. (2000). Poor judgment in spite of high intellect: Neurological evidence for emotional intelligence. In R. Bar-On and J. D. A. Parker (Eds.), *Handbook of emotional intelligence*. San Francisco: Jossey-Bass, pp. 192-214.

[27] Bar-On, R., Tranel, D., Denburg, N. L., & Bechara, A. (2003). Exploring the neurological substrate of emotional and social intelligence. *Brain, 126*, 1790-1800.

[28] Lane, R. D., & McRae, K. (2004). Neural substrates of conscious emotional experience: A cognitive-neuroscientific perspective. In B. M. Amsterdam and J. Benjamins (Eds.), *Consciousness, emotional self-regulation and the brain*, pp. 87-122.

[29] Bar-On, R., Tranel, D., Denburg, N. L., & Bechara, A. (2005). Exploring the neurological substrate of emotional and social intelligence. In J. T. Cacioppo and G. G. Bernston (Eds.), *Key readings in social psychology: Social neuroscience*. New York, NY: Psychology Press, pp. 223-237.

[30] Bechara, A., & Bar-On, R. (2006). Neurological substrates of emotional and social intelligence: Evidence from patients with focal brain lesions. In J. T. Cacioppo, P.S. Visser, and G. L. Pickett (Eds.), *Social neuroscience: People thinking about thinking people*. Cambridge, MA: MIT Press, pp. 13-40.

[31] Bechara, A., Damasio, A., & Bar-On, R. (2007). The anatomy of emotional intelligence and the implications for educating people to be emotionally intelligent. In R. Bar-On, J. G. Maree, & M. Elias (Eds.), *Educating people to be emotionally intelligent*. Westport, CT: Praeger, pp. 273-290.

[32] Davies, M., Stankov, L., & Roberts, R. D. (1998). Emotional intelligence: In search of an elusive construct. *Journal of Personality and Social Psychology, 75*, 989-1015.

[33] Zeidner, M., Matthews, G., & Roberts, R. D. (2001). Slow down, you move too fast: Emotional intelligence remains an "elusive" intelligence. *Emotion, Vol. 1 (No. 3)*, 265-275.

[34] Matthews, G., Roberts, R. D., Zeidner, M. (2003). Development of emotional intelligence: A skeptical – but not dismissive – perspective. *Human Development, 46*, 109-114.

[35] Gardner, H. (1983). *Frames of mind*. New York: Basic Books.

[36] Saarni, C. (1990). Emotional competence: How emotions and relationships become integrated. In R. A. Thompson (Ed.), *Socioemotional development. Nebraska symposium on motivation (vol. 36)*. Lincoln, NE: University of Nebraska Press, pp. 115-182.

[37] Bar-On, R. (1988). *The development of a concept of psychological well-being*. Unpublished doctoral dissertation, Rhodes University, South Africa.

[38] Bar-On, R. (1997b). *The Emotional Quotient Inventory (EQ-i): Technical manual*. Toronto, Canada: Multi-Health Systems, Inc.

[39] Bar-On, R. (2000). Emotional and social intelligence: Insights from the Emotional Quotient Inventory (EQ-i). In R. Bar-On and J. D. A. Parker (Eds.), *Handbook of emotional intelligence*. San Francisco: Jossey-Bass, pp. 363-388.

[40] Spielberger, C. (Ed.) (2004). *Encyclopedia of Applied Psychology*. Academic Press.

[41] Mayer, J. D., & Salovey, P. (1997). What is emotional intelligence: In P. Salovey, & D. Sluyter (Eds.). *Emotional development and emotional intelligence: Implications for educators*. New York: Basic Books, pp. 3-31.

[42] Mayer, J. D., Salovey, P., & Caruso, D. R. (2002). *Mayer-Salovey-Caruso Emotional Intelligence Test (MSCEIT)*. Toronto, Canada: Multi-Health Systems, Inc.

[43] Goleman, D. (1998). *Working with emotional intelligence*. New York: Bantam Books.

[44] Boyatzis, R. E., Goleman, D., & HayGroup (2001). *The Emotional Competence Inventory (ECI)*. Boston: HayGroup.

[45] Bar-On, R. (1997a). *The Emotional Quotient Inventory (EQ-i): A test of emotional intelligence*. Toronto, Canada: Multi-Health Systems, Inc.

[46] Bar-On, R., & Handley, R. (2003a). *The Bar-On EQ-360*. Toronto, Canada: Multi-Health Systems.

[47] Bar-On, R., & Handley, R. (2003b). *The Bar-On EQ-360: Technical manual*. Toronto, Canada: Multi-Health Systems.

[48] Bar-On, R., & Handley, R. (2003c). *The Bar-On Emotional Quotient Interview (EQ-interview)*. Toronto, Canada: Multi-Health Systems.

[49] Bar-On, R. (2005). The impact of emotional intelligence on subjective well-being. *Perspectives in Education, 23 (2)*, 41-61.

[50] Bar-On, R. (2006). The Bar-On model of emotional-social intelligence. *Psicothema, 18*, supl., 13-25.

[51] Bar-On, R. (2004). The Bar-On Emotional Quotient Inventory (EQ-i): Rationale, description, and summary of psychometric properties. In G. Geher (Ed.), *Measuring emotional intelligence: Common ground and controversy*. Hauppauge, NY: Nova Science Publishers, pp. 111-142.

[52] Plake, B. S., & Impara, J. C. (Eds.). (1999). *Supplement to the thirteenth mental measurement yearbook*. Lincoln, NE: Buros Institute for Mental Measurement.

[53] Geher, G. (Ed.) (2004). *Measuring emotional intelligence: Common ground and controversy*. Hauppauge, NY: Nova Science Publishers.

[54] Stewart-Brown, S., & Edmunds, L. (2007). Assessing emotional intelligence in children: A review of existing measures of emotional and social competence. In R. Bar-On, J. G. Maree, & M. Elias (Eds.), *Educating people to be emotionally intelligent*. Westport, CT: Praeger, pp. 241-257.

[55] Van Rooy, D. L., & Viswesvaran, C. (2007). Assessing emotional intelligence in adults: A review of the most popular measures. In R. Bar-On, J. G. Maree, & M. Elias (Eds.), *Educating people to be emotionally intelligent*. Westport, CT: Praeger, pp. 259-272.

[56] Idler, E. L., Kasl, S. V., & Lemke, J. H. (1990). Self-evaluated health and mortality among elderly in New Haven, Connecticut, and Iowa and Washington counties, Iowa.1982-1986. *American Journal of Epidemiology, 131*, 91-103.

[57] Idler, E. L., & Kasl, S. V. (1991). Health perceptions and survival: Do global evaluations of health status really predict mortality. *Journal of Gerontology, 46*, S55-S65.

[58] Balty, D. (1999). Self-perceived health and 5-year mortality risks among elderly in Shanghai, China. *American Journal of Epidemiology, 150*, 219.

[59] Bosworth, H. B., Siegler, I. C., Brummett, B. H., Barefoot, J. C., Williams, R. B., Clapp-Channing, N. E., & Mark, D. B. (1999). The association between self-rated health and mortality in a well-characterized sample of coronary artery disease patients. *Medical Care, 37*, 1226-1236.

[60] Lesser, G. T. (2000). Social and productive activities in elderly people: Self rated health is an important predictor of mortality. *BMJ, 320*, 185.

[61] Shadbolt, B., Barresi, J., & Craft, P. (2002). Self-rated health as a predictor of survival among patients with advanced cancer. *Journal of Clinical Oncology, 20* (10), 2514-2519.

[62] Monselise, A., Bar-On, R., Chan, L. J. Y., Leibushor, N, McElwee, K. J., & Shapiro, J. (2011). Examining the relationship between alopecia areata, androgenetic alopecia and emotional intelligence. Submitted to the *Journal of the American Academy of Dermatology*.

[63] Dunkley, J. (1996). *The psychological well-being of coronary heart disease patients before and after an intervention program*. Unpublished master's thesis. University of Pretoria, South Africa.

[64] Krivoy, E., Weyl Ben-Arush, M., Bar-On, R. (2000). Comparing the emotional intelligence of adolescent cancer survivors with a matched sample from the normative population. *Medical & Pediatric Oncology, 35* (3), 382.

[65] Fredrickson, B. L. (2004). The broaden-and-build theory of positive emotions. *Philosophical Transactions of the Royal Society of London: Biological Sciences, 359*, 1367-1377.

[66] Isen, A. M., & Daubman, K. A. (1984). The influence of affect on categorization *Journal of Personality and Social Psychology, 47*, 1206-1217.

[67] Isen, A. M., Rosenzweig, A. S., & Young, M. J. (1991). The influence of positive affect on clinical problem solving. *Medical Decision Making, 11*, 221-227.

[68] Estrada, C. A., Isen, A. M., & Young, M. J. (1997). Positive affect facilitates integration of information and decreases anchoring in reasoning among physicians. *Organizational Behavior and Human Decision Process, 72*, 117-135.

[69] Isen, A. M., Daubman, K. A., & Nowicki, G. P. (1987). Positive affect facilitates creative problem solving. *Journal of Personality and Social Psychology, 52*, 112-1131.

[70] Isen, A. M. (1990). The influence of positive and negative affect on cognitive organization: Some implications for development. In N. Stein, B. Leventhal & T. Trabasso (Eds.), *Psychological and biological approaches to emotion*. Hillsdale, NJ: Erlbaum, 75-106.

[71] Ryff, C. D. (1989). Happiness is everything, or is it? Explorations on the meaning of psychological well-being. *Journal of Personality and Social Psychology, 57*, 1069-1081.

[72] Helliwell, J. F., & Putnam, R. D. (2004). The social context of well-being. *Philosophical Transactions of the Royal Society of London: Biological Sciences, 359*, 1435-1446.

[73] Oswald, A. J. (1997). Happiness and economic performance. *Economic Journal., 107*, 1815-1831.

[74] Clark, A. E. (2003). Unemployment as a social norm: Psychological evidence from panel data. *Journal of Labor Economics, 21*, 323-351.

[75] Huppert, F. A., & Baylis, N. (2004). Well-being: Towards an integration of psychology, neurobiology and social science. *Philosophical Transactions of the Royal Society of London: Biological Sciences, 359*, 1447-1451.

[76] Huppert, F. A., Baylis, N., & Keverne, B. (2004). Introduction: Why do we need a science of well-being. *Philosophical Transactions of the Royal Society of London: Biological Sciences, 359*, 1331-1332.

[77] Diener, E. (2000). Subjective well-being: The science of happiness and a proposal for a national index. *American Psychologist, 55*, 34-43.

[78] Helliwell, J. F. (2001). Social capital, the economy and well-being. In K. Banting, A. Sharpe & F. St-Hilaire (Eds.), *The review of economic performance and social progress*. Montreal and Ottawa: Institute for Research on Public Policy and Centre for the Study of Living Standards, pp. 43-60.

[79] Donovan, N., Halpern, D., & Sargeant, R. (2003). *Life satisfaction: The state of knowledge and implications for government*. London: Cabinet Office Strategy Unit.

[80] Nesse, R. M. (2004). Natural selection and the elusiveness of happiness. *Philosophical Transactions of the Royal Society of London: Biological Sciences, 359*, 1333-1347.

[81] Brackett, M. A., & Mayer, J. D. (2003). Convergent, discriminant, and incremental validity of competing measures of emotional intelligence. *Personality and Social Psychology Bulletin, 29* (9), 1147-1158.

[82] Patrikakou, E. N., & Weissberg, R. P. (2007). School-family partnerships to enhance children's social, emotional and academic learning. In R. Bar-On, J. G. Maree, & M. Elias (Eds.), *Educating people to be emotionally intelligent*. Westport, CT: Praeger, pp. 49-61.

[83] Saarni, C. (2007). The development of emotional competence: Pathways for helping children to become emotionally intelligent. In R. Bar-On, J. G. Maree, & M. Elias (Eds.), *Educating people to be emotionally intelligent*. Westport, CT: Praeger, pp. 15-35.

[84] Stern, R., & Elias, M. J. (2007). Emotionally intelligent parenting. In R. Bar-On, J. G. Maree, & M. Elias (Eds.), *Educating people to be emotionally intelligent*. Westport, CT: Praeger, pp. 37-48.

[85] Freedman, J, (2003). Key lessons from 35 years of social-emotional education: How Self-Science builds self-awareness, positive relationships, and healthy decision-making. *Perspectives in Education, 21*(4), 69-80.

[86] Cohen, J., & Sandy, S.V. (2007). The social, emotional and academic education of children: Theories, goals, methods and assessments. In R. Bar-On, J. G. Maree, & M.

Elias (Eds.), *Educating people to be emotionally intelligent*. Westport, CT: Praeger, pp. 63-77.

[87] Hayes, N. M. (2007). The Comer School Development Program: A pioneering approach to improving social, emotional and academic competence. In R. Bar-On, J. G. Maree, & M. Elias (Eds.), *Educating people to be emotionally intelligent*. Westport, CT: Praeger, pp. 95-107.

[88] McCown, K., Jensen, A. L., & Freedman, J. (2007). The Self-Science approach to social-emotional learning. In R. Bar-On, J. G. Maree, & M. Elias (Eds.), *Educating people to be emotionally intelligent*. Westport, CT: Praeger, pp. 109-121.

[89] Zins, J. E., Elias, M. J., & Greenberg, M. T. (2007). School practices to build social-emotional competence as the foundation of academic and life success. In R. Bar-On, J. G. Maree, & M. Elias (Eds.), *Educating people to be emotionally intelligent*. Westport, CT: Praeger, pp. 79-94.

[90] Sheehy, J. M., Bennett, B. L., & Bar-On, R. The impact of emotional intelligence on academic performance. Submitted to the *South African Journal of Psychology*.

[91] Sjölund, M., & Gustafsson, H. (2001). *Outcome study of a leadership development assessment and training program based on emotional intelligence*. An internal report prepared for the Skanska Management Institute in Stockholm, Sweden.

[92] Langhorn, S. (2004a). *The role of emotions in service encounters*. An unpublished doctoral dissertation submitted to the University of Luton (UK).

[93] Langhorn, S. (2004b). How emotional intelligence can improve management performance. *International Journal of Contemporary Hospitality Management*, (16), 220-230.

[94] Slaski, M., & Bardzil, P. (2002). Emotional intelligence: Fundamental competencies for enhanced service provision. In S. Tax et al. (Eds.), *Quality in service: Crossing borders*. Vitoria, BC: University of Victoria, pp. 3-6.

[95] Slaski, M., & Cartwright, S. (2002). Health, performance and emotional intelligence: An exploratory study of retail managers. *Stress and Health, Vol. 18*, 63-68.

[96] Slaski, M., & Cartwright, S. (2003). Emotional intelligence training and performance and its implications for stress, health and performance. *Stress and Health, Vol. 19*, 233-239.

[97] Bar-On, R., Handley, R., & Fund, S. (2005). The impact of emotional and social intelligence on performance. In Vanessa Druskat, Fabio Sala, and Gerald Mount (Eds.), *Linking emotional intelligence and performance at work: Current research evidence*. Mahwah, NJ: Lawrence Erlbaum, pp. 3-19.

[98] Bharwaney, G. (2007). Coaching executives to enhance emotional intelligence and increase productivity. In R. Bar-On, J. G. Maree, & M. Elias (Eds.), *Educating people to be emotionally intelligent*. Westport, CT: Praeger, pp. 183-197.

[99] Boyatzis, R. E. (2007). Developing emotional intelligence through coaching for leadership, professional and occupational excellence. In R. Bar-On, J. G. Maree, & M. Elias (Eds.), *Educating people to be emotionally intelligent*. Westport, CT: Praeger, pp. 155-168.

[100] Lennick, D. (2007). Emotional competence development and the bottom line: Lessons from American Express Financial Advisors. In R. Bar-On, J. G. Maree, & M. Elias (Eds.), *Educating people to be emotionally intelligent*. Westport, CT: Praeger, pp. 199-210.

[101] Taylor, G. J., & Taylor-Allan, H. L. (2007). Applying emotional intelligence in understanding and treating physical and psychological disorders: What we have learned from alexithymia. In R. Bar-On, J. G. Maree, & M. Elias (Eds.), *Educating people to be emotionally intelligent.* Westport, CT: Praeger, pp. 211-223.

[102] Stohl, L., Dangerfield, D., Christensen, J., Justice, D., & Mottonen, D. (2007). Applying emotional intelligence in treating individuals with severe psychiatric disorders: A psychotherapeutic model for educating people to be emotionally intelligent. In R. Bar-On, J. G. Maree, & M. Elias (Eds.), *Educating people to be emotionally intelligent.* Westport, CT: Praeger, pp. 225-240.

[103] Bar-On, R., Maree, J. G., Elias, M. J. (Eds.), (2007). *Educating people to be emotionally intelligent.* Westport, CT: Praeger.

[104] Brackett, M. A., Alster, B., Wolfe, C. J., Katulak, N. A., & Fale, E. (2007). Creating an emotionally intelligent school district: A skills-based approach. In R. Bar-On, J. G. Maree, & M. Elias (Eds.), *Educating people to be emotionally intelligent.* Westport, CT: Praeger, pp. 123-137.

[105] Maree, J. G., & Mokhuane, Q. E. M. (2007). First steps in developing a community-based teacher training program designed to educate children to be emotionally intelligent. In R. Bar-On, J. G. Maree, & M. Elias (Eds.), *Educating people to be emotionally intelligent.* Westport, CT: Praeger, pp. 139-153.

4

Clinical Perspectives in Emotional Intelligence

Michel Hansenne
University of Liège, Department of Psychology
Belgium

1. Introduction

Emotional intelligence (EI) is the ability to recognize and express emotions in yourself, and the ability to understand the emotions of others (Salovey & Mayer, 1990). Research devoted to EI has now split off into two distinct perspectives. Both perspectives share the idea that cognitive abilities are not the unique predictor of successful adaptation but that emotional competencies have to be taken into consideration. However, these perspectives markedly differ regarding their conceptualization of such emotional competencies and their assessment. On the one hand, ability models (Mayer & Salovey, 1997) conceive EI as an ability encompassing four dimensions: (a) emotions identification; (b) emotions utilization; (c) emotions understanding; and (d) emotions regulation. In this ability perspective, EI is assessed via intelligence-like tests which comprise correct and wrong responses. On the other hand, trait models (Petrides & Furnham, 2001) consider EI as a multifaceted construct encompassing 13–15 (depending on the model) emotion-related behavioral dispositions thought to affect the ways an individual would cope with demands and pressures (e..g, self-control, well-being, emotional sensibility and sociability). In this trait perspective, EI is evaluated via personality-like questionnaires. While ability tests capture maximal performance like intelligence tests, trait tests aim to capture typical performance (Petrides & Furnham, 2003). Therefore, one can say that ability EI assess what an individual could do, and trait EI what he really do.

Recently the scientific community becomes interested in EI, in order to discern what is true among the huge number of claims on this topic. Indeed, there is still controversy about whether EI represents an entity that differs from what psychologists in the field of intelligence, personality, and applied psychology already know under other names. But now, several lines of evidence suggest the existence of the influence of EI on quality of life, educational attainment, and occupational success. Therefore, since the theoretical foundations of EI are now well recognized, clinical researches are of interest. In this chapter, the main results concerning the relationships between EI and well-being will be reported. After that, some findings on EI and both anxious and depressive states will be developed. Finally, some recent data supporting the possibility to increase EI with specific interventions will be presented.

2. Emotional intelligence and well-being

A vast amount of research has documented a positive association between trait EI and well-being related variables (Zeidner et al., 2009), even if as for other outcomes, it is important to distinguish theoretically and replicated findings from anecdotal ones (Matthews et al., 2002). More particularly, interpersonal abilities are expected to be related to better social and personal relationships, whereas intrapersonal skills are expected to be related to life satisfaction and subjective well-being. Indeed, a better emotional regulation should lead to lower perception of stress and a better quality of life, and subjects with higher EI should report elevated psychological well-being and happiness. Some data demonstrated that subjects that can manage others' emotions seem to respond less intensively to stressful situations, they express more empathy and they have a better social support that protects them from negative feelings. In addition, positive correlations between EI and subjective happiness and life satisfaction were found.

A study reported by Ciarrochi et al. (2001) investigated the relationship between trait EI as assessed by the Schutte's scale (Schutte et al., 1998) and different outcomes theoretically linked to EI among a large sample of adolescents. The results showed first that trait EI, as expected, was positively correlated to self-esteem and negatively with trait anxiety. Second, the authors reported positive associations between EI and the amount of social support, the satisfaction with social support and parental warmth. Interestingly, when self-esteem and trait anxiety were controlled, the relationships remained significant except for parental warmth, meaning that EI explained over these variables some important outcomes. In addition, the amount of social support from friends and extended family was more related to EI than the amount of social support from parents and siblings. The question of the direction of these associations is still open: are individuals with higher EI able to develop and maintain strong social support, or are individuals with relevant social support become better in EI?

The same findings, in addition with health-related measures, were found in a large sample of young adults (Austin et al., 2005). EI was assessed by the revised version of the scale of Schutte (Austin et al., 2004), which proposes three factors: optimism/mood regulation, appraisal of emotion, and utilisation of emotion. The results showed that total EI score was positively correlated with the social network size, the satisfaction with social support, the temporal satisfaction with life, and negatively correlated with the units of alcohol per week, but that EI was not associated with self-rated heath compared to others and nor with the number of visits to family doctor the last six months. Moreover, total EI score was negatively correlated with alexithymia. Regression analyses showed that when personality was controlled EI was a significant predictor of social network size, but didn't play a role as a significant predictor for other outcomes. In sum, the finding showed that EI has limited incremental validity, only for social network size, although other studies have reported incremental validity of EI over personality for life satisfaction and loneliness (Palmer et al., 2002; Saklofske et al., 2003). More recently, findings from a study reported by Austin et al. (2010) showed that lower scores of EI were associated with higher level of stress among undergraduate students assessed at the start of the semester and before the pre-exam period, and that EI mediated the effects of personality on stress and subjective well-being.

Another field of investigation of the association between EI and psychological outcomes involves well-being in itself. Last years, substantial literature extends the concept of well-being outside the domain of ill-being state (Cavanagh et al., 2011). Indeed, the majority of previous studies were focused on the therapeutic strategies developed to increase well-being in depressive or anxious patients as well as in diverse somatic disorders, but now efforts are allocated to ameliorate well-being in normal subjects. This recent interest comes from the development of positive psychology (Peterson, 2006; Wood et al., 2010). There are two main approaches to the study of well-being: the subjective well-being (SWB) approach and the psychological well-being (PWB) one (Ryan & Deci, 2001). First, SWB is defined in relation to life experiences that make the life either enjoyable or unpleasant. In another words, some life experiences are more favorable to induce and maintain well-being. SWB is strongly associated to individual differences related to positive and negative affect, or more particularly to the affective style described by Davidson (2004). A positive affective style means a positive bias towards life experiences and emotional experiences in which individuals allocate more automatic and controlled attention in the direction of positive life experiences and positive emotions (e.g., more recall of positive personal experiences or positive rather than negative words in a free recall test and more positive projection in the future), and this affective style is associated with higher left frontal brain activity as compared to right frontal brain activity. In contrast, individuals with a negative affective style are characterized by a negative bias towards personal life and emotional experiences, and exhibited higher right frontal brain activity as compared to left frontal one.

Second, PWB is considered as a predictor of the strength and the duration of the SWB, and comprises some characteristics that favor the SWP, as self-acceptance, life's goals, environmental mastering, autonomy, supportive relationships, and personal growth (Cloninger, 2004). Recent findings showed that PWB is a strongly predictor of SWB after controlling for personality and demographic measures (Burns & Machin, 2010).

There are four ways to consider a link between EI and well-being (Zeidner & Olnick-Shemesh, 2010). First, since individuals with higher EI are more aware of their emotion and that they are more able to regulate their emotion, they should exhibit lower distress and therefore higher well-being. Second, since these individuals report greater social skills and higher social network quality, this can help them to improve their well-being. Third, understanding our emotions and those of others induce a better environmental and social adaptation, leading to a higher well-being. Finally, individuals with higher EI experience more positive than negative emotions, which play a role to a better well-being.

Mikolajczak et al. (2010) investigated the link between affective style and EI among a sample of young adults. Affective style was assessed by the alpha power band of the electroencephalogram recorded over frontal electrodes. More precisely, an asymmetry index was created from the five frontal electrodes pairs (right/left) by subtracting the natural logarithm of the right site from the natural logarithm of the left homologous site. The results revealed that individuals with higher trait EI as assessed by the Trait Emotional Intelligence Questionnaire (TEIQue, Petrides & Furnham, 2003) had significantly higher left-sided mean frontal asymmetry scores than individuals with lower trait EI. This result was mainly explained by the factor sociability and to a lesser extent by factors self-control and well-being. Therefore, according to the hypothesis, the pattern of resting electroencephalographic activity recorded in the frontal areas was significantly associated with EI.

Zeidner and Olnick-Shemesh (2010) point out that the significant relationships found between EI and well-being measures are limited to trait EI measures and that the results obtained with ability EI measures are not conclusive. As Mikolajczak et al. (2008) argued, ability EI assess what an individual could do, and trait EI what he really do. Consequently, knowing what is better to do doesn't allow an individual to improve his or her well-being. In their prospective study, Zeidner and Olnick-Shemesh (2010) demonstrated that ability EI is not related to either cognitive or affective facets of SWB.

3. Emotional intelligence in depression and anxiety

Despite the link between EI and well-being, few studies have examined the relationship between EI and both depression and anxiety. However, a better emotional regulation should have direct implications to prevent depressive states since EI is associated with higher psychological well-being and happiness (Austin et al., 2005; Furnham & Petrides, 2003). Therefore, it could be postulated that EI should be reduced in depressive patients. Moreover, some findings among normal (non-depressed) subjects suggest such an association between depression and EI.

When developing the first measure of EI based on a comprehensive model of EI, Schutte et al. (1998) reported on a large group of university students and adults significant positive correlations between EI score and optimism, and negative ones between pessimism and depressive tendencies. Moreover, Dawda and Hart (2000) assessed the convergent validity of the Bar-On Emotional Quotient Inventory (EQ-i) and found, logically based on EI construct, that EI exhibited strong negative correlations with the Beck Depression Inventory (BDI), and more particularly the intrapersonal EQ composite score (i.e., the ability to express and experience emotions). Ciarrochi et al. (2002) showed also that subjects that can manage others' emotions seem to respond less intensively to stressful situations and exhibit less suicidal ideation, less depression, and less hopelessness. Moreover, they express more empathy and they have better social support that protects them from negative feelings. In contrast, subjects higher on emotional perception reported greater depression, hopelessness, and suicidal ideation.

This later finding implying that some facets of EI (i.e., emotion perception) could be considered as a vulnerability factor for depression was replicated in a further study examining the link between EI and depression as regards to cultural variables (Fernandez-Berrocal et al., 2005). These authors assessed the cultural influences on the relationship between EI and depression, and more particularly the influence of individualistic/collectivistic cultures and Masculinity/Femininity dimension. Indeed, individualistic cultures are characterized by greater relevance of own emotions and higher quality of live (i.e., greater positive than negative emotions), while in collectivistic cultures less attention is allocated to the emotional dimension of the individual. Moreover, feministic nations reported more emotional expression than the masculinity ones. The results showed that emotional perception was positively associated with the BDI score, but that emotional regulation was correlated negatively with depression, and that these associations were more intense in feministic countries. In contrast, the individualistic/collectivistic division didn't influence the results. In other words, emotional perception without regulation has rather negative consequences. This finding was extended to job performance (Quoidbach & Hansenne, 2009). Indeed, in this study health care quality of nursing teams was positively correlated with emotion regulation of the team, but emotion appraisal was negatively correlated with the health care quality provided by teams.

In addition to the abovementioned studies, Martinez-Pons (1997) showed that EI correlated positively with life satisfaction, but negatively with depressive symptoms, suggesting that individuals with higher EI report greater life satisfaction and fewer depressive-related symptoms than those with lower EI. Saklofske et al. (2003) also reported negative correlations corresponded to theoretical expectations between EI and social, family, and romantic loneliness as well as between EI and depression-proneness (i.e., the tendency towards developing depressive feelings), and positive correlations between EI and subjective happiness and temporal, past and concurrent life satisfaction among undergraduate students. The persistence of significant associations with these measures when personality is controlled suggests that EI displays incremental validity, implying some degree of explanatory power for these measures over and above those provided by personality trait scores. Schmidt and Andrykowski (2004) demonstrated that EI was associated with lower distress and lower avoidance of the disease among a sample of women with breast cancer, and that higher EI could act as a buffer against the negative impact of a toxic social environment. Moreover, Brown and Schutte (2006), when examining the relationship between EI and subjective fatigue among university students, demonstrated that higher EI was associated with less fatigue, probably because EI allows individuals to develop coping strategies, such as healthier mood, as well as more adaptive ways of interpreting the world and a better social support to ameliorate the effects of physical stresses. Finally, Extremera and Fernandez-Berrocal (2006) using the Trait Meta-Mood Scale (TMMS) reported that low levels of emotional clarity (i.e., understanding owns emotions) and mood repair (i.e., emotional regulation) were related to high levels of depression, but that in contrast, high level of emotional attention (i.e., amount of attention toward owns emotions) was related to depression.

Fisher et al. (2010) investigated the relationship between EI as assessed by the TMMS and both arousal and apprehensive anxieties as well as depression within an emotion-word Stroop task. In addition, Event-Related Brain Potentials (ERPs) were recorded to assess the temporal information processing of the emotional words (see Hansenne, 2006 for a review on ERPs). From a behavioral point of view, the authors reported that both clarity and repair but not attention facets of the TMMS were negatively correlated with both anxious apprehension and arousal as well as with anhedonic depression. Hierarchical regressions showed that only anxious arousal accounted for the variance in clarity and that anhedonic depression was the only predictor for the variance of mood repair. ERPs results showed that P200 amplitude (i.e., an index of automatic attention) was related to attention of emotion and to apprehensive anxiety without an effect of the valence of the word: individuals with higher scores of attention of emotion and with higher apprehensive anxiety exhibited higher P200 amplitude, meaning more attentional allocation to the stimuli. P300 latency (i.e., an index of the time of stimulus conscious processing) was related to emotional clarity and apprehensive anxiety for the negative word, meaning that individuals with higher scores of emotional clarity and with higher apprehensive anxiety processed slower negative words. Taken together, these results demonstrated that attention to emotion and apprehensive anxiety are associated with enhanced automatic processing of information, and that emotional clarity and apprehensive anxiety are associated with increased time to categorize the negative stimuli. In other words, some facets of EI in combination with apprehensive but neither arousal anxiety nor anhedonic depression modify the processing of emotional stimuli.

These studies suggest that emotional regulation dimension's of EI is the core feature of the association between EI and depression, and that emotional perception could be considered as a vulnerability factor for depression. Although these findings are robust they are observed mainly on control subjects and not on depressive ones. Therefore, one step further is to examine the association between EI and depression among major depressive disorder patients. Such study could investigate the impact of EI on depressive severity and to assess whether EI in depression is state or/and trait dependent. Hansenne and Bianchi (2009) investigated EI in a group of depressive inpatients at the beginning of the hospitalization and among a subsample of these patients when they were in a period of remission. Remission was defined by clinical assessment and by a score lower than 7 on the 17-item of the Hamilton Depressive Rating Scale (HDRS), and a score lower than 2 on item 1. EI was assessed by the modified version of Schutte's scale (Schutte et al., 1998) proposed by Austin et al. (2004). The results showed that depressed patients (time 1, beginning of the hospitalization) had lower EI total scores and lower scores for the subscale optimism/mood regulation, as well as for appraisal of emotions as compared to the control group (Table 1). As compared to the depressed state (time 1), patients in remission (time 2) had higher scores on the total EI scale as well as on optimism/mood regulation subscale (Table 2). Comparisons between patients in remission and the group of control participants showed that the two groups didn't differ for either the total EI score or the sub-scores. Stepwise regression conducted among depressed patients at time 1 showed that the HDRS score was not explained by total EI score or the sub-scores.

	Depressive Inpatients	Controls	P
Optimism/Mood regulation	41.1 + 7.2	47.9 + 5.5	<0.001
Appraisal of emotions	30.2 + 7.6	38.2 + 5.8	<0.001
Utilisation of emotions	19.0 + 3.9	20.2 + 2.9	NS
EI total	131.7 + 18.1	153.2 + 14.6	<0.001

Table 1. Comparisons between depressed patients and controls for EI

The main findings of Hansenne and Bianchi (2009) study's are that depressed patients exhibit lower total EI score and lower subscale scores on optimism/mood regulation and appraisal of emotions. Interestingly, patients in remission have higher scores on the total EI scale as well as on the subscale optimism/mood regulation as compared with their scores during the depressed state. These results suggest a state but not a trait effect because patients in remission do not show differences from controls, but when patients are ill, the total score and the scores of two subscales (i.e., optimism/mood regulation and appraisal of emotions) are lower in the clinical group than in controls. The results also show that the subscale optimism/mood regulation is more particularly dependent of the clinical state since it is modified in the remission phase as compared with the acute phase of the depressive episode. This is the first study that investigated the relationships between EI and depression and the findings could suggest important clinical implications. Since optimism/emotional regulation is the core dimension found in depression, therapeutic strategies based on EI construct could be useful as an important part of the psychological treatment. However, since the score of this dimension is only affected by the clinical state, one cannot conclude that optimism/emotional regulation is an enduring emotional deficit in remitted depression, and in consequence that this dimension couldn't be considered as a vulnerability factor as some dimensions of personality (e.g., the dimension of harm avoidance, Hansenne & Bianchi, 2009). Nevertheless, the introduction of a therapeutic strategy designed to enhance the ability to maintain a positive mood and to reduce a negative one could be very important during the depressive episode, as suggested by Palmer et al. (2002). Training of this type might help to prevent future depressive relapses, as well as improving the quality of the clinical recovery from the depressive episode.

	Depressive Inpatients	Remitted Depressives	P
Optimism/Mood regulation	41.1 ± 4.8	45.4 ± 4.8	0.01
Appraisal of emotions	33.4 ± 7.7	34.9 ± 6.3	NS
Utilisation of emotions	18.6 ± 3.6	19.2 ± 3.8	NS
EI total	134.8 ± 18.4	144.5 ± 16.8	0.02

Table 2. Comparisons of EI between depressed patients and remitted depressive patients

Since EI is related to well-being and consecutively to self-esteem, besides to depressive states, anxiety could be logically related to lower emotion regulation and higher emotional perception. Fernandez-Berrocal et al. (2006) investigated the link between EI and anxiety in a sample of adolescents from 14 to 19 years old. The results showed that the score of the State-Trait Anxiety Inventory is negatively correlated to two facets of EI's TMMS scale; mood repair and emotional clarity. More exactly, regression analysis demonstrated that adolescents which report higher abilities to discriminate and understand their emotion, as well as higher skills to regulate their emotional state, exhibited lower anxiety independently to the level of self-esteem.

Concerning anxious disorders, some data have reported associations between several facets of EI and social phobia as well as generalized anxiety disorder (GAD). GAD is an anxious disorder characterized mainly by exaggerate worries about usual activities, and some theoretical models assume that individuals with GAD avoid emotional processing of various stimulations by the use of worries because they are unable to cope with their overwhelming emotions. In consequence GAD implies an avoidance of intense emotions through worries, which means a deficit of emotional regulation as a core feature of this disorder. Worries let the individual to process emotion in an abstract and conceptual level and avoid intense negative emotions. Indeed, empirical findings show that individuals with GAD exhibit greater emotional experience for negative but not for positive emotions than controls, and have poorer abilities to identify and describe their emotional experience, as well as to modulate their negative emotions (Mennin et al., 2005). In another words, the deficit is mainly localized in term of excessive emotion perception but without emotion awareness. In contrast, Novick-Kline et al. (2005) using a questionnaire based on emotional scenarios that elicited specific emotion with five levels of increasing difficulty found that, conversely to previous researches, individuals with GAD exhibit greater emotional awareness than controls. However, since this questionnaire requests a conceptual processing level rather than an automatic one, the results can be considered as congruent with the findings of Mennin et al. (2005). Finally, Turk et al. (2005) reported that individuals with GAD exhibited greater emotion intensity and higher negative emotion expression than individuals with social anxiety disorder.

Social phobia (SP) is mainly characterized by the fear of social situations in which the individual could be judged, leading to high level of discomfort. These subjects consider their social performance as very negative, and allocate their attention to no-relevant information that justifies their anxious state. So, avoidance strategies to cope with social anxiety are usually utilized. Several lines of evidence suggest that SP is associated to atypical responses to other's emotions, and more particularly individuals with SP exhibit higher neural responses to diverse emotional facial expressions (Amir et al., 2005; Straube et al., 2005). The deficit of emotional processing in SP is directly related to some aspects of EI. Therefore, investigating the relationship between EI and SP could add some relevant information to this disorder. It could be argued that the fear of social situations found in SP could reveal a reduced ability to interpret these situations due to a reduced EI. This hypothesis was recently investigated in a sample of SP patients (Jacobs et al., 2008). In this study, EI was assessed by the Mayer-Salovey-Caruso Emotional Intelligence Test (MSCEIT) which considers four branches of EI; perceiving emotion, using emotion, understanding emotion, and managing emotion. In addition to the MSCEIT, the Liebowitz Social Anxiety Scale (LSAS), the Beck Anxiety Inventory (BAI), and the Global Assessment of Functioning (GAF) scale were completed by the patients. The results showed that individuals with SP exhibited MSCEIT scores within the normal range of normal scores. Moreover, as compared to control participants, SP patients reported only a trend toward lower scores of perceiving emotion, but the scores of the three other branches didn't differ from the control group. Therefore, SP seems not characterized by deficit in EI. However, correlations between LSAS and MSCEIT scores revealed interesting findings: significant negative correlations between the severity of social anxiety as assessed by the LSAS and both the perceiving and using emotions branches but not significant correlations with the two other branches (i.e., understanding and managing emotions).

These results are interesting since the significant correlations were observed on the experiential aspect of EI, and not on the strategic one, meaning that social anxiety is strongly related to lower perception of emotional information. Strategic EI involves the ability to reason about emotions and their management, and is related to semantic knowledge about emotions, and reflects more conscious processing of emotion. Therefore, these skills are not related to social anxiety. In contrast, experiential EI (i.e., using and perceiving emotions) is strongly related to social anxiety, and specifically because the severity of anxiety as assessed by the BAI doesn't explain the associations. This finding means that a core feature of social anxiety is really related to a deficit in the perception of own and other emotional states. In other words, individuals with reduced experiential EI could be more influenced by social misinterpretations, leading to an increase of social anxiety symptoms. Summerfeldt et al. (2011) confirm and extend these findings. They showed that SP is mainly characterized by a lower interpersonal EI score (i.e., understanding and identification of others' emotions) as compared to controls, but that panic disorder and obsessive-compulsive disorder didn't differ from controls. In addition they reported that intrapersonal EI (i.e., understanding and identification of owns emotions) was reduced within the three clinical groups as compared to controls, but with a greater level in SP patients.

Finally, a recent study investigated the link between social intelligence conceived as a broad concept including EI and social anxiety (Hampel et al., 2011). The authors considered social intelligence from a theoretical model that comprises five cognitive abilities: social understanding, social memory, social perception, social flexibility, and social knowledge. A measure of three of these facets called the Magdeburg Test of Social Intelligence has been validated. These performance based measures consist of a rating of emotion perceived by the participants throughout scenario description, video or picture of social interaction. As expected, social perception, social memory, and social understanding predict negatively the level of social anxiety.

4. Increasing emotional intelligence

Interventions designed to improve EI have recently flourished particularly among children's, managers, and subjects with affective difficulties. Despite the huge expansion of EI development methods and the preliminary evidence for their effectiveness, very few EI programs are based on a solid theoretical model and even fewer have been rigorously tested (Matthews et al., 2007). Although validated programs for kids have emerged with positive outcomes (Zins et al., 2007), programs for adults have been less successful due to several drawbacks. First, these trainings lack a clear theoretical and methodological rationale and use a miscellany of techniques whose psychological bases are sometimes questioning. Second, they usually target only some EI dimensions (e.g., emotion identification but not emotion management) and add a number of skills which are not considered as parts of EI, such as problem solving, alcohol or drugs prevention, and reduction of violence. Third, when evaluations of these programs exist, they are often limited to subjective impression right after the training given by teachers for EI training at school or by the director for EI training at work, without considering the long-term effects. Finally, none of the EI trainings' evaluations to date included a control group.

Thus, in spite of the proliferation of trainings, important questions have remained unanswered: is it possible to meaningfully improve adults' EI? Do the changes last? Do they lead to subsequent alterations in personality? In addition, crucially, which benefits in terms of well-being, health, social relationships, and work success are expected from such EI improvement?

Recent studies (Nélis et al., 2009, 2011) aim to answer those questions while avoiding the shortcomings that have detracted from previous research. To this end, an 18-hour intervention was designed that focused on teaching theoretical knowledge about emotions and on training participants to apply specific emotional skills in their everyday lives. The EI intervention consisted of either three 6-hour sessions (a session on each of 2 consecutive days and the last session 2 weeks later) or six 3-hour sessions (one session per week for 6 weeks). This interval between sessions gave participants time to apply their learning in their daily life. Sessions were centered on the four core emotional competencies: identification, understanding, regulation, and utilisation (Mayer & Salovey, 1997; Saarni, 1999). Each session was designed to enhance a specific emotional competence: understanding emotions, identifying one's own emotions, identifying others' emotions, regulating one's own emotions, regulating others' emotions, and using positive emotions to promote well-being. The content of each session consisted of short lectures, role-playing games, group discussions, and work in dyads. Participants were also provided with a personal diary in which they had to daily report one emotional experience. These emotional experiences had to be analyzed in light of the theory presented in session. Finally, various readings were also proposed. The detailed outline of the sessions is presented in Table 3.

Outline of EI Training Sessions	
Session 1: Understanding Emotions	Welcome-Explanation of the sessions and introduction to the use of the personal diary Introduction to the importance of emotions and explanation of key concepts (emotions, EC) Video clips illustrating the importance of emotions Summary
Session 2: Identifying Emotions	Review of previous session Identifying one's emotions using three doors (i.e., physiological activation, cognitions, and action tendencies): theory and practice Identifying other's emotions through nonverbal communication Identifying other's emotions through facial expression decoding: drill with the METT program Summary and homework
Session 3: Listening to Other's Emotions	Review of previous session and homework Basic communication rules Active listening Empathic listening Role play on active listening Summary
Session 4: Expressing Emotions to Others	Review of previous session How to express emotions: facts — emotions — needs — positive solutions Role play on the expression of emotions How to manage a conflict? Theory and role play Summary and homework
Session 5: Managing Emotions	Review of previous session and homework Coping strategies and their effectiveness: theory and group discussion Positive reappraisal: role play and drill Mind-body connections and relaxation exercises Summary
Session 6: Enhancing Emotions	Review of previous session The importance of positive emotions: theory and group discussion Using the power of positive emotions: promoting positive feelings (e.g., gratefulness) Savoring: theory and exercises Summary-Questions-Evaluation

Table 3. Outline of EI training

After the in-class training, an e-mail-based follow-up was set up to optimize knowledge transfer in daily life. Participants have received two e-mails per week for 6 weeks (12 e-mails total). Each e-mail included a theoretical reminder of the notions discussed in class and a related practical exercise. E-mails were kept as short and simple as possible to increase the chances they were read and put into practice.

In the first study (Nélis et al., 2009), participants of the experimental and control groups completed measures of trait EI, emotion regulation, emotion comprehension, and personality prior to the intervention, at the end of the intervention, and 6 months later. The findings indicated that compared to the control group, the training group showed a significant improvement in emotion understanding, emotion regulation, and overall EI directly after the intervention (Figure 1). Analysis of the change dynamics further revealed that these initial changes remained stable over a 6-month period. That the effect was significant on all these three measures of emotional competences suggests that the training didn't only increase emotion-related knowledge and abilities but also, and more crucially, the use of these knowledge and abilities in daily life. Finally, the intervention led to an immediate increase in extraversion (Figure 2) as well as a progressive increase in agreeableness and a progressive decrease in neuroticism (Figure 3), which all reached significance 6 months after training. Moreover, mediation analysis revealed that these changes were partly mediated by the increase in EI. The more participants learned to understand and manage their emotions, the more sociable and emotionally stable they became. These results suggest that personality traits that have been shown to be relatively stable over time can be modified through intensive training. These findings dovetail with previous studies, demonstrating that clinical interventions can actually change person.

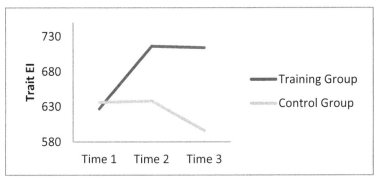

Fig. 1. Comparisons of trait EI between the training and the control group before the training (Time 1), just after the training (Time 2) and six months after the training (Time 3)

In the second study (Nélis et al., 2011), the authors examined whether changes in EI resulted in observable changes in EI correlates, namely psychological well-being, subjective health, quality of social relationships, and work success. To ensure that the benefits of the training were attributable to the changes in EI and not to unrelated factors such as conforming to the experimenter's expectations, developing a social network, becoming involved in a new activity, and so forth, the efficiency of the EI training was assessed with two control groups: one composed of people who didn't participate in the training program, and another one composed of people following an improvisation drama training. Consistent with the previous findings, results showed that EI can increase after a brief training. Moreover, that EI didn't increase in the drama improvisation and control group suggests that these improvements were specific to the training and cannot be explained by experimenter demand, expectation of improvement, or other group processes. More importantly the results showed that developing EI leads to a wide array of positive consequences. Participants in the EI training group reported a significant improvement of their physical health, mental health, happiness, life satisfaction, and global social functioning. Likewise, employability also increased following the EI intervention, as a diverse panel of human resource professionals was more likely to hire participants after the training.

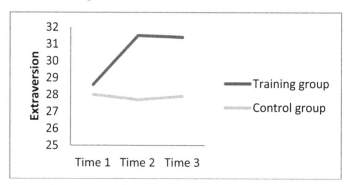

Fig. 2. Comparisons of extraversion between the training and the control group before the training (Time 1), just after the training (Time 2) and six months after the training (Time 3)

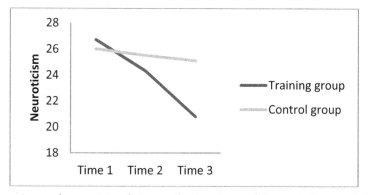

Fig. 3. Comparisons of neuroticism between the training and the control group before the training (Time 1), just after the training (Time 2) and six months after the training (Time 3)

Another recent study (Di Fabio & Kenny, 2011) reports identical positive findings of an EI intervention on different psychological characteristics. This study assessed the efficacy of a training program focused on EI among Italian high school students. The training was elaborated on an ability-based model of EI and the procedure comprised an experimental and a control group like in the Nélis et al.'s studies (Nélis et al., 2009, 2011). The training was divided into four sessions of 2 hour and a half each, weekly. Each session focused on one of the four branches of the MSCEIT (i.e., perceiving emotions, facilitating thought, understanding emotion, and managing emotion). The results showed significant increasing of the scores of the MSCEIT within the experimental group after the intervention, and also increasing scores of the Schutte's et al. (1998) scale. Moreover, the results showed that EI training decreased levels of indecisiveness and career decision difficulties.

Overall, these findings are promising because they demonstrate that, with a proper methodology relying on the latest scientific knowledge of emotion and emotional processing, EI can be enhanced, which in turn, improves people's lives. Not only can people improve their emotional competencies as adults, but learning to identify, understand, express, manage, and use emotions to one's advantage can also be beneficial for them. These findings bring hope to people who have not had the opportunity to develop their EI during their personal development. With motivation, effort, and guidance, such individuals can still improve their EI later in life, and thereby enhance their adjustment in many domains of life. Applications of this intervention in health, educational, and organizational settings offer a promising approach to developing and promoting effective life skills.

5. Conclusions

Theoretical models of EI are now well-validated and robust findings give to this concept a real place into the study of individual differences as personality and intelligence. Even if researches are needed to increase the knowledge of EI, there are sufficient empirical data to explore and investigate clinical applications of EI in different settings.

Indeed, EI is clearly associated to well-being related outcomes and can explain negative states like anxiety and depression. The core feature is emotional regulation. Since appropriate trainings of EI have shown promising results to promote well-being and to reduce negative states, the challenge now is to implement those training not only to enhance emotional well-being in normal individuals but also to reduce poorer emotional regulation leading to negative states like anxiety and depression.

6. References

Amir, N., Klumpp, H., Elias, J., Bedwell, J.S., Yanasak, N., & Miller, L.S. (2005). Increasing Activation of the Anterior Cingulate Cortex during Processing of Disgust Faces in Individuals with Social Phobia. *Biological Psychiatry*, Vol.57, No.9, (May 2005), pp. 975-981, ISSN 0006-3223

Austin, E., Saklofske, D.H., Huang, S.H.S., & McKenney, D. (2004). Measurement of Trait Emotional Intelligence: Testing and Cross-Validating a Modified Version of Schutte et al.'s (1998) Measure. *Personality and Individual Differences*, Vol.36, No.3, (February 2004), pp. 555-562, ISSN 0191-8869

Austin, E., Saklofske, D.H., & Egan, V. (2005). Personality, Well-Being, and Health Correlates of Trait Emotional Intelligence. *Personality and Individual Differences*, Vol.38, No.3, (February 2005), pp. 547-558, ISSN 0191-8869

Austin, E., Saklofske, D.H., & Mastoras, S.M. (2010). Emotional Intelligence, Coping and Exam-Related Stress in Canadian Undergraduate Students. *Australian Journal of Psychology*, Vol.62, No.1, (March 2010), pp. 42-50, ISSN 0004-9530

Burns, R.A., & Machin, M.A. (2010). Indentifying Gender Differences in the Independent Effects of Personality and Psychological Well-Being on Two Broad Affect Components of Subjective Well-Being. *Personality and Individual Differences*, Vol.48, No.1, (January 2010), pp. 22-27, ISSN 0191-8869

Brown, R.F., & Schutte, N.S., (2006). Direct and Indirect Relationships between Emotional Intelligence and Subjective Fatigue in University Students. *Journal of Psychosomatic Research*, Vol.60, No.6, (June 2006), pp. 585-593, ISSN 0022-3999

Cavanagh, S. R., Urry, H.L., & Shin, L.M. (2011). Mood-Induced Shifts in Attentional Bias to Emotional Information Predict Ill- and Well-Being. *Emotion*, Vol.11, No2, (April 2011), pp. 241-248, ISSN 1528-3542

Ciarrochi, D.R., Deane, F.P., & Anderson, S. (2001). Measuring Emotional Intelligence in Adolescents. *Personality and Individual Differences*, Vol.31, No.7, (November 2001), pp. 1105-1119, ISSN 0191-8869

Ciarrochi, D.R., Deane, F.P., & Anderson, S. (2002). Emotional Intelligence Moderates the Relationship Between Stress and Mental Health. *Personality and Individual Differences*, Vol.32, No.2, (January 2002), pp. 197-209, ISSN 0191-8869

Cloninger, C.R. (2004). *Feeling Good: The Science of Well-Being*, Oxford University Press, ISBN 0-195-05137-8, New York

Davidson, R.J. (2004). Well-Being and Affective Style: Neural Substrates and Biobehavioural Correlates. *Philosophical Transactions of the Royal Society of London Series B-Biological Sciences*, Vol.359, No.1449, (September 2004), pp. 1395-1411, ISSN 0962-8436

Dawda, D., & Hart, S.D. (2000). Assessing Emotional Intelligence: Reliability and Validity of the Bar-On Emotional Quotient Inventory (EQ-i) in University Students. *Personality and Individual Differences*, Vol.28, No.4, (April 2000), pp. 797-812, ISSN 0191-8869

Di Fabio, A., & Kenny, M.E. (2011). Promoting Emotional Intelligence and Career Decision Making Among Italian High School Students. *Journal of Career Assessment*, Vol.18, No1., (January 2011), pp. 21-34, ISSN 1069-0727

Extremera, N., & Fernandez-Berrocal, P. (2006). Emotional Intelligence as Predictor of Mental, Social, and Physical Health in University Students. *Spanish Journal of Psychology*, Vol.9, No.1, (May 2006), pp. 45-51, ISSN 1138-7416

Fernandez-Berrocal, P., Salovey, P., Vera, A., Extremera, N., & Ramos, N. (2005). Cultural Influences on the Relation between Perceived Emotional Intelligence and Depression. *International Review of Social Psychology*, Vol.18, No.1, (January 2005), pp. 91-107, ISSN 0992-986X

Fernandez-Berrocal, P., Alcaide, R., Extremera, N., & Pizarro, D. (2006). The Role of Emotional Intelligence in Anxiety and Depression among Adolescents. *Individual Differences Research*, Vol.4, No.1, (January 2006), pp. 16-27, ISSN 1541-745X

Fisher, J.E., Sass, S.M., Heller, W., Levin Silton, R., Edgar, J.C., Stewart, J.L., & Gregory A. Miller, G.A. (2010). Time Course of Processing Emotional Stimuli as a Function of Perceived Emotional Intelligence, Anxiety, and Depression. *Emotion*, Vol.10, No.4, (August 2010), pp. 486-497, ISSN 1528-3542

Furnham, A., & Petrides, K.V. (2003). Trait Emotional Intelligence and Happiness. *Social Behavior and Personality*, Vol.31, No.8, (December 2003), pp. 815-824, ISSN 0301-2212

Hampel, S., Weis, S., Hiller, W., & Witthöft, M. (2011). The Relations between Social Anxiety and Social Intelligence: A Latent Variable Analysis. *Journal of Affective Disorders*, Vol.25, No.4, (May 2011), pp. 545-553, ISSN 0887-6185

Hansenne, M. (2006). Event-Related Brain Potentials in Psychopathology: Clinical and Cognitive Perspectives. *Psychologica Belgica*, Vol.54, No.1-2, (April 2006), pp. 5-36, ISSN 0033-2879

Hansenne, M., & Bianchi, J. (2009). Emotional Intelligence and Personality in Major Depression: Trait versus State Effects. *Psychiatry Research*, Vol.166, No.1, (March 2009), pp. 63-68, ISSN 0165-1781

Jacobs, M., Snow, J., Geraci, M., Vythilingam, M., Blair, R.J.R., Charney, D.S., Pine, D.S., & Blair. K.S. (2008). Association between Level of Emotional Intelligence and Severity of Anxiety in Generalized Social Phobia. *Journal of Anxiety Disorders,* Vol.22, No8, (December 2008), pp. 1487-1495, ISSN 0887-6185

Martinez-Pons, M., (1997). The Relation of Emotional Intelligence with Selected Areas of Personal Functioning. *Imagination, Cognition and Personality,* Vol.17, No.1, (January 1997), pp. 3–13, ISSN 0276-2366

Matthews, G., Zeidner, M., & Roberts, R. D. (2002). *Emotional Intelligence. Science and Myths,* The MIT press, ISBN 0-262-63296-9, Cambridge, MA.

Matthews, G., Zeidner, M., & Roberts, R. D. (2007). *The Science of Emotional Intelligence: Knowns and Unknowns,* Oxford University Press, ISBN 978-0-19-518189-0, New York

Mayer, J. D., & Salovey, P. (1997). What is Emotional Intelligence, In: *Emotional Development and Emotional Intelligence: Educational Implications,* P. Salovey & D. Sluyter (Eds.), 3-31, Basic Books, ISBN 0-465-09587-9, New York, NY

Mennin, D.S., Heimberg, R.G., Turk, C.L., &Fresco, D.M. (2005). Preliminary Evidence for an Emotion Dysregulation Model of Generalized Anxiety Disorder. *Behaviour Research and Therapy,* Vol.43, No.10, (October 2005), pp. 1281-1310, ISSN 0005-7967

Mikolajczak, M., Nélis, D., Hansenne, M., & Quoidbach, J. (2008). If you Can Regulate Sadness, you Can Probably Regulate Shame: Associations between Trait Emotional Intelligence, Emotional Regulation and Coping Efficiency across Discrete Emotions. *Personality and Individual Differences,* Vol.44, No.6, (April 2008), pp. 1356-1368, ISSN 0191-8869

Mikolajczak, M., Bodarwe, K., Laloyaux, O., Hansenne, M., & Nélis, D. (2010). Association between Frontal EEG Asymmetries and Emotional Intelligence among Adults. *Personality and Individual Differences,* Vol.48, No.2, (January 2010), pp. 177-181, ISSN 0191-8869

Nélis, D., Quoidbach, J., Mikolajczak, M., & Hansenne, M. (2009). Increasing Emotional Intelligence: (How) is it Possible? *Personality and Individual Differences,* Vol.47, No.1, (July 2009), pp. 36-41, ISSN 0191-8869

Nélis, D., Quoidbach, J., Hansenne, M., Kotsou, I., Weitens, F., Dupuis, P., & Mikolajczak, M. (2011). Increasing Emotional Competence Improves Psychological and Physical Well-Being, Social Relationships, and Employability. *Emotion,* Vol.11, No.2, (April 2011), pp. 354-366, ISSN 1528-3542

Novick-Kline, P., Turk, C.L., Mennin, D.S., Hoyt, E.A., & Gallager, C.L. (2005). Level of Emotional Awareness as a Differentiating Variable between Individuals with or without Generalized Anxiety Disorder. *Anxiety Disorders,* Vol.19, No.5, (October 2005), pp. 557-572, ISSN 0887-6185

Palmer, B., Donaldson, C., & Stough, C. (2002). Emotional Intelligence and Life Satisfaction. *Personality and Individual Differences,* Vol.33, No.7, (November 2002), pp. 1091-1100, ISSN 0191-8869

Peterson, C. (2006). *A Primer in Positive Psychology.* Oxford University Press, ISBN 978-0-19-518833-2, New York

Petrides, K.V., & Furnham A. (2003). Trait Emotional Intelligence: Psychometric Investigation with Reference to Established trait taxonomies. *European Journal of Psychology,* Vol.15, No.6, (November 2001), pp. 425-448, ISSN 0890-2070

Petrides, K.V., & Furnham A. (2003). Trait Emotional Intelligence: Behavioural Validation in Two Studies of Emotion Recognition and Reactivity to Mood Induction. *European Journal of Psychology,* Vol.17, No.1, (February 2003), pp. 39-57, ISSN 0890-2070

Quoidbach, J., & Hansenne, M. (2009). The Impact of Trait Emotional Intelligence on Nursing Team Performance and Cohesiveness. *Journal of Professional Nursing*, Vol.25, No.1, (January 2009), pp. 23-29, ISSN 8755-7223

Ryan, R.M., & Deci, E.L. (2001). On happiness and human potentials: A review of research on hedonic and eudaimonic well-being. *Annual Review of Psychology*, Vol.52, (January 2001), pp. 141-166, ISSN 0066-4308

Saarni, C. (1999). *The Development of Emotional Competence*, Guilford Press, ISBN 1-57230-433-2, New York, NY

Salovey, P., & Maycr, J.D. (1990). Emotional Intelligence. *Imagination, Cognition and Personality*, Vol.9, No.3, (September 1990), pp. 185-211, ISBN 0276-2366

Saklofske, D.H., Austin, E., & Minski, P.S. (2003). Factor Structure and Validity of a Trait Emotional Intelligence Measure. *Personality and Individual Differences*, Vol.34, No.4, (March 2003), pp. 707-721, ISSN 0191-8869

Schmidt, J.E., & Andrykowski, M.A. (2004). The Role of Social and Dispositional Variables Associated with Emotional Intelligence in Adjustment to Breast Cancer: an Internet-Based Study. *Health Psychology*, Vol.23, No.3, (May 2004), pp. 259-266, ISSN 0278-6133

Schutte, N.S., Malouff, J.M., Hall, L.E., Haggerty, D.J., Cooper, J.T., Golden, C.J., & Dornheim, L. (1998). Development and Validation of a Measure of Emotional Intelligence. *Personality and Individual Differences*, Vol.25, No.2, (August 1998), pp. 167-177, ISSN 0191-8869

Straube, T., Mentzel, H.J., & Miltner, W.H. (2005). Common and Distinct Brain Activation to Threat and Safety Signals in Social Phobia. *Neuropsychobiology*, Vol.52, No.3, (April 2005), pp. 163-168, ISSN 0302-282X

Summerfeldt L.J., Kloosterman, P.H., Antony M.M., & McCabe R.E., & Parker, J.D.A. (2011). Emotional Intelligence in Social Phobia and Other Anxiety Disorders. *Journal of Psychopathology and Behavioral Assessment*, Vol.33, No.1, (March 2011), pp. 69-78, ISSN 0882-2689

Turk, C.L., Heimberg, R.G., Luterek, J.A., Mennin, D.S., & Fresco, D.M. (2005). Emotion Dysregulation in Generalized Anxiety Disorder: A Comparison with Social Anxiety Disorder. *Cognitive Therapy and Research*, Vol.29, No.1, (February 2005), pp. 89-106, ISSN 0147-5916

Wood, A.M., Froh, J.J., & Geraghty, A.W.A. (2010). Gratitude and well-being: A review and theoretical integration. *Clinical Psychology Review*, Vol.30, No.7, (November 2010), pp. 890-905, ISSN 0272-7358

Zeidner, M., Matthews, G., & Robert, R. (2009). *What we Known about Emotional Intelligence. How it Affects Learning, Work, Relationship, and our Mental Health*, MIT Press, ISBN 978-0-262-25501-0, Cambridge, MA.

Zeidner, M., & Olnick-Shemesh, D. (2010). Emotional Intelligence and Subjective Well-Being Revisited. *Personality and Individual Differences*, Vol.48, No.4, (March 2010), pp. 431-435, ISSN 0191-8869

Zins, J. E., Payton, J. W., Weissberg, R. P., & Utne O'Brien, M. (2007). Social and emotional learning for successful school performance, In: *The Science of Emotional Intelligence: Knowns and Unknowns*, G. Matthews, M. Zeidner, & R. D. Roberts, (Eds.), 376-395, Oxford University Press, ISBN 978-0-19-518189-0, New York

5

A Meta-Analytic Review of Quantitative Studies on Emotional Intelligence and Leadership

Hui-Wen Vivian Tang[1] and Mu-Shang Yin[2]
[1]Department of Applied English, Ming Chuan University
Taoyuan,
[2]Department of Travel Management, Hsing Wu Institute of Technology
Taipei,
Taiwan

1. Introduction

Ever since Daniel Goleman (1998) maintained that emotional intelligence is the "sine qua non" of leadership, the link between emotional intelligence and leadership has become a topic of widespread interest in leadership research. The overriding focus of the leadership literature has been on emotional intelligence as hypothesized competencies or traits of individual leaders to affect leadership behaviors, effectiveness or emergence (e.g., Leban and Zulauf, 2004; Hawkins and Dulewicz, 2007; Rego *et al.*, 2007). Many studies have found that leaders' emotional intelligence explains a high proportion of variance in leadership effectiveness and a variety of organizational outcomes (e.g., Carmeli, 2003; Ozcelik et al., 2008). A significant range of literature also provides empirical evidence to support the notion that emotional intelligence is a predictor of transformational leadership (Barbuto and Burbach, 2006; Leban and Zulauf, 2004; Mandell and Pherwani, 2003; Duckett and Macfarlane, 2003). Despite all the evidence supporting the positive value of emotional intelligence on leadership, several studies have produced contradictions regarding the necessity of emotional intelligence for leadership behavior, practices or effectiveness by arguing that more data based on defensible methodologies are needed to prove the validity of the EI/leadership link (Antonakis, 2003; Antonakis *et al.*, 2009; Locke, 2005).

EI constructs have been generalized into two competing models: the ability-based model and the trait-based (or mixed) model (Conte, 2005; Day *et al.*, 2002). The ability-based model conceptualized by Mayer and Salovey (1997) defines emotional intelligence as a type of intelligence reflecting the ability to process emotional information. The trait-based model of emotional intelligence was endorsed by Goleman and Bar-On (Goleman, 1998; Bar-On, 1997); emotional intelligence is defined as a set of non-cognitive attributes, encompassing five broad skill areas: intrapersonal skills, interpersonal skills, adaptability, stress management and general mood (Conte, 2005; Van der Zee and Wabeke, 2004). Previous studies and anecdotal evidence have verified the claim that transformational leadership style could be predicted from trait-based emotional intelligence (Harms and Credé, 2010; Barbuto and Burbach, 2006; Brown and Moshavi, 2005; Mandell and Pherwani, 2003). A number of studies have also been carried out, indicating the ability-based EI to be a determinant of transformational leadership (Daus and Ashkanasy, 2005; Coetzee and Schaap, 2004; Walter and Bruch, 2007). Despite all the above, further doubt has been casted on validation issues with the various EI constructs prior to operational uses in scientific investigations (Cartwright and Pappas, 2009; Landy, 2005; Walter *et al.*, 2011).

With a wide range of literature supporting the significant role of EI in leadership effectiveness and various leadership outcomes, developing EI skills and competencies is thus crucial to leadership development. Empirical studies on interventions of emotional intelligence have provided convincing evidence relating to the positive results of teaching emotional intelligence on individuals' life success and work performance. Accordingly, EI can be learned and developed successfully among employees and managers through well-designed EI training activities and programmes (Perks and Bar-On, 2010; Meyer et al., 2004; Latif, 2004); however, speculation does exist on the content of such interventions and the nature of EI training outcomes (Zeidner, Roberts, & Matthews, 2002). The issue whether emotional intelligence can be taught is as important as the question of whether emotional intelligence competencies relate to leadership in the research community.

Meta-analytic studies which have examined literature on the relationships between various facets of leadership and emotional intelligence have been found over the period of 2001 to 2010. These synthesized studies, such as Mills' (2009) meta-analysis on whether a consistent, research-driven link can be established between the concept of emotional intelligence and effective leadership, have provided evidence that emotional intelligence may have immense significance and relevance for leadership effectiveness. Another meta-analytic investigation is a dissertation performed by Whitman (2009) on potential process mechanisms that may account for the EI-leadership effectiveness relationship further ascertained that mixed model EI appears to be a better predictor of leadership than ability EI. Similar results were found in Harms and Credé's (2010) meta-analysis containing 62 independent samples derived from existing literature from 1982 to 2009. It was revealed that trait-based (mixed) model of EI has more promise as a predictor of leadership effectiveness than did ability-based measures. Despite the fact that EI may contribute to successful leadership at some level, results of Harms and Credé's meta-analytic estimate suggested that EI being the core determinant of transformational leadership were overstated. The aforementioned meta-analytic studies which quantitatively reported their findings in terms of standardized effect sizes have continued to spur research interest in whether emotional intelligence had a significant effect on leadership.

Two meta-analytic reviews were found to qualitatively examine the linkage of emotional intelligence and nurse leadership. The two integrative reviews undertaken by Akerjordet and Severinsson (2008, 2010) revealed that emotionally intelligent nurse leadership is associated with favorable work climate characterized by resilience, innovation and change. However, controversies do exist in knowledge regarding the nature of EI and the current state of the art in the conceptual development of EI as abilities, skills and personality dispositions (Akerjordet and Severinsson, 2008, 2010).

Meta-analytical investigation is therefore needed as a common practice to resolve conflicts found in similar research approach (Rosenthal and DiMatteo, 2001; Dixon-Woods *et al.*, 2005). Through systematic review of literature on emotional intelligence and leadership, the study aims at providing a detailed synthesis of what have been investigated and what are in need of further exploration in EI and leadership research. The methodology employed in this qualitative meta-analytic review is inspired by Kun and Demetrovics (2010), Gooty *et al.* (2010) and Walter et al (2011). In the qualitative investigation conducted by Gooty et al. (2010), a selective, qualitative review of affect, emotions, and emotional competencies in leadership studies was adopted to examine theory, methods and quality of affect-based scholarship in leadership. The present study was also informed by a comprehensive attempt by Kun and Demetrovics (2010) who qualitatively reviewed and critically discussed literature on the relationship of emotional disregulation and addictive disorders. In an effort to ascertain whether EI is the sine qua non of leadership, Walter et al. (2011) critically reviewed recent empirical studies aiming at constructively framing EI's role in three criteria of leadership research: leadership emergence, leadership effectiveness and leadership behavior. In a similar vein, the present study follows research procedure employed by Gooty *et al.* (2010), Kun and Demetrovics (2010) and Walter et al. (2011) in the design and reporting of this systematic review.

The primary objective of the study is to assess research methods/designs and data analysis procedures employed by researchers investigating the relationship between EI and leadership over the period 2001-2010. The contributions of research on the linkage between the two constructs using quantitative approach were reviewed in terms of data analysis techniques, research design, measures used to assess EI, and subject matters in relation to leadership. The purpose was to provide the breadth of knowledge available on the potential utility of EI for predicting leadership effectiveness. The second purpose of the study was to identify research gaps and formulate research questions that could drive further endeavor in exploring topics relevant to the EI-leadership relationship.

2. Literature search

To provide a composite knowledge of the diversity of the theories, measures, samples, and contexts that have been employed by research studies on emotional intelligence and leadership, this study made extensive search for relevant research articles from the following six academic databases: *Academic Search Premier,* Show all*Education Research Complete, ERIC, PsycARTICLES, Psychology and Behavioral Sciences Collection, PsycINFO.* The focus was on scholarly articles employing quantitative approaches to examine studies exploring the relevance of emotional intelligence to leadership from January 2001 through December 2010. *Emotional intelligence and leadership* were the two keywords used to execute the electronic search. The electronic search was supplemented by a manual search for further studies found on reference lists shown up by the electronic search. Up to 116 articles were found with topics related to emotional intelligence and leadership. Inclusion and exclusion criteria formulated to identify articles for further examinations were: (1) Papers should be quantitative research studies related to emotional intelligence of leaders, supervisors, or managers in all professions; (2) Papers included should go through peer-review process and published between 2001 to 2010; (3) Articles focusing mainly upon multiple intelligence, general intelligence or social intelligence were excluded; (4) The present analysis is restricted to English language publications. For the purpose of this research, all articles using pure quantitative research methods focusing on the relevance of EI to leadership were reviewed. A total of 43 articles were included in the final data analysis. Major categories being analyzed include:

- Statistical/mathematical techniques used
- Research design used
- EI measure used
- Subject matters investigated in relation to leadership

3. Statistical/mathematical techniques & research design used

In 1980s', commonly employed data analysis procedures to study educational psychology and educational phenomena were ANOVA, correlation, *t*-test, chi-square, non-parametric and factor analysis. The trends and shifts of data analysis procedures during the last decades were well summarized by Hsu (2005). In general, there is a continuous drop of experimental research and the trends of frequently used data analysis procedures remain steady. By surveying articles published by the *American Educational Research Journal* (*AERJ*), *Journal of Experimental Education* (*JEE*) and *Journal of Educational Research* (*JER*), Hsu (2005) synthesized that the most frequently used statistical procedures in educational research during 1971 to 1998 in rank order were descriptive statistics, ANOVA/ANCOVA, correlation, regression, *t*-test, and psychometric statistics. ANOVA, chi-square, correlation, multiple regression and *T* test were found to be the most frequently employed statistical techniques to assess statistical power in applied psychology and management research published between 1992 and 1994.

To explore current trends of quantitative studies in emotional intelligence and leadership, categorization for plotting statistical techniques was based on reviews of literature on applied psychology, management and educational research designs (Elmore and Woehlke, 1998; Hsu, 2005; Gooty *et al.* 2010). The coding process included statistical techniques used in each article and categorizing techniques used in each article. Since a single article may employ more than one statistical technique, the total coded techniques would exceed the total number of article reviewed. The focus is on inferential statistical techniques used in conducting research on the relevance of emotional intelligence to leadership; therefore, when an article employed a specific technique more than once as different data analysis procedures, it was coded as one technique. For instance, if a research used 3 independent sample *t*-tests in one study, it was counted as one statistical technique. However, subsets under a category were treated as separate techniques. Therefore, if an article used both linear regression and hierarchical regression analyses, it was coded as two statistical techniques under the category of regression. Another instance was that if an article employed both one-sample *t*-test and independent sample *t*-test, they were counted as two subsets of techniques under the category of *t*-test.

After coding and categorizing statistical techniques used in articles employing quantitative approach, we found that during the period of 2001 to 2010 the most frequently used technique was correlational analysis; 28 analyses (33.7%) were coded and categorized into that category. Regression analysis ranked the second frequently used techniques, with a total number of 24 analyses (28.9%). Factor analysis ranked the third, with a total of 11 analyses (13.2%), followed by *t* test (7 analyses; 8.4%), ANOVA/ANCOVA and others (4 analyses respectively; 4.6%), meta-analysis and psychometric theory (2 analyses respectively; 2.3%). The results are presented in Tables 1, & 2.

Statistical Techniques	Frequency of techniques used by years									
Years/	2001	2002	2003	2004	2005	2006	2007	2008	2009	2010
No.of articles	3	5	6	3	3	7	5	3	4	6
Chi-square	0	0	0	0	0	0	0	0	0	0
correlation	2	4	3	2	1	4	3	3	1	5
t-test	1	0	2	1	0	0	1	2	0	0
ANOVA/ ANCOVA	0	0	0	0	0	1	1	0	0	2
Multivariate	0	0	0	0	0	0	1	0	0	0
Psychometric theory	1	0	0	0	0	0	0	0	1	0
Regression	1	4	4	1	2	6	2	1	1	2
Factor analysis (SEM)	0	2	0	2	1	1	1	1	2	1
Meta-analysis	0	0	0	0	0	0	0	0	1	1
Others	0	0	1	0	1	0	0	1		1

Table 1. Major Statistical/mathematical techniques used in EI-leadership research (2001-2010)

Statistical Techniques	Total Techniques used	
Number of & % of techniques (total)	# 83	%
Chi-square	0	0%
correlation	28	33.7%
t-test	7	8.4%
ANOVA/ ANCOVA	4	4.8%
Multivariate	1	1.2%
Psychometric theory	2	2.4%
Regression	24	28.9%
Factor analysis (Structural equation modeling)	11	13.2%
Meta-analysis	2	2.4%
Others	4	4.8%

Table 2. Major Statistical/mathematical techniques used in EI-leadership research (Total 2001-2010)

In studying emotional intelligence in relation to leadership, more emphasis has been given to non-experimental research designs than experimental ones. After classifying the 43 research studies included in the final analysis, only 2 out of the 43 (4.5%) were experimental research. Forty-one research studies reviewed in the study (95.0%) employed non-experimental approach, which obviously outweighed the number of experimental research. The two experimental exploratory studies confirmed EI can be learned and developed through deliberate training and interventions (Groves *et al.*, 2008; Meyer *et al.*, 2004). Forty-one studies using non-experimental designs are tabulated below in Table 3.

Research Design	Non-experimental
Descriptive study	5(10.6%)
Correlational study	9 (20.0%)
Correlational predictive study	23 (48.9%)
Casual-comparative study	4 (8.5%)
Psychometric testing/model testing	4(8.5%)
Secondary data analysis/meta analysis	2 (4.2%)
Total	47 research designs used by 41 articles

Table 3. Studies by Research Design (Non-Experimental)

Since an article may involve the application of multimethod analysis, the total number of research designs may exceed the total number of articles reviewed in the present study. Among the 40 non-experimental research articles, 47 research designs were found. Correlational predictive (23 entries, 48.9%) and correlational analyses (9 entries, 20.0%) were the most popular research designs, with a total of 32 studies, followed by descriptive study, with a total of 5 studies (10.6%). It is important to note that descriptive statistics was excluded if they were used to present frequencies, percentages, averages of demographic variables; only those involved with analyzing data collected from surveys and reported in findings were counted as studies using descriptive statistics.

4. EI measures used

As noted in the introduction section, the ability-based model and the trait-based (or mixed) model are the two most prominent theoretical constructs for creating EI measures. Researchers in Mayer and Salovey's ability-based tradition have developed various comprehensive measures, including the Multifactor Emotional Intelligence Scale (MEIS; Mayer et al. 2000), the Mayer, Salovey and Caruso Emotional Intelligence test or MSCEIT, Version 2.0 (Mayer *et al.* 2002), the Levels of Emotional Awareness Scale or LEAS (Lane *et al.* 1990), the Emotional Accuracy Research Scale or EARS (Mayer and Geher, 1996), the WLEIS measure (Wong and Law EI Scale, 2002), and self-rated emotional intelligence scale (SREIS; Brackett et al., 2006). Examples of widely used trait-based (or mixed) EI measures include Bar-On's Emotional Quotient Inventory or EQ-I (Bar-On 1997), Emotional Quotient (EQ) questionnaire (Goleman, 1999), Emotional Competence Inventory (ECI, a 360-degree instrument by Boyatzis *et al.* 2000), the Swinburne University Emotional Intelligence Test or SUEIT (Palmer and Stough 2001), trait meta-mood scale (TMMS; Salovey *et al.*, 1995) and the Emotional Intelligence Question (EIQ; Dulewicz and

Higgs 1999). The ability-based model has been under criticism with low reliability and with slight correlations with cognitive ability; whereas the trait-based (or mixed) model was found to lack discriminant validity and overlap with existing personality trait measures (Conte, 2005; Oboyle et al., 2011).

Tables 4 and 5 present a summary of 46 EI measures used by the 43 articles reviewed in the present study. Since one article may use more than one EI measure, the sum of EI measures used is not expected to equal the total number of articles examined in the study. The trait-based (mixed) model of EI appears to be predominant in articles published from 2001 to 2010, with an overall percentage of 39% (18 articles). Twelve entries of EI measures (26%) were classified as ability-based measures of EI, whereas 16 EI measures (35%) were "others". Among all the measures used, the most frequently used ones were the ability-based MSCEIT, the trait-based EQ-i and SUEIT , with 6 entries each (13%), followed by the ability-based WLEIS (5 entries, 11%). The classified models of EI measures used from 2001 to 2010 were presented in Tables 4, showing that the trait-based measures were the predominant constructs used to examine EI and leadership during 2001 to 2006, with an exception of 2004 when it was the first time the ability-based measures exceeded the trait-based measures. The trait-based and ability-based constructs seem to have leveled off during 2007 to 2010. Ever since the ability-based model entered the leadership research community in 2003, the two theoretical constructs became competing models in examining quantitative studies in relation to EI and leadership.

EI Measures	Frequency of measures used by years									
Years/ No. of measures	2001 3	2002 5	2003 7	2004 3	2005 3	2006 9	2007 5	2008 3	2009 3	2010 5
Ability-based	0	0	3	2	0	3	1	1	1	1
Trait-based	2	3	4	1	1	5	1	1	0	1
Others	1	2	1	0	2	1	3	1	2	3

Table 4. EI measures used (2001-2010)

Table 5 depicts total numbers of different EI models based on which various EI measures were created. Among all the measures classified as "others", the Leadership Dimensions Questionnaire developed by Dulewicz and Higgs in 2004 had been used in two studies published in 2005 and 2007 respectively (Hawkins and Dulewicz, 2007; Dulewicz et al., 2005). The LDQ was used to measure 15 leadership competences clustered under the three dimensions of intellectual competencies (IQ), managerial competencies (MQ), and emotional competencies (EQ) of leaders or managers in the two studies. The above two studies provided empirical evidences to support the positive effect of EQ on leadership performance.

New models of EI have emerged during 2001 to 2010. For example, a nonverbal measure of the ability to recognize emotional expressions displayed by others was developed in 2001 by Morand. Psychometric properties of the emotional intelligence self-description inventory (EISDI), a measure developed based on the ability-based model of EI, was examined and improved for operational use with fully employed business students in the United States (Groves *et al.*, 2008). In 2008, a newly developed 16-item measure of EI was validated for use with supervisor–subordinate dyads in Hong Kong. The issue of translation and psychometric validation of a measure before adapted across cultures was investigated in two studies. In 2004, the Trait Meta-Mood Scale (TMMS; Salovey, Mayer, Goldman, Turvey) was cross-culturally validated for use with management students in Hong Kong (Law *et al.*, 2004). In 2010, a standardized forward-backward translation procedure was conducted ensure the quality of the translated version of Emotional Skills Assessment Process (ESAP) developed in the United States before administering it on academic leaders in Taiwan (Tang *et al.*, 2010).

EI Measures Used	Total	Percent
No. & % of EI Measures (total)	46	100%
Ability-based	12	26%
MSCEIT	6	13%
WLEIS	5	11%
SREIS	1	2%
Trait-based (Mixed)	18	39%
EQ-i	6	13%
SUEIT	6	13%
TMMS	3	7%
EIQ	2	4%
ECI	1	2%
Others	16	35%

Table 5. EI measures used (Total 2001-2010)

5. Subject matters investigated in relation to leadership

Leadership was first conceptualized into leadership emergence and leadership effectiveness, the two criteria based on which the bulk of leadership researchers in favor of trait theory have made investigations linking personality traits to leadership. Accordingly, traits within a Big Five framework may yield differential associations with leadership across the study settings (Bono and Judge, 2004; De Hoogh et al., 2005; Judge et al., 2002). In model of the aforementioned studies, subject matters in relation to leadership, or leadership criteria, are used in the present study as an organizing framework to estimate leadership-EI relations. As mentioned earlier, the critical review by Walter *et al.* (2011) was of assistance in informing the present review in classifying subject matters in relation to leadership. For the purpose of offering more generalizability as to subject matters investigated, quantitative studies reviewed in the present study will be classified based on three distinct leadership criteria employed by Walter *el al.* (2011): leadership emergence, behavior, and effectiveness. Leadership emergence refers to the degree an individual is viewed by others as a leader when limited information about that individual's performance is known. Leadership effectiveness, on the other hand, represents a leader's performance in exerting influence on and giving guidance to the activities toward achievement of goals. Performance of a leader is often measured in terms of team, group, or organizational effectiveness. Studies on leadership behavior are described as predominately focusing on transformational leadership behaviors of idealized influence, inspirational motivation, individualized consideration, and intellectual stimulation. Bernard Bass's assessment tool, the Multifactor Leadership Questionnaire (MLQ), is a typical measure used to assess transformational leadership behaviors. However, several studies could hardly be classified into the three leadership criteria. Examples include the two experimental studies examining the possibilities and impacts of EI interventions, validation studies on measurement tools developed for leaders, and meta-analytic studies on EI's role in leadership. The present study therefore suggests that there is a forth criterion classified as "others" used to accurately code experimental, construct validation and meta-analytic studies on EI-leadership relationships.

Leadership criteria	Frequency of leadership criteria focused by years									
Years/ No. of articles	2001 3	2002 5	2003 6	2004 3	2005 3	2006 7	2007 5	2008 3	2009 4	2010 6
Emergence	1	1	2	0	1	0	2	0	0	2
Effectiveness	1	2	1	0	1	2	2	2	1	0
Behavior	0	2	2	1	1	4	1	0	1	3
Others	1	0	1	2	0	1	0	1	2	1

Table 6. Subject matters investigated coded based on leadership criteria (2001-2010)

Leadership criteria focused	Total	Percent
No. & % of articles (total)	45	100%
Emergence	9	20.0%
Effectiveness	12	26.6%
Behaviors	15	33.3%
Others	9	20.0%

Table 7. Subject matters investigated coded based on leadership criteria (Total)

In Tables 6 and 7, subject matters in relation to leadership coded into the four leadership criteria are presented, showing the number of articles in each criterion and the total percentage of the articles they represent, for each year and overall. Articles coded under the four criteria appear to be evenly distributed throughout the past ten years. The most commonly studied criterion is leadership behavior, with a total of 15 articles (33.3%), followed by leadership effectiveness (12 articles; 26.6%), leadership emergence (9 articles;

20%) and others (9 articles; 20%). Among those coded as others, two meta-analytic studies were found providing syntheses of the literature on the theoretical and empirical basis of emotional intelligence and it's linkage to leadership. The two experimental studies were conducted to support the notion that EI can be learned, enhanced and developed through proper training techniques (Groves *et al.*, 2008; Meyer *et al.*, 2004). New EI constructs or measures were established with a focus on particular groups of leaders, such as servant leadership and managers in Hong Kong (Barbuto and Wheeler, 2005; Wong and Low, 2002). In 2001, one way of measuring emotional intelligence validated by Morand (2001) is to combine psychological with perception measures. It is worth pointing out that Morand, in developing a composite measure of emotional intelligence (2001), used Ekman and Friesen's (1975) *The Face of Emotion* encompassing a set of 17 photos and Merabian and Epstein's empathy scale to conceptualize a nonverbal perception measure of skill at nonverbal communication to assess individuals' recognitions of emotional expressions displayed by others. This perspective is somewhat in contrast to the prevailing psychological-based Likert-scale EI measurements developed to conceptualize and assess emotional intelligence.

6. Conclusions

This study identified and tabulated research methods and data analysis procedures from studies on leadership and EI relationships over the past 10 years. In addition, it also identified the types of EI measures used and subject matters in relation to leadership investigated. Percentages of frequently used statistical/mathematical techniques, research designs, types of EI measures used and subject matters focused were presented annually so that their trends and practices can be assessed. The results were synthesized from 43 studies conducted between 2001 to 2010 retrieved from six academic databases.

Correlational analysis, regression analysis and factor analysis were identified as frequently employed techniques in research on leadership-EI research. Correlational predictive and correlational analyses research, two most dominant research designs used, overweight casual-comparative research design using ANOVAs or *t* tests frequently seen in educational and management studies. In addition, research studies on leadership and EI relations employing quantitative methodologies show preference of non-experimental research designs to experimental ones and this preference has remained steady in the research community.

With regard to EI measured used, the majority of them, based on either ability or trait-based models, are heavily reliant on the assessment of self-perceived EI. Despite the increasing number of particular EI instruments developed during the decade, self-reported approach has been widely adopted in framing the newly created constructs of EI. Only a few studies reviewed in the present studies incorporate multi-rater assessments, such as LDQ, ECI and WLEIS, to provide a more accurate and complete evaluation of an individual's EI competences (Hawkins and Dulewicz, 2007; Wang and Huang, 2009; Barbuto and Wheeler, 2006). The vast dominance of self-reported measures developed for use in exploring the links between leadership and EI may be seen as problematic since socially desirable self and self-knowledge may cause faking goods, which in turn would bring distortion.

With regard to leadership criteria researched, the research community has more or less neglected the subject of leadership development, such as the effects of incorporating EI training in leadership development programs. The impact of EI interventions on leadership development is still at the exploratory stage. The two experimental studies reviewed in the present study have thus far provided empirical evidence suggesting that EI can be heightened among groups of student samples. More research efforts are needed to demonstrate whether EI abilities can be taught, learned, and developed among those holding leadership or management roles. In addition, the empirical shortening in the area of potential effects of an EI training program on leaders' work-related outcomes will provide an avenue for further investigation.

7. Limitations and overall implications

Several important limitations must be considered. First, studies included in the present meta-analytic review are highly selective. Quantitative studies published from 2001 to 2010 that explicitly focused on leadership and emotional intelligence were collected and coded; therefore, many peripheral themes, such as emotional labor and emotional literacy, are left out. Such narrow focus helped clearly delineate a predictor of leadership criterion. To expand the present research effort, further studies can adopt a broad literature search using keyword combinations around leadership (leaders, team leadership, management/leadership effectiveness, management/leadership outcomes, leader-member exchange) and emotional intelligence (emotion, emotional labor, emotional literacy, emotional learning).

The current study is also limited by the focus on elite journals from databases in management, psychology and education. To increase the number of studies and avoid publication bias, future studies may identify possible sources of data via searches of Dissertation Abstracts and Internet searches for additional unpublished data sources. A third limitation of the current study lies in the lack of inter-observer agreement on specific coding variables (Clarke *et al.*, 2002). To ensure a high level of accuracy and coding consensus, coding variables could be performed by experienced experts or trained graduate students working independently on coding sheets provided by the authors (Clarke *et al.*, 2002; Van Rooy and Visweswaran, 2004).

In 2010, Harms and Crede conducted a meta-analysis on transformational leadership and emotional intelligence and found that the claim that EI serves as a core competence for transformational leadership was overstated. It was noted that the majority of studies used in their investigation were from unpublished sources; the lack of methodological rigor in data source may yield weak results in their findings. Findings from the present analysis on published peer-reviewed quantitative studies lead to the similar conclusion: the 15 research studies coded under the subject area of "leadership behavior" using transformational leadership measures indicate that EI contribute to transformational leadership at some level, but different studies found significant relationships between distinct areas of EI and distinct components of transformational leadership across cultures and research settings (e.g. Corona, 2010; Tang *et al.*, 2010; Polychroniou, 2009; Sunindijo et al., 2007).

In conclusion, there was obviously still a pressing need among the leadership research community for valid experimental research designs in the area of EI interventions for leaders. The potential application of EI as a pedagogical tool into leadership education may offers a new approach to improving various leadership outcomes. It is also recommended that multiple ratings or 360-degree feedbacks on leaders' EI and leadership competences should be applied to provide a more holistic conceptualization of the nature of this relationship. With regard to cross-cultural adaptation of EI or leadership measures, dominant among the EI measures in use are those developed in English and later translated for use with samples in cultures other than English speaking countries. Appropriate translation and rigorous validation process therefore may have detrimental effects on the study results (Wang *et al.*, 2006; Guillemin *et.al.*, 1993; Jones and Kay, 1992). EI measures reviewed in the present studies have been widely applied to Hong Kong, Greece, Portugal, Singapore, Taiwan and Thailand (Law *et al.*, 2004; Polychroniou, 2009; Rego *et al.*, 2007; Tang *et al.*, 2010; Sunindijo *et al.*, 2007). However, there is some lack of clarity regarding appropriate translation and rigorous validation process before those measures were operationally used in other cultures. Trans-cultural validation of EI assessment tools is therefore required in leadership research in order to develop more refined measures of the construct utilized to investigate the full potential of EI on leadership practices in different countries.

8. Acknowledgement

This study is an extension of a research project sponsored by National Science Council, Taiwan (Grant No:NSC 100-2410-H-130-028-)

9. References

Akerjordet, K. and Severinsson, E. (2008), Emotionally intelligent nurse leadership: a literature review study. *Journal of Nursing Management, 16*(5), 565–577

Akerjordet, K. and Severinsson, E. (2010), The state of the science of emotional intelligence related to nursing leadership: an integrative review. *Journal of Nursing Management, 18* (4), 363–382

Antonakis, J. (2003), Why 'emotional intelligence' does not predict leadership effectiveness: A comment on Prati, Douglas, Ferris, Ammeter, and Buckley, *The International Journal of Organizational Analysis, 11*, 355-361.

Antonakis, J., Ashkanasy, N., & Dasborough, M. (2009). Does leadership need emotional intelligence? *The Leadership Quarterly, 20*, 247-261.

Barbuto, J. E. and Burbach, M. E. (2006), The emotional intelligence of transformational leaders: A field study of elected officials, *Journal of Social Psychology, 146* (1), 51-64.

Barbuto, J.E. and Wheeler, D.W. (2005).Scale development and construct clarification of servant leadership, *Group & Organization Management 31*(3), 300-326

Bar-On, R. (1997). *Bar-On Emotional Quotient Inventory: Technical manual*. Multi-Health Systems, New York: NY.

Bono, J. E. and Judge, T. A. (2004). Personality and Transformational and Transactional Leadership: A Meta-Analysis, *Journal of Applied Psychology, 89*(5), 901-910

Brown, F.W. and Moshavi, D. (2005), Transformational leadership and emotional intelligence: a potential pathway for an increased understanding of interpersonal influence, *Journal of Organizational Behavior,* Vol. 26 No. 7, pp. 867-71.

Carmeli, A. (2003), The relationship between emotional intelligence and work attitudes, behavior and outcomes: An examination of senior managers, *Journal of Managerial Psychology, 18* (7/8), 788-811.

Cartwright, S. and Pappas, C. (2008), Emotional intelligence, its measurement and implications for the workplace. *International Journal of Management Reviews, 10* (2), 149–171

Clarke, S., Dunlap, G., & Stichter, J. P. (2002). A descriptive analysis of intervention research in emotional and behavioral disorders from 1980 through 1999. *Behavior Modification, 26,* 659-683.

Conte, J. M. (2005), A review and critique of emotional intelligence measures" *Journal of Organizational Behavior, 26* (4), 433-40.

Corona, M.G.. (2010). The relationship between emotional intelligence and transformational leadership: A Hispanic American examination, *The Business Journal of Hispanic Research, 4*(1), 22-34

Day, A., Newsome, S. and Catano, V. M., (2002), Emotional intelligence and leadership, (CFLI Contract Research Report #CR01-0078). *Kingston, ON: Canadian Forces Leadership Institute.*

De Hoogh, A. H. B., Den Hartog, D. N. and Koopman, P. L. (2005), Linking the Big Five-Factors of personality to charismatic and transactional leadership; perceived dynamic work environment as a moderator. *Journal of Organizational Behavior, 26*(7), 839–865

Dixon-Woods, M., Agarwal, S., Jones, D., Young, B., & Sutton, A. (2005). Synthesizing qualitative and quantitative evidence: a review of possible methods. *Journal of Health Services Research & Policy, 10*(1), 45-53.

Duckett, H, and Macfarlane, E. (2003). Emotional intelligence and transformational leadership in retailing, *Leadership & Organization Development Journal,24* (6), 309 – 317

Dulewicz, C., Young, M., & Dulewicz, V. (2005). The relevance of emotional intelligence for leadership performance. *Journal of General Management, 30*(3), 71-86.

Elmore, P. B,and Woehlke, P. L. (1998), *Twenty years of research methods employed in "American Educational Research Journal," "Educational Researcher" and "Review of Educational Research."* Paper presented at the Annual Meeting of the American Educational Research Association, San Diego, California.

Goleman, D. (1998). What makes a leader? *Harvard Business Review, 76,* 92–103.

Goleman, D. (1998). *Working with emotional intelligence. Bantam Books*: New York.

Goody, J., Connelly, S., Griffith, J, and Gupta, A. (2010). Leadership, affect and emotions: A state of the science review, *Leadership Quarterly, 21*(6), 979-1004

Groves, K.S., McEnrue, M.P., and Shen, W. (2008). Developing and measuring the emotional intelligence of leaders, *Journal of Management Development, 27* (2), 225 – 250

Guillemin, F., Bombardier, C., & Beaton, D. (1993). Cross-cultural adaptation of healthrelated quality of life measures: Literature review and proposed guidelines. *Journal of Clinical Epidemiology, 446*, 1417-1432.

Harms, P.D. and Credé, M. (2010). Emotional intelligence and transformational and transactional leadership: a meta-analysis, *Journal of Leadership and Organization Studies, 17*, 5-17.

Hawkins, J. and Dulewicz, V. (2007), The Relationship between Performance as a Leader and Emotional Intelligence, intellectual and Managerial Competences. *Journal of General Management, 33*(2), 57-58.

Hsu, T.C. (2005). Research methods and data analysis procedures used by educational researchers, *International Journal of Research & Method in Education, 28*(2), 109-133.

Jones, E.G., & Kay, M. (1992). Instrumentation in cross-cultural research. *Nursing Research, 41*(3), 86-188.

Judge, T. A., Bono, J. E., Ilies, R. and Gerhardt, M.W. (2002). Personality and leadership: A qualitative and quantitative review, *Journal of Applied Psychology, 87*(4), 765-780

Kun, B. and Demetrovics, Z. (2010). Emotional intelligence and addictions: A systematic review, *Substance Use & Misuse, 45*(7-8),1131–1160

Landy, F. J. (2005), Some historical and scientific issues related to research on emotional intelligence. *Journal of Organizational Behavior, 26*(4), 411–424

Latif, D. A. (2004). Using emotional intelligence in the planning and implementation of a management skills course. *Pharmacy Education, 4*(2), 81- 89.

Law, K. S., Wong, C.S. and Song, L.J. (2004). The construct and criterion validity of emotional intelligence and its potential utility for management studies, *Journal of Applied Psychology, 89*(3), 483-496

Leban, W. and Zulauf, C. (2004). Linking emotional intelligence abilities and transformational leadership styles, *Leadership & Organization Development Journal, 25*(7), 554 – 564

Locke, E.A. (2005), Why emotional intelligence is an invalid concept, *Journal of Organizational Behavior, 26* (4), 425-31.

Mandell, B. and Pherwani, S. (2003), Relationship between emotional intelligence and transformational leadership style: A gender comparison, *Journal of Business & Psychology, 17* (3), 387-404.

Morand, D.A. (2001). The emotional intelligence of managers: Assessing the construct validity of a nonverbal measure of "people skills", *Journal of Business and Psychology, 16*(1), 21-33.

Meyer, B. B., Fletcher, T. B., & Parker, S. J. (2004). Enhancing emotional intelligence in the health care environment: An exploratory study. *Health Care Manager, 23*(3), 225-234.

Mayer, J.D., & Salovey, P. (1997). What is emotional intelligence? In P. Salovey & D. Sluyter (Ed.). *Emotional development, emotional literacy, and emotional intelligence* (pp. 3-31). Basic Books: New York.

Mills, L.B. (2009). A meta-analysis of the relationship between emotional intelligence and effective leadership, *Journal of Curriculum and Instruction, 3*(2), 22-38

O'Boyle, E. H., Humphrey, R. H., Pollack, J. M., Hawver, T. H. and Story, P. A. (2011), The relation between emotional intelligence and job performance: A meta-analysis. *Journal of Organizational Behavior, 32*(5), 788–818

Ozcelik, H., Langton, N. and Aldrich, H. (2008), Doing well and doing good: The relationship between leadership practices that facilitate a positive emotional climate and organizational performance, *Journal of Managerial Psychology, 23* (2), 186-203.

Perks, J., & Bar-On, R. (2010). Coaching for Emotionally Intelligent Leadership. In J. Passmore (Ed.), *Coaching for leadership.* London, UK: Kogan Page.

Polychroniou, P.V. (2009). Relationship between emotional intelligence and transformational leadership of supervisors: The impact on team effectiveness, *Team Performance Management, 15* (7/8), 343 - 356

Rego, A., Sousa, F., Pina e Cunha, M., Correia, A. and Saur-Amaral, I. (2007), Leader Self-Reported Emotional Intelligence and Perceived Employee Creativity: An Exploratory Study. *Creativity and Innovation Management, 16*(3), 250–264.

Rosenthal, R., & DiMatteo, M. R. (2001). Meta-analysis: Recent developments in quantitative methods for literature reviews. *Annual Review of Psychology, 52*(1), 59-82

Sunindijo, R.Y., Hadikusumo, B.H.W. and Ogunlana, S. (2007). Emotional intelligence and leadership styles in construction project management, *Journal of Management in Engineering 23*(4), 166-171.

Tang, H.W.,Yin, M.S., & Nelson, D.B., (2010). The relationships between leadership effectiveness and emotional intelligence: A cross-cultural study of academic leaders in Taiwan and the USA. , *Journal of Managerial Psychology.25(8), 899-926.* (Special Issue on Intercultural Competency, SSCI).

Van der Zee, K. and Wabeke, R. (2004), Is trait-Emotional Intelligence simply or more than just a trait? *European Journal of Personality, 18* (4), 243-63.

Van Rooy, D. L., & Viswesvaran, C. (2004). Emotional intelligence: A meta-analytic investigation of predictive validity and nomological net. *Journal of Vocational Behavior, 65,* 71-95.

Walter, F., & Bruch, H. (2007), Leadership: The role of leaders' positive mood and emotional intelligence. In C. E. J. Härtel, N. M. Ashkanasy, & W. J. Zerbe (Eds.), *Research on Emotion in Organizations (Vol. 3): Functionality, Intentionality and Morality:* pp. 55-85. Amsterdam: Elsevier.

Walter, F., Cole, M.S. and Humphrey, R.H. (2011). Emotional Intelligence: Sine Qua Non of Leadership or Folderol? *Academy of Management Perspectives, 25* (1), 43-59.

Wang, Y.S. and Huang, T.C. (2009). The relationship of transformational leadership with group cohesiveness and emotional intelligence, *Social Behavior and Personality: an international journal 37*(3), 379-392

Wang, W.L., Lee, H.L., & Fetzer, S.J. (2006). Challenges and strategies in instrument translation, *Western Journal of Nursing Research, 28*(3), 310-321.

Wong, C., Law, K. S. (2002). The effects of leader and follower emotional intelligence on performance and attitude: An exploratory study. *Leadership Quarterly*, 13(3), 243-274.

Zeidner, M., Roberts, R.D., & Mattews, G. (2002). Can emotional intelligence be schooled? A critical review. *Educational Psychologist, 37*(4), 215-231

6

Emotional Intelligence: The Most Potent Factor of Job Performance Among Executives

Reza Gharoie Ahangar
Department of Management and Economics, Science and Research Branch,
Islamic Azad University
Iran

1. Introduction

Nowadays, we observe that some organizations are successful and others are not. One of the reasons can be related to the ability of the organization's executives. The important factor which has a significant role in the success of an executive is emotion. Emotions are an important part of any person's life which seriously affects all aspects of life. Each emotion has a motivating characteristic, a personal meaning, and an expression reflected in behaviors (Çeçen, 2006). The term emotion encompasses an item, which is Emotional Intelligence (EI). Emotional Intelligence (EI) is often measured as an Emotional Intelligence Quotient (EQ), the term (EQ) was coined by (Bar-On, 1988) and can be traced to early studies in the 1920s (Bar-On & Parker, 2000). The concept of 'social intelligence' was introduced by (Thorndike, 1920), who defined it, as the ability to understand and manage people to act wisely in human relations. The concept of EI grew out of this particular definition, which influenced how EI was understood and conceptualized. In the early 1980s, scholars began to systematically conceptualize the idea of EI. Notably, (Gardner, 1983), a psychologist at Harvard University, initiated the theory of multiple intelligences and proposed that intrapersonal and interpersonal intelligence are as important as the type of intelligence typically measured by Intelligence Quotient (IQ) and related tests and after that (Salovey & Mayer, 1990) introduced the term EI and defined it as the ability to deal with emotions. Then the concept of EI was made popular by (Goleman, 1995) with his famous book Emotional Intelligence: Why It can matter More Than IQ. Daniel Goleman explains that IQ is considered to account for approximately 20% of the factors that determine life success, and he argues that EI can account for the remaining factors. The importance of emotional intelligence is emphasized because human relations in organizations are affected by emotional factors more than by rational factors (Jung & Yoon, In Press). There are many definition of EI; (Salovey & Mayer, 1990) defined emotional intelligence as "the subset of social intelligence that involves the ability to monitor one's own and others' feelings and emotions, to discriminate among them and to use this information to guide one's thinking and actions". Salovey & Mayer (1997), revised the definition to complement it. They defined emotional intelligence as "the ability to perceive accurately, appraise, and express emotion; the ability to access and/or generate feelings when they facilitate thought; the ability to understand emotion and emotional knowledge; and the ability to regulate emotions to promote emotional and intellectual growth". Martinez (1997), refers to emotional intelligence as being: an array of non-cognitive skills, capabilities and competencies that influence a person's ability to cope with environmental demands and pressures. Another definition is given by (Bar-On, 1997) that EI is a kind of multiple-level ability that crosses over self emotions and social composition, and had focused on non cognitive capabilities that influence one's ability to succeed in life (For example, Bar-On et al., 2007). Research has indicated that individuals with higher level of EI are more likely to experience performance related success than individuals with lower levels of EI (Goleman, 1996; Schutte et al., 1998). Schmidt & Hunter (2000), defined intelligence as the "ability to grasp and reason correctly with abstractions (concepts) and solve problems". Mayer & Cobb (2000), explain that Emotional intelligence consists of these "four branches of mental ability": I) Emotional identification, perception and expression II) Emotional facilitation of thought III) Emotional understanding IV) Emotional management For most people, including senior executives, it was thought that those with a higher Intelligence Quotient (IQ) were the most important aspect of a company's success, but we can see Emotional Intelligence has become a vital part of how today's executives meet the significant challenges they face. Emotionally intelligent individuals can handle and perform efficiently in problems and emergencies, as (Scott-ladd, 2004) argued that emotional intelligence (EI) in employees is self-awareness and an ability to deal with any exceptional uncertainty. Emotional intelligence (EI) is the capability to identify own and others feelings and utilize this awareness to facilitate own-self and others (Berman, 2008). Emotional Intelligence (EI) refers to abilities concerning recognition and regulation of emotions in self and others, and to use this information to guide one's thinking and actions (Giardini & Frese, 2008; Mayer, Salovey, & Caruso, 2008). Two main conceptualizations of EI are explored and there is growing consensus on two models: (i) the "ability model", measuring maximal performance (Mayer et al., 2000b) and (ii) the "trait model", measuring typical performance (Petrides & Furnham, 2000, 2001). The first model, perceives EI as a form of pure intelligence that is, EI concerns an individual's capacity to reason about emotions and to process emotional information to enhance cognitive processes and regulate behavior. (Petrides et al., 2007) delineated trait EI, or emotional self-efficacy, assesses an individual's belief in their emotional abilities, and is defined as "A constellation of emotional self-perceptions located at the lower levels of personality hierarchies". The second model, ability approach uses maximum performance measures to assess individual differences in the interface of emotion with cognitive processes (Mayer et al., 2000b). The ability measure of EI correlates only modestly with other forms of cognitive ability (Mayer, Roberts, & Barsade, 2008) used an ability performance-based test to assess emotional intelligence and reported mixed results with positive effects found only in a few of the emotional abilities examined. Emotional Intelligence can help executives in an ever more difficult leadership role, one that fewer and fewer people seem capable of fulfilling. Moreover, in the middle of the "Talent War," especially at the highest levels in organizations, emotional intelligence can give developing executives a competitive edge.

2. Literature review

2.1 Components of emotional intelligence

In 1998, in Working with Emotional Intelligence, Goleman set out a framework of emotional intelligence (EI) that reflects how an individual's potential for mastering the skills of Self-Awareness, Self-Management are personal competence, Social Awareness, and Relationship

Management are social competence that related to the job success. The first component of emotional intelligence is Emotional Self-Awareness, which contains of Emotional self-awareness, Accurate self-assessment, and Self-confidence. It is means, knowing what one feels, or Knowing one's internal states, preferences, resources, and intuitions. (Mayer & Geher, 1996) mentioned that emotional intelligence is different from general intelligence and that the former is differential intelligence that needs to be investigated in the future. John Mayer (for example, Mayer & Stevens, 1994) uses the term meta-mood, the affective analogue of meta-cognition, for key aspects of Emotional Self-Awareness. The second component of EI, Self-Management, that contains of Emotional self-control, Transparency, Adaptability, and Achievement orientation. The means of this factor is the ability to regulate distressing affects like anxiety and anger and to inhibit emotional impulsivity, or managing one's internal states and resources. The third EI component is Social Awareness that means awareness of others' feelings, needs, and concerns, which encompasses the competency of Empathy, also involves the amygdala. Studies of patients with discrete lesions to the amygdala show impairment of their ability to read nonverbal cues for negative emotions, particularly anger and fear, and to judge the trustworthiness of other people (Davidson et al., 2000). Other items are organizational awareness and service orientation. Lastly, the fourth EI component is Relationship Management, or Social Skill, poses a more complex picture, or adeptness at inducing desirable responses in others. In a fundamental sense, the effectiveness of our relationship skills hinges on our ability to attune ourselves to or influence the emotions of another person. This factor encompasses Developing others, Inspirational leadership, Change catalyst, Influence, Conflict management, and Teamwork and collaboration. (Mayer & Salovey, 1997) indicated that emotional intelligence as composed of four distinct dimensions: 1) Appraisal and expression of emotion in the self. 2) Appraisal and recognition of emotion in others. 3) Regulation of emotion in the self. 4) Use of emotion to facilitate performance. (Bar-On, 1997) conceptualized EI as a non-cognitive ability; involving five broad skill areas that help an individual become more effective in dealing with environmental demands and pressures: Intrapersonal Skills, this related to identify, understand and express oneself, Interpersonal Skills, this related to be aware of, to understand, and relate to others, Adaptability is related to strong emotions and control one's impulses, Stress Management is related to control of stress with confront of different situation, and General Mood is related to adapt to change and to solve problems of personal or a social nature. (Davies et al., 1998) proposed that EQ has four abilities: Self-emotional appraisal, others' emotional appraisal, regulation of emotion, and use of emotion. (Salovey et al., 2000) have argued that EI components are related to a number of coping processes, such as rumination, social support networks and the disclosure of trauma. Wong & Law (2002), have argued that Emotional intelligence consists of four aspects: others' emotional appraisal, use of emotion, self-emotion appraisal, and regulation of emotion. (Cote & Miners, 2006) divided emotional intelligence into emotion perception, emotion utilization, emotion understanding, and emotion control. Goleman (2006), revealed EI concerns the ability of a person to maintain self-control, enthusiasm, persistence and self-encouragement, as shown in five major dimensions: knowing your emotions, managing your own emotions, motivating yourself, recognizing and understanding other people's emotions, and managing relationships.

2.2 Job performance and role of emotional intelligence

Organizations are settings that require interpersonal interaction. Most of these interactions are related to the performance of job duties. According to (Savoie & Brunet, 2000), team performance assessment should include at least four different measures: (a) group experience quality, that is, the degree upon which group experience contributes to well-being and personal growth of team member; (b) team output, which relies on objective, measurable, and quantifiable performance criteria, for example, number of mistakes, waste ratio, or in the present context, percentage of technical acts meeting hygiene and safety standards; (c) team viability, that is, the capability of the team to continue to function as a unit; and (d) team legitimacy which relates to the appraisal of team's effectiveness by external actors who have close ties with it (managers, clients, suppliers, etc.) Emotions can influence thought processes by promoting different information processing strategies (Forgas, 1995; Schwarz, 1990). For example, positive emotions tend to promote heuristic processing (Schwarz, 1990) and may be useful for creative tasks (Isen et al., 1987) and short-term memory tasks (Gray, 2004), whereas negative emotions promote deeper processing (Bless et al., 1990; Schwarz, 1990) and better spatial task performance (Gray, 2004). Emotion and cognition can be integrated to influence performance on a variety of tasks (Gray, 2004). Austin (2004), examined the relationships between trait emotional intelligence (EI) and tasks involving the recognition of facial expressions of emotion. Two facial expression recognition tasks using the inspection time (IT) paradigm assessed speed of emotional information processing. Results show that, general emotion-processing ability contributes to performance on these tasks. Quoidbach & Hansenne (2009), investigated the relationships between EI, performance, and cohesiveness in 23 nursing teams. Results showed that, EI provided an interesting new way of enhancing nursing teams' cohesion and patient/client outcomes. Among psychologists, Emotional intelligence (EI) is proposed as an important predictor of key organizational outcomes including job satisfaction (Daus & Ashkanasy, 2005; Van Rooy & Viswesvaran, 2004). Kafetsios & Zampetakis (2008), tested the extent to which positive and negative affect at work mediate personality effects (Emotional Intelligence) on job satisfaction. Results indicated that positive and negative affect at work substantially mediate the relationship between EI and job satisfaction with positive affect exerting a stronger influence. Lyons & schneider (2005), examined the relationship of ability-based EI facets with performance under stress. They expected high levels of EI would promote challenge appraisals and better performance, whereas they found low EI levels would foster threat appraisals and worse performance. Mishra & Mohapatra (2010), mentioned yet, there is some evidence to suggest that a high EI is desirable in the work place, and if it is, can it be taught? (Matthews et al., 2002) Note that this may be changing as there is now some evidence that EI can be measured and that it does improve performance in the work place (O'Boyle et al., 2010). Kim (2010), investigated how salespersons' emotional intelligence affects adaptive selling and positive emotional expression during the process of interaction with customers, and how such adaptive selling and positive emotional expression affects the quality of service perceived by customers. The results show those greater salespersons' emotional intelligence results in better adaptive selling and positive emotional expression. He found that a person with positive emotional intelligence in work has better sales. Nooraei & Arasi (2011), determined possible relationship between faculty's social competencies and their academic performance in Iran; results indicated that the social competencies elements are significantly associated with the level of faculties' academic performance. This finding shows the important of EI in academic setting. Khajehpour (2011), investigated the relationship between emotional intelligence, parental involvement and academic performance of 300 high school Students in Tehran, Iran. Results showed that both emotional intelligence and parental involvement could predict academic achievement in high school students. Similarly, there were significant positive relationship between emotional intelligence and academic achievement. Some research revealed emotions, such as excitement or enthusiasm, could stimulate employees to provide better customer service, complete their work assignments, or contribute to the organization. Conversely, negative emotions, such as anxiety, could facilitate employees' ability to focus on their work tasks. Employees with high emotional intelligence should be more adept at regulating their own emotions and managing others' emotions to foster more positive interactions, which could lead to more organizational citizenship behaviors that contribute to performance (Mossholder et al., 1981; Wong & Law, 2002) Teams with a high level of EI had a preference for collaborative conflict resolution strategies, whereas teams with low EI preferred avoiding strategies (Jordan & Troth, 2002). Rapisarda (2002), also found a positive relationship between "empathy" (a sub dimension of EI) and performance in student teams. (Jordan et al., 2002) reported that self-learning student teams with lower average EI scores initially performed at a lower level than teams with high scores did, but eventually achieved the same level of performance over the 10 weeks of their study. Feyerherm & Rice (2002), demonstrated a relationship between EI and customer service teams. According to these authors, two of Mayer and Salovey's factors ("understanding emotions" and "managing emotions") were positively correlated with some performance measures related to customer service. Research has demonstrated that trait-based EI enhances performance in interviewing (Fox & Spector, 2000), management (Slaski & Cartwright, 2002), academics (Petrides et al., 2004), and teams (Jordan et al., 2002), and on cognitive tasks (Shutte et al., 2001) and contextual performance. The high EI person is more likely to have possessions of sentimental attachment around the home and to have more positive social interactions, particularly if the individual scored highly on emotional management. Such individuals may also be more adept at describing motivational goals, aims, and missions (Mayer et al., 2004). (Seibert et al., 2001) discussed that Emotional intelligence may contribute to work performance (as reflected in salary, salary increase, and company rank) by enabling people to nurture positive relationships at work, work effectively in teams, and build social capital. Work performance often depends on the support, advice, and other resources provided by others. Emotional intelligence may also contribute to work performance by enabling people to regulate their emotions so as to cope effectively with stress, perform well under pressure, and adjust to organizational change.

2.3 Emotional intelligence and job performance in the executives

Focusing on EI as an important factor that related to performance, researchers presents reviews a number of studies of the drivers of workplace performance. Numerous studies have found that EI is associated with a number of positive outcomes in the workplace, affecting variables such as leadership (Scott- Halsell et al., 2008), resistance to stress (Bar-On et al., 2000; Mikolajczak et al., 2007), work attitude (Carmeli, 2003), job satisfaction and performance (Kafetsios & Zampetakis, 2008; Law et al., 2008; Wong & Law, 2002), employees' creativity (Zhou & George, 2003) and career achievements (Dulewitz & Higgs, 1999). In recent years, different researches suggested that, IQ is not the only factor of managers' success and performance improvement, but also there is another factor called emotional intelligence that results in outstanding performance at work. Some researchers have found that emotional intelligence has a positive and significant relation with performance (Goleman, 1998; Mount, 2006). (Mayer et al., 2000a) suggested that EI may influence work-related outcomes (e.g., job performance) and interpersonal interactions (e.g., job interviews). Goleman (1995, 1998), claimed that EI predicts life and work success. Goleman (1998), also claimed that, because EI affects almost every aspect of work life, employees who are high in EI are "star performers." Publishers of EI tests advocate the use of EI tests for personnel selection, claiming that research has demonstrated a strong correlation between EI and job performance, and also he demonstrates that managers who do not develop their emotional intelligence have difficulty in building good relationships with peers, subordinates, superiors and clients. Carmeli (2003), has shown that managers with high EI produce positive work attitudes and altruistic behaviors and that their employees enjoy higher job satisfaction and performance (Wong & Law, 2002). Managers with high EI can facilitate the performance of their employees by managing employees' emotions that foster more creativity, resilience, and enables employees to act successfully (Fredrickson, 2003; Zhou & George, 2003). Furthermore, managers with high EI should be more adept at nurturing more positive interactions between employees that could foster more cooperation (Barsade, 2002), coordination (Sy et al., 2005). The high EI individual, relative to others, is less apt to engage in problem behaviors, and avoids self-destructive, negative behaviors. Dulewicz & Higgs (2000), demonstrates clearly that EI impacts on work success. Work success was defined in this review as advancement in one's work organization. Some research suggests that emotional intelligence is important for work settings (Carmeli, 2003; Jordan et al., 2002). Researchers assert that employees' EI can predict work related outcomes, such as job satisfaction and job performance (Bachman et al., 2000; Prati et al., 2003; Wong & Law, 2002). Furthermore, theorists posit that managers' EI can significantly impact these work outcomes (George, 2000; Goleman et al., 2002). A study by (Day & Carroll, 2004) shows the positive relation of ability-based EI on performance. (Sy et al., 2006) examined the relationships among employees' emotional intelligence, their manager's emotional intelligence, employees' job satisfaction, and performance. They found that employees' emotional intelligence was positively associated with job satisfaction and performance. In addition, manager's emotional intelligence had a more positive correlation with job satisfaction for employees with low emotional intelligence than for those with high emotional intelligence. Emotional intelligence is conceptually relevant for predicting employees' work performance because organizations require interpersonal interactions to accomplish goals, and because most jobs require the ability to manage emotions. EI has the potential to be a strong predictor of performance. Linking EI with performance can provide organizations with a valid alternative for selecting and assessing employees. Enhancing EI skills enables managers to regulate their emotions and motivate themselves more effectively. (Patnaik et al., 2010) investigates the relationship between emotional intelligence and work performance of executives working in the Cooperative bank and Gramya Banks in Odisha. Their study revealed High EQ is necessary for better performance in the banking sector. But, high EQ cannot be the only requirement for good performance on the job. (Song et al., 2010) Studied about whether emotional intelligence (EI) has incremental validity over and above traditional intelligence dimensions. They found support for the notion that EI has a unique power to predict academic performance, and also revealed that EI is related to the quality of social interactions with peers. Clarke (2010), examined a contribution specifically to the project management field by studying the effects of training on a sample of project managers in the UK, and identifying whether changes occur in their emotional intelligence and relevant project management competences. Using a pre/post test research design, positive effects were found 6 months later in the emotional ability, understanding emotions as well as the two project manager competences. (Shahzad et al., 2011) investigated impact of EI on employee's performance among telecom employees in Pakistan. The results revealed that a positive relationship exits between social awareness and relationship management and employee's performance, also they found Telecom sector needs to consider meaningful features of EI as a strong predictor for efficient performance of employees. Chaudhry & Usman (2011), examined the relationship between employees' emotional intelligence and their performance in Pakistan. The results revealed a moderately high correlation between emotional intelligence and organizational citizenship behavior. It was also established that employees' job performance can be predicted significantly based upon their emotional intelligence scores. (Tsai et al., 2011) analyzed the impacts among the emotional intelligence and leadership style, self-efficacy and organizational commitment of employees in the banking industry in Taiwan. They found that a supervisor's emotional intelligence has a significant positive influence on his/her personal leadership style, that a supervisor with high emotional intelligence is able to perform excellent leading skills to elevate the employee self-efficacy, and that employees self-efficacy results in a significant positive influence on organizational commitment. Jung & Yoon (2011), studied the interrelationships among the emotional intelligence of employees in a deluxe hotel. The results showed that as elements of emotional intelligence, others' emotion appraisal, use of emotion, and self-emotion appraisal significantly affected counterproductive work behaviors, whereas self-emotion appraisal and use of emotion affected organizational citizen behaviors. Focusing on these literature reviews, we can find that there is relation between Emotional Intelligence with job performance of executives or any person that has a responsibility in a company, organization, or society, and EI may improve the manager performance in work and increases organizational success, therefore the findings of this research will show this matter.

2.4 Aim and hypothesis

The aim of the current study is to explore the relationship between emotional intelligence and job performance among executives. Therefore the objective of this research is drawing links between EI and performance at work place. The study helps the executives at their organization to develop and explore the concept of EI to ensure high level of performance resulting in increased achievement of organizational and individual goals.

Accordingly, based on the foregoing literature review, we propose:

H1: Executives' EI associates positively with job performance for employees with low EI than for employees with high EI.

H2: Executives' EI associates positively with their job performance.

H3: Executives' scores on EI significantly predict their job performance.

3. Method

3.1 Participants

A number of executives from north, south, east, and west of Iran organizations have been chosen as the subjects of the study through purposive sampling. A total of 500 questionnaires were distributed conveniently to executives in various organizations, out of which 218 questionnaires were returned, and a total of 18 questionnaires were excluded from the study due to incompleteness. Therefore the participants in this study were 200 male and female executives that 73% were male, working in Iran organizations, and having graduation degree in engineering and master's degree in management have been selected. The majority (92%) of the executives were in the age range 40-60 years with the remaining 8% being in the age range 20–30 years,

3.2 Measures

In this study, Job Performance is dependent variable and Emotional Intelligence is independent variable and to measure the emotional intelligence of the sample of executives, we used Emotional intelligence scale constructed by (Schutte et al., 1998). Participants fulfilled a Persian version of the Schutte Emotional Intelligence Scale. The tool contains 33 items using a 5-point Likert scale, where 1 represents 'strongly disagree' and 5 'strongly agree'. Total score may range from 33 to 165. The high scores indicate employees' higher ability to recognize and manage emotions. In this content (Austin et al., 2004) reported a good internal consistency of the scale with a Cronbach alpha of .85. The reliability of the scale was .88 therefore, is appropriate. The items of the scale are directly related to the concept of emotional intelligence. It includes self-awareness, empathy, self motivation, emotional stability, managing relations, integrity, self-development, value-orientation, commitment and altruistic behavior. This measure was chosen because it is readily available, widely used and suitable for an Iranian sample, and also a recent study showed that the scale is more appropriate for Iranian respondents (Khajehpour, 2011). For the purpose of data analysis, several statistical tools and method were utilized from the statistical package for social sciences (SPSS) version 16. To assess the relationship between EI and performance, we performed **T-tests, ANOVA, and Regression.**

4. Results

Present study investigates the effect of emotional intelligence on the work performance of executives. Significance of mean differences on work performance dimensions of emotionally high and low intelligence groups of executives was determined.

Table1 shows the difference between the mean scores of high and low emotionally intelligence executive groups on all the dimensions of job performance is in favor of high emotionally intelligence group of executive except one dimension that is dependability. The T-values are significant at .01 levels for Quality of work performance, Speed on the job, Quantity of work, Capacity of work, Ability to work without supervision, Ability to handle different jobs, Ability to get along with others, Initiative on the job and Overall job performance dimensions of job performance. T-value of Amount of effort expended on job, Care in handling company, Attendance and punctuality, Planning Ability dimensions of job performance are significant at .05 levels. The result of T-tests shows that have significant effect on high and low emotionally intelligence executive groups. This result supports the first hypothesis of the study.

N.	Dimensions of Job Performance	Groups	N	Mean	SD	t
1	Quality of work performance	High EI	100	4.4	.517	2.89**
		Low EI	100	4.1	.568	
2	Amount of effort expended on job	High EI	100	4.6	.528	2.69*
		Low EI	100	3.9	.632	
3	Speed on the job	High EI	100	4.7	.516	3.80**
		Low EI	100	3.9	.422	
4	Quantity of work	High EI	100	4.3	.527	3.54**
		Low EI	100	3.8	.482	
5	Capacity of work	High EI	100	4.3	.517	3.65**
		Low EI	100	3.8	.317	
6	Care in handling company	High EI	100	4.5	.516	2.69*
		Low EI	100	3.7	.789	
7	Ability to work without supervision	High EI	100	4.8	.483	3.81**
		Low EI	100	3.7	.675	
8	Ability to handle different jobs	High EI	100	4.7	.422	4.16**
		Low EI	100	3.5	.632	
9	Dependability	High EI	100	4.7	.843	1.64*
		Low EI	100	3.9	.789	
10	Ability to get along with others	High EI	100	4.6	.517	2.88**
		Low EI	100	3.9	.568	
11	Attendance and punctuality	High EI	100	4.7	.422	2.50*
		Low EI	100	4.1	.633	
12	Planning Ability	High EI	100	4.7	.483	2.87*
		Low EI	100	3.7	.738	
13	Initiative on the job	High EI	100	4.5	.483	3.58**
		Low EI	100	3.8	.632	
14	Overall work performance	High EI	100	4.7	.317	6.61**
		Low EI	100	3.6	.422	

*$P > .05$
**$P > .01$

Table 1. Mean and SD of high and low emotionally intelligent groups of executives on various dimensions of job performance.

Model	Sum of Squares	Df	Mean Square	F	Sig.
Regression	32.228	1	32.228	125.890	.000[a]
Residual	50.652	198	0.256		
Total	82.880	199			

a. Predictors: (Constant), Emotional Intelligence

Table 2. Prediction of Job Performance through Scores on Emotional Intelligence.

Table 2 ANOVA, shows that employees' EI is positively related with performance as measured through Job Performance, it is reveals the presence of a significant positive correlation between total EI scores and Job Performance (p < 0.01). The results of the current research support the first hypothesis. Also results in Table 2 show a significant P-value =0.000 (less than 0.05) for the prediction relation between EI and Job Performance. Thus, the second hypothesis asserting that executives' scores on emotional intelligence significantly predict the future is supported. Table 3 proves only the presence of a prediction relation between EI and the dependent variable (Job Performance).

	Un-standardized Coefficients		Standardized Coefficients	t	Sig.
	B	Std. Error	Beta		
Emotional Intelligence	0.823	0.048	0.682	18.259	.000

a. Dependent Variable: Job Performance

Table 3. Regression Coefficients (a).

The strength of the relationship is shown in Table 3 with the help of the values of intercept (0.872) and slope for EI regression line (0.823). This suggests that for a one unit increase in emotional intelligence, the respective manager can significantly predict a 0.823 increase in their performance, whereas a slope of 0.682 for EI is produced when the test utilizes standardized independent and dependent variables. To measure the strength of a prediction relation through 'Beta' may indicate some inflated results. Consequently a conservative measure 'coefficient of determination' was calculated. Employees' scores on emotional intelligence exhibit nearly high positive association (r = 0.682) with their organizational citizenship behavior.

R	R Square	Adjusted R Square	Std. Error of the Estimate
0.682 a	0.465	0.464	0.3281

a. Predictors: (Constant), Emotional Intelligence

Table 4. Model Summery of Regression for Emotional Intelligence and Job Performance.

The presence of a strong positive association between executives' EI and performance suggested that executives' future performance could be predicted on the basis of their EI scores. The second hypothesis of the study implies that employees' EI scores significantly predict their Job Performance. A regression analysis was applied, because, Job Performance as a single continuous dependent variable and EI as a single continuous independent variable are involved in this case. The test produced the significance values for hypothesis testing regarding individual regression parameters. Table 4 indicates an 'R2' value of 0.465 that shows nearly 50% of the variance in Job Performance, can be accounted for by executive's score on EI. This result supports the third hypothesis of the study that executives' EI score significantly predict their job performance.

5. Discussion and conclusion

This study investigates empirically the relationship between emotional intelligence and job performance between Iranian executives. Based on the findings of previous research, a significant positive correlation was expected between EI and performance. The results indicated nearly high positive correlation (r =0.682) between the independent (EI) and dependent (Job Performance) variables. Therefore, finding of this research revealed that there is a significant relationship between emotional intelligence and performance. The result that EI has a predictive effect on job performance concurs with the findings of the previous researchers (Goleman, 1995). Proponents of EI have claimed that EI is an important predictor of all areas of workplace performance; particularly for managers (e.g., Goleman, 1998). Also Goleman's research shows that emotional well-being is the strongest predictor of academic achievement and success in life. According with several studies (Lopes et al., 2006; Sy et al., 2006) the results demonstrated convincingly that EI is an important personality-level predictor of work affectivity and job satisfaction. Our study provides some preliminary support for researchers who have proposed the importance of EI for leaders and executives (e.g., Boal & Hooijberg, 2000; Day, 2000; Hooijberg et al., 1997; Sternberg, 1997). Executives, in particular, need high EI because they represent the organization to the public, they interact with the highest number of people within and outside the organization and they set the tone for employee morale, says Goleman. The success of an individual working within an organization is a function of emotional intelligence. Much of this success depends on the abilities of individuals to motivate them and to accomplish tasks by forming teams from a loose network of fellow workers with specific talents and expertise. Leaders with empathy are able to understand their employee's needs and provide them with constructive feedback. According to (Mayer et al., 2000), individuals who score highly on the Emotional Perception scale will be able to identify how family members and colleagues are feeling, and will also be skilled at interpersonal interactions. Therefore, high EI people may simply have a response style of viewing themselves, others, and neutral stimuli in a manner consistent with positive affectivity. The results also support other researches (e.g., Law et al., 2004; Sy et al., 2006; Wong & Law, 2002) indicating that employees' with higher EI have higher job performance, suggesting that employees with high EI are more adept at using their emotions to facilitate job performance. Employees with high EI seem to be more aware of how certain emotions can influence their behaviors and work outcomes and more adept at regulating their emotions in such a manner that they are aligned with the requirements of the task. This finding is supported by (Stein, 2002) which discussed about the EI factor: The sample group scored slightly higher than average on total EI. In order from most to least above the norms, the group scored above average on independence, assertiveness, optimism, self-actualization, and self-regard. Highly emotionally intelligent executives are more punctual and take maximum initiatives on the job, they put much amount of efforts to expended their job and have better work performance as compared to their counterparts. The finding is according to (Dulewicz et al., 2003) that found managers' emotional intelligence correlated positively with quality of work life and morale, also (Brackett et al., 2004) concluded that low scores on EI were associated with poor quality peer relations. (Suliman & Al-Shaikh, 2007) revealed that employees with higher levels of EI were found to report higher levels of readiness to create and innovate. Results also favor the same and this finding was also supported by (Tischler et al., 2002) he examined the linking emotional intelligence, spirituality and work place performance and displayed a positive relationship between emotional intelligence and work place success and also by (Cooper & Sawaf, 1997; Megerian & Sosik, 1996; Wright and Staw, 1999). The findings of the study revealed that

Emotional intelligence has a positive effect on the job performance among executives. The executives having higher emotional intelligence show better quality of job performance as compared to their counterparts. Emotional intelligence is an effective determinant of job performance. The study of the relationship between *emotional intelligence* and *job performance* among *executives* can be the first study which has been done in Iran. The current study is therefore a reflection of the kinds of research that are the current focus within the area of emotional intelligence and performance. The fact that emotional intelligence is significantly related to executive's performance may have valuable implications for their recruiters, trainers, and supervisors, and governments.

6. Limitation, future research, and implication

Several limitations of the study could be mentioned. The first is the size of the sample. Although, we gather questionnaires from different parts of Iran, but having larger sample size (N= 200) would have strengthened the impact of the study's results. The second is that it may be unreasonable to generalize these results to the other country. Lastly, data collection was also a limitation because information on particular variable could be collected through a limited number of top executives who are usually busy. In the future, we suggest that researchers consider the importance of the influence of emotional intelligence on performance; this study can be conducted in other countries to identify if the geographical environment or cultural characteristics may change the results. For instance, researchers would like to do a survey related to Emotional Intelligence among international executives; such as Iranian, Japanese, and American executives. Results of this study also have certain practical implication. In today's society using emotion as a tool to achieve organizational objectives, the rate of emotional executives is gradually increasing. Therefore, it is necessary to draw up an effective plan to promote emotional intelligence through continuous education and training for executives within a company and choose a manager with high EI.

7. Acknowledgment

The author would like to thank the Islamic Azad University, Science and Research Branch of Iran for financially supporting this research.

8. References

Austin, E. J. (2004). An investigation of the relationship between trait emotional intelligence and emotional task performance, *Personality and Individual Differences* 36 (2004) 1855–1864.

Austin, E. J., Saklofske, D. H., Huang, S. H. S., & McKenney, D (2004). Measurement of trait emotional intelligence: Testing and cross-validating a modified version of Schutte et al.'s (1998) measure. *Personality and Individual Differences*, 36, 555–562.

Bachman, J., Stein, S., Campbell, K., & Sitarenios, G. (2000). Emotional intelligence in the collection of debt.*International Journal of Selection and Assessment, 8*, 176–182.

Bar-On R (1997).*The Emotional Quotient Inventory (EQ-i): A Test of Emotional Intelligence.* Toronto, Canada: Multi-Health Systems.

Bar-On, R. (1988). The development of a concept of psychological well-being. *Unpublished Doctoral Dissertation*, Rhodes University, South Africa.

Bar-On R, Parker JDA (2000). The Handbook of Emotional Intelligence: *Theory, Development, Assessment, and Application at Home, School, and in the Workplace.* Jossey-Bass, San Francisco, CA.

Bar-On R, Maree JG, Elias MJ (2007). *Educating People to Be Emotionally Intelligence.* Westport Connecticut, London: Praeger.

Barsade, S. G. (2002). The ripple eVect: Emotional contagion and its inXuence on group behavior. *Administrative Science Quarterly*, 47, 644–675.

Berman EM, West JP (2008). Managing Emotional Intelligence in U.S. Cities: A Study of Social Skills among Public Managers. *Pub. Adm. Rev.*, 68 (4): 742 – 758.

Bernaud & C. Lemoine (Eds.), Traité de psychologie du travail et des organisations. Paris: Dunod.

Bless, H., Bohner, G., Schwarz, N., & Strack, F. (1990). Mood persuasion: A cognitive response analysis, *Personality and Social Psychology Bulletin*, 16, 331–345.

Boal, K. B., & Hooijberg, R. (2000). Strategic leadership research: moving on. *The Leadership Quarterly Yearly Review of Leadership*, 11 (4), 515–550.

Brackett MA, Mayer JD, Warner RM (2004). Emotional intelligence and its relation to everyday behavior. *Person. Individual Diff.*, 36: 1387- 1402.

Carmeli, A. (2003). The relationship between emotional intelligence and work attitudes, behavior and outcomes, *Journal of Managerial Psychology*, 18(8), 788–813.

Çeçen AR (2006). The development of skills in managing emotions scale: validity and reliability studies [Development of emotions manegement skills scale: The studies of validity and reliability]. *Turk. J. Couns. Guid.*, 3(26): 101-113.

Chaudhry, A. A, Usman, A. (2011). An investigation of the relationship between employees' emotional intelligence and performance, *African Journal of Business Management* Vol.5 (9), pp. 3556-3562.

Clarke, N. (2010). The impact of a training programme designed to target the emotional intelligence abilities of project managers, *International Journal of Project Management* 28 (2010) 461–468.

Cooper R. & Sawaf A. (1997). *Executive EQ: Emotional Intelligence in Business.* London, Orion.

Cote, S., Miners, C.T.H., 2006. Emotional intelligence, cognitive intelligence and job performance. *Administrative Science Quarterly* 51 (1), 1–28.

Daus, C. S., & Ashkanasy, N. M. (2005). The case for the ability-based model of emotional intelligence in organizational behaviour. *Journal of Organizational Behavior*, 26, 453–466.

Davidson, R.J., Jackson,D.C. & Kalin,N.H.(2000). Emotion, plasticity, context and regulation: Perspectives from affective neuroscience. *Psychological Bulletin*, 126, 890-906.

Davies M, Stankov L, Roberts RD (1998). Emotional intelligence: In search of an elusive construct. *J. Pers. Soc. Psych.* 75, 989–1015.

Day, D. V. (2000). Leadership development: a review in context. *The Leadership Quarterly Yearly Review of Leadership*, 11 (4), 581–614.

Day, A. L., & Carroll, S. A. (2004). Using an ability-based measure of emotional intelligence to predict individual performance, group performance, and group citizenship behaviours. *Personality and Individual Differences*, 36, 1443–1458.

Dulewitz V, Higgs M (1999). Can emotional intelligence be measured and developed? *Leadership Org. Dev. J.*, 20(5): 242-252.

Dulewicz, Higgs, M (2000), *Emotional Intelligence, A Review and Evaluation Study*, Henley Management College, Henley-on-Thames.

Dulewicz V, Higgs M, Slaski M (2003). Measuring emotional intelligence: Content, construct and criterion-related validity. *J. Manage. Psychol.*, 18(5): 406-420.

Forgas, J. P. (1995). Mood and judgment: The affect infusion model (AIM). *Psychological Bulletin*, 117, 39–66.

Feyerherm, A. E., & Rice, C. L. (2002). Emotional Intelligence and Team Performance: The good, the bad and the ugly. *International Journal of Organizational Analysis*, 10, 343–362.

Fox, S., & Spector, P. E. (2000). Relations of emotional intelligence, practical intelligence, general intelligence, and trait affectivity with interview outcomes: It's not all just "g". *Journal of Organizational Behavior*, 21, 203–220.

Fredrickson, B. L. (2003). Positive emotions and upward spirals in organizations. In K. S. Cameron, J. E. Dutton, & R. E. Quinn (Eds.), *Positive organizational scholarship: Foundations of a new discipline*. San Francisco: Barrett Koehler.

Gardner H (1983). *Frames of Mind: The Theory of Multiple Intelligences*. New York: Basic Books.

George, J. M. (2000). Emotions and leadership: The role of emotional intelligence. *Human Relations*, 53, 1027–1055.

Giardini A, Frese M (2008). Linking service employees' emotional competence to customer satisfaction: A multilevel approach. *J. Organ. Behav.*, 29: 155-170.

Goleman D., (1995). *Emotional intelligence. Why it can matter More Than IQ*, New York: Bantam Books.

Goleman D., (2006). *Emotional Intelligence, 10th Anniversary ed.*, Bantam Books, New York.

Goleman D., (1998). *Working with Emotional Intelligence*. New York: Bantam Books.

Goleman, D., Boyatzis, R., & McKee, A. (2002). *Primal leadership: Realizing the power of emotional intelligence*. Boston, MA: Harvard Business School Press.

Gray, J. R. (2004). Integration of emotion and cognitive control. *Current Directions in Psychological Science*, 13, 46–48.

Hooijberg, R., Hunt, J. G., & Dodge, G. E. (1997). Leadership complexity and development of the leaderplex model. *Journal of Management*, 23 (3), 375–408.

Hyo Sun Jung, Hye Hyun Yoon, The effects of emotional intelligence on counterproductive work behaviors and organizational citizen behaviors among food and beverage employees in a deluxe hotel, *International Journal of Hospitality Management*; xxx (2011) xxx–xxx , Article In Press.

Isen, A. M., Daubman, K. A., & Nowicki, G. P. (1987). Positive affect facilitates creative problem solving. *Journal of Personality and Social Psychology*, 52, 1122-1131.

Jordan, P. J., Ashkanasy, N. M., Hartel, C. E., & Hooper, G. S. (2002). Workgroup emotional intelligence: Scale development and relationship to team process, effectiveness, and goal focus. *Human Resource Management Review*, 12, 195–214.

Jung, H. S., Yoon, H. H. (2011). The effects of emotional intelligence on counterproductive work behaviors and organizational citizen behaviors among food and beverage employees in a deluxe hotel, *International Journal of Hospitality Management* xxx (2011) xxx–xxx, Article in Press.

Kafetsios K, Zampetakis LA (2008). Emotional intelligence and job satisfaction: Testing the mediatory role of positive and negative affect at work., *Personality and Individual Differences* 44(3): 710-720.

Khajehpour, M. (2011). Relationship between emotional intelligence, parental involvement and academic performance of high school students, *Procedia Social and Behavioral Sciences* 15 (2011) 1081–1086.

Kim, S. H. (2010). The effect of emotional intelligence on salesperson's behavior and customers' perceived service quality, *African Journal of Business Management* Vol. 4(11), pp. 2343-2353.

Law KS, Wong CS, Huang GH, Li X (2008). The effects of emotional intelligence on job performance and life satisfaction for the research and development scientists in China. *Asia Pacif. J. Manage.*, 25(1): 51-69.

Lopes, P. N., Grewal, D., Kadis, J., Gall, M., & Salovey, P. (2006). Evidence that emotional intelligence is related to job performance and affect and attitudes at work. *Psicothema*, 18(1), 132–138.

Lyons, J. B., Schneider, T. R. (2005). The influence of emotional intelligence on performance, *Personality and Individual Differences* 39 (2005) 693–703.

Martinez, M.N (1997), "The smarts that count", *HR Magazine*, Vol. 42 No.11, pp.72-8.

Matthews, G., Zeidner, M., & Roberts, R. (2002). *Emotional Intelligence: Science & Myth.* Cambridge, Massachusetts: The MIT Press.

Mayer, J. D., & Cobb (2000), Educational policy on emotional intelligence: Does it make sense? *Educational Psychology Review,* 12, 163-183.

Mayer J. D., Geher, G (1996). "Emotional Intelligence and the Identification of Emotion," *Intelligence*, 22(2): 89-113.

Mayer JD, Salovey P (1997). *What is emotional intelligence? In Emotional development and emotional intelligence*: Implications for educators, Peter Salovey, David Sluyter, eds., New York: Basic Books, pp. 3-31.

Mayer, J. D., Salovey, P., & Caruso, D. R. (2000a). *Test manual for the Mayer, Salovey, Caruso Emotional Intelligence Test: research version 1.1 (3rd ed)*. Toronto, Canada: MHS.

Mayer, J. D., Salovey, P., & Caruso, D. R. (2000b). *Models of emotional intelligence.* In R. Sternberg (Ed.), Handbook of intelligence (pp. 396–422). Cambridge: Cambridge University Press.

Mayer, J.D., Salovey, P., Caruso, D.R. (2004), "Emotional intelligence: theory, findings, and implications", *Psychological Inquiry*, Vol. 15 No.3, pp.197-215.

Mayer, J.D., Roberts, R.D., Barsade, S.G., (2008). Human abilities: emotional intelligence. *Ann. Rev. Psych.* 59, 507–536.

Mayer J.D., Salovey P., Caruso D.R. (2008). Emotional intelligence: New ability or eclectic traits? *Am. Psychol.*, 63: 503-517.

Mayer, J. D., & Stevens, A. (1994). An emerging understanding of the reflective (meta-) experience of mood. *Journal of Research in Personality, 28, 351-373*

Megerian, L.E., & Sosik, J.J (1996). An affair of the heart: Emotional intelligence and transformational ledership. *The journal of leadership studies, 3(3), 31-48.*

Mikolajczak M, Menil C, Luminet O (2007). Explaining the protective effect of trait emotional intelligence regarding occupational stress: exploration of emotional labour processes. *J. Res. Pers.*, 41(5): 1107–1117.

Mishra P. S & Mohapatra A. K Das, (2010). Relevance of Emotional Intelligence for Effective Job Performance: An Empirical Study, *VIKALPA*, Vol. 35, No 1. pp. 53-61.

Mossholder, K. W., Bedian, A. G., & Armenakis, A. A. (1981). Group process-work outcome relationships: A note on the moderating impact of self-esteem. *Academy of Management Journal, 25,* 575–585.

Mount G (2006). The role of emotional intelligence in developing international business capability: EI provides traction. In Druskat V. Sala F. Mount G *Linking emotional intelligence and performance at work.* NJ: Erlbaum.

Nooraei, M, Arasi, I. S. (2011). Emotional intelligence and faculties' academic performance: The social competencies approach, *International Journal of Education Administration and Policy Studies* Vol. 2(4), pp. 45-52.

O'Boyle, E. H., Humphrey, R. H., Pollack, J. M., Hawver, T. H., Story, P. A. (2010). The relation between emotional intelligence and job performance: A meta-analysis. *Journal of Organizational Behavior,* 2010; DOI: 10.1002/job.714

Quoidbach, J., Hansenne, M.(2009) The Impact of Trait Emotional Intelligence on Nursing Team Performance and Cohesiveness, *Journal of Professional Nursing,* Vol 25, No 1 (January–February), 2009: pp 23–29.

Patnaik, C. M, Satpathy, I, Pradhan, P. K. (2010). A study to assess emotional intelligence and performance of Managers in Cooperative and Gramya Banks in Orissa, *Asian Journal of Management Research,* pp. 10-20, ISSN 2229 - 3795.

Petrides, K. V., & Furnham, A. (2000). On the dimensional structure of emotional intelligence. *Personality and Individual Differences,* 29, 313–320.

Petrides, K. V., & Furnham, A. (2001). Trait emotional intelligence: Psychometric investigation with reference to established trait taxonomies. *European Journal of Personality,* 15, 425–448.

Petrides, K. V., Frederickson, N., & Furnham, A. (2004). The role of trait emotional intelligence in academic performance and deviant behavior at school. *Personality and Individual Differences,* 36, 277–293.

Petrides, K. V., Pita, R., & Kokkinaki, F. (2007). The location of trait emotional intelligence in personality factor space. *British Journal of Psychology,* 98, 273–289.

Prati, L. M., Douglas, C., Ferris, G. R., Ammeter, A. P., & Buckley, M. R. (2003). Emotional intelligence, leadership effectiveness, and team outcomes. *International Journal of Organizational Analysis,* 11, 21–41.

Rapisarda, B. A. (2002). The impact of emotional intelligence on work team cohesiveness and performance. *International Journal of Organizational Analysis,* 10, 363–379.

Salovey, P., Bedell, B. T, Detweiller, J. B., & Mayer, J. D. (2000). *Coping intelligently: emotional intelligence and the coping process.* In C. R. Snyder (Ed.), Coping: the psychology of what works (pp. 141–164). New York: Oxford University Press.

Salovery P, Mayer JD (1990). Emotional intelligence. *Cog. Pers.,* 9(3):185-211.

Salovey P, Mayer JD (1997). *What is emotional intelligence? In Emotional development and emotional intelligence: Implications for educators,* Peter Salovey, David Sluyter, eds., New York: Basic Books, pp. 3-31.

Savoie, A., & Brunet, L. (2000). Les équipes de travail: Champ d'intervention privilégié pour les psychologies. In J.-L. Bernaud & C. Lemoine (Eds.), Traité de psychologie du travail et des organisations. Paris: Dunod.

Schwarz, N. (1990). Feelings as information: Informational and affective functions of affective states. In E. T. Higgins & R. M. Sorrentino (Eds.). *Handbook of motivation and cognition: Foundations of social behavior* (Vol. 2, pp. 527–561). New York: Guilford.

Schmidt FL, Hunter JE (2000). *Select on intelligence, in E. A. Locke (ed.)*, The Blackwell handbook of organizational principles. (p. 3–14). Oxford: Blackwell.

Schutte, N.S., Malouff, J.M.Hall, L.E.Haggerty, D.J.Cooper, J.T.Golden, C.J & Dornheim,L (1998). Development and validation of a Measure of Emotional Intelligence. *Personality and Individual Differences*, 25(2), pp 167177.

Scott-Ladd B, Chan CCA Chan (2004). Emotional intelligence and participation in decision-making: strategies for promoting Organizational learning and change. *Strateg. Chang.*, 13(2): 95–105.

Scott-Halsell S, Shumate SR, Blum S (2008). Using a model of emotional intelligence domains to indicate transformational leaders in the hospitality industry. *J. Hum. Res. Hosp. To.*, 7(1): 99-113.

Shahzad, K., Sarmad, M., Abbas, M., Amanullah Khan, M. (2011). Impact of Emotional Intelligence (EI) on employee's performance in telecom sector of Pakistan, *African Journal of Business Management*, Vol.5 (4), pp. 1225-1231.

Shutte, N. S., Schuettpelz, E., & Malouff, J. M. (2001). Emotional intelligence and task performance. *Imagination, Cognition, and Personality*, 20, 347–354.

Slaski, M., & Cartwright, S. (2002). Health, performance and emotional intelligence: An exploratory study of retail managers. *Stress and Health*, 18, 63–68.

Song, L. J., Huang, G. H., Peng, K. Z., Law, K. S., Wong, C. M., Chen, Z. (2010). The differential effects of general mental ability and emotional intelligence on academic performance and social interactions, *Intelligence* 38 (2010) 137–143.

Stein, S. (2002). The EQ factor: *Does emotional intelligence make you a better CEO?* Special Report: Innovator's Alliance, Ontario, Canada, NOV 25th.

Suliman AM, Al-Shaikh FN (2007). Emotional intelligence at work: Links to conflict and innovation. *Empl. Relations*, 29(2): 208-220.

Sy, T., Cote, S., & Saavedra, R. (2005). The contagious leader: Impact of the leader's mood on the mood of group members, group aVective tone, and group processes. *Journal of Applied Psychology, 90*, 295–305.

Sy, T., Tram, S., O'Hara, L. A. (2006). Relation of employee and manager emotional intelligence to job satisfaction and performance, *Journal of Vocational Behavior* 68 (2006) 461–473.

Thorndike EL (1920). *Intelligence and its uses*. Harpers Mag., 140: 227- 235.

Tischler L, Biberman J, McKeage R. 2002. Linking emotional intelligence, spirituality and workplace performance: definitions, models and ideas for research. *Journal of Managerial Psychology* 17(3): 203–218

Tsai, M. T., Tsai, C. L. Wang, Y. C. (2011). A study on the relationship between leadership style, emotional intelligence, self-efficacy and organizational commitment : A case study of the Banking Industry in Taiwan, *African Journal of Business Management* Vol. 5(13), pp. 5319-5329.

Van Rooy, D. L., & Viswesvaran, C. (2004). Emotional intelligence: A meta-analytic investigation of predictive validity and nomological net. *Journal of Vocational Behavior*, 65(1), 71–95.

Wong, C., & Law, K. S. (2002). The eVect of leader and follower emotional intelligence on performance and attitude: An exploratory study. *Leadership Quarterly, 23*, 243–274.

Wong CS, Law KS (2002). The effects of leader and follower emotional intelligence on performance and attitude: an exploratory study. *Leadership Quarterly*, 13(3): 243-274.

Wright, T.A. & Staw, B.M. (1999). Affect and favorable work outcomes: Two longitudinal tests of the happy-productive worker thesis. *Journal of Organizational Behavior, 20, 123.*

Zhou, J., & George, J. M. (2003). Awakening employee creativity: The role of leader emotional intelligence. *Leadership Quarterly*, 14(5), 545–568.

7

Emotional Intelligence and Leadership – A Case for Quality Assurance Managers in Kenyan Universities

Laban Peter Ayiro and James K. Sang
*Department of Educational Management and Policy Studies, Moi University, Eldoret
Kenya*

1. Introduction

The notion of quality is hard to define precisely, especially in the context of tertiary education where institutions have broad autonomy to decide on their own visions and missions. Any statement about quality implies a certain relative measure against a common standard; in tertiary education, such a common standard does not exist. Various concepts have evolved to suit different contexts ranging from quality as a measure for excellence to quality as perfection, quality as value for money, quality as customer satisfaction, quality as fitness for purpose, and quality as transformation (in a learner) (SAUVCA 2002). Some institutions have adopted the International Standards Office (ISO) approach in some of their activities. Depending on the definition selected, quality implies a relative measure of inputs, processes, outputs or learning outcomes. Institutions, funders, and the public need some method for obtaining assurance that the institution is keeping its promises to its stakeholders. This is the primary goal of quality assurance. The leadership of the quality assurance directorates in universities has therefore come into sharp focus.

The emergence of theories of emotional intelligence has added a new dimension to thinking about leadership. Its importance in the work place has been highlighted (Cooper and Sawaf, 1997; Morris, 1999; Mayer and Salovey, 2002) particularly in terms of work success (Goleman, 1998; Higgs and Dulewicz, 1999; Pickard, 1999; Cherniss, 2000) through the management of own and others' emotions in the working environment (Caruso and Wolfe, 2001). While it has been noted that successful people in a variety of careers develop emotional intelligence skills they have learnt intuitively and often use without conscious awareness (Merlevede et al., 2001) there is little evidence on how emotional intelligence impacts on leaders in university settings in Kenya. This led to this study on the usefulness of emotional intelligence on the leadership of quality assurance directorates and how this can help them manoeuvre the uncharted terrain of ensuring quality of teaching and evaluation in Kenyan universities.

2. Emotional intelligence

2.1 Theory of emotional intelligence by Goleman (1998)

At this first level of conceptualization, scholars embrace a broad definition of emotional intelligence, which views EI as an integration of emotion and reason. Psychologists of this line of thought focus on EI as a wide array of competencies and suggest that it explains individual difference in social and emotional skills (Goleman, 1995) and can be fostered in schools (Payne, 1985). Goleman's theory is an example that reflects the aforementioned perspectives. Goleman, (1998) set out a framework of EI, often referred to as the mixed model which combines traits with social behaviours and competencies (Brown *et al*. 2006). It is composed of four domains: self-awareness, self-management, social awareness and relationship management (Boyatzis *et al.* 2000). Each domain contains a group of competencies, such as adaptability, communication and conflict management (Goleman, 1998). The measure for Goleman's EI model is the Emotional Competencies Inventory (ECI). The recent version (2.0) contains 72 statements about the EI-related behaviours (Boyatzis & Sala, 2004). These items were constructed based on emotional competencies identified by Daniel Goleman (1998), and on competencies from Hay/McBer's *Generic Competency Dictionary* (1996), as well as Richard Boyatzis's Self-Assessment Questionnaire (SAQ) (Sala 2002). The internal consistency of the instrument is 'adequate', but there is 'little evidence' of the test–retest reliability (Goleman *et al.* 1999). The reason may be that Goleman's EI theory is primarily competency-based and the 'crucial EI competencies can indeed be learned' (Goleman, 1995). So, it is likely that people's EI competencies and skills change over time. There are also limitations of the validity of the inventory, but overall it 'shows promise' (Goleman *et al.* 1999).

Mayer *et al.* (2000) pointed out that the meaning of EI in this category, such as defined by Goleman, was the broadest among the three categories of EI theories. It conveys some aspects of the cultural spirit during the 1980s and 1990s, which called for an integration of both emotion and rationality. However, such broad definitions and the associated measures may not be held up as 'scientific' ones.

2.2 The theoretical foundation of the Bar-On model

The Bar-On model provides the theoretical basis for the Emotional Quotient Inventory(EQ-i), which was originally developed to assess various aspects of this construct as well as to examine its conceptualization. According to this model, *emotional-social intelligence is a cross-section of interrelated emotional and social competencies, skills and facilitators that determine how effectively we understand and express ourselves, understand others and relate with them, and cope with daily demands.* The emotional and social competencies, skills and facilitators referred in this conceptualization include the five key components described above; and each of these components comprises a number of closely related competencies, skills and facilitators which are described in the Appendix. Consistent with this model, to be emotionally and socially intelligent is to effectively understand and express oneself, to understand and relate well with others, and to successfully cope with daily demands, challenges and pressures. This is based, first and foremost, on one's intrapersonal ability to be aware of oneself, to understand one's strengths and weaknesses, and to express one's feelings and thoughts non-destructively. On the interpersonal level, being emotionally and socially intelligent encompasses the ability to be aware of others' emotions, feelings and needs, and to establish and maintain cooperative, constructive and mutually satisfying relationships. Ultimately, being emotionally and socially intelligent means to effectively manage personal, social and environmental change by realistically and flexibly coping with the immediate situation, solving problems and making decisions. To do this, we need to manage emotions so that they work for us and not against us, and we need to be sufficiently optimistic, positive and self-motivated.

Description of the instrument used to develop the Bar-On model (the EQ-i)

To better understand the Bar-On model of emotional social intelligence (ESI) and how it developed, it is important to first describe the Emotional Quotient Inventory (the EQ-i) which has played an instrumental role in developing this model. For the purpose of the present discussion, it is also helpful to stress that the Bar-On model is operationalized by the EQ-i.

The EQ-i is a self-report measure of emotionally and socially intelligent behavior that provides an estimate of emotional-social intelligence. The EQ-i was the first measure of its kind to be published by a psychological test publisher (Bar-On, 1997a), the first such measure to be peer-reviewed in the *Buros Mental Measurement Yearbook* (Plake & Impara, 1999), and the most widely used measure of emotional-social intelligence to date (Bar-On, 2004). A detailed description of the psychometric properties of this measure and how it was developed is found in the *Bar-On EQ-i Technical Manual* (Bar-On, 1997b) and in Glenn Geher's recent book titled *Measuring Emotional Intelligence : Common Ground and Controversy* (2004).

In brief, the EQ-i contains 133 items in the form of short sentences and employs a 5-point response scale with a textual response format ranging from "very seldom or not true of me" (1) to "very often true of me or true of me" (5). A list of the inventory's items is found in the instrument's technical manual (Bar-On, 1997b). The EQ-i is suitable for individuals 17 years of age and older and takes approximately 40 minutes to complete.

The individual's responses render a total EQ score and scores on the following 5 composite scales that comprise 15 subscale scores: Intrapersonal (comprising Self-Regard, Emotional Self-Awareness, Assertiveness, Independence, and Self-Actualization); Interpersonal (comprising Empathy, Social Responsibility, and Interpersonal Relationship); Stress Management (comprising Stress Tolerance and Impulse Control); Adaptability (comprising Reality-Testing, Flexibility, and Problem-Solving); and General Mood (comprising Optimism and Happiness). A brief description of these emotional-social intelligence competencies, skills and facilitators measured by the 15 subscales is found in the Appendix as was previously mentioned.

Scores are computer-generated. Raw scores are automatically tabulated and converted into standard scores based on a mean of 100 and standard deviation of 15. This resembles IQ (Intelligence Quotient) scores, which was Bar-On ,intention when he coined the term "EQ" ("Emotional Quotient") during his doctoral studies (1988). Average to above average EQ scores on the EQ-i suggest that the respondent is effective in emotional and social functioning. The higher the scores, the more positive the prediction for effective functioning in meeting daily demands and challenges. On the other hand, low EQ scores suggest an inability to be effective and the possible existence of emotional, social and/or behavioral problems.

The EQ-i has a built-in correction factor that automatically adjusts the scale scores based on scores obtained from two of the instrument's validity indices (Positive Impression and Negative Impression). This is an important feature for self-report measures in that it reduces the potentially distorting effects of response bias thereby increasing the accuracy of the results.

2.3 Mayer–Salovey–Caruso model of emotional intelligence

Credited for inventing the term emotional intelligence, Salovey and Mayer (1990: 189) describe it as 'a type of social intelligence that involves the ability to monitor one's own and others' emotions, to discriminate among them, and to use the information to guide one's thinking and actions'. Taylor and Bagby (2000: 45) referred to this definition as 'encompass[ing] emotional self awareness and empathy', stating it did not take into account 'thinking about feelings', although they recognized that 'the definition clearly refers to the ability to use emotional information to guide cognition and behaviour'. Emotional quotient (EQ), the term used in relation to the assessment of emotional intelligence, was originated by Bar-On (1985). Taylor and Bagby (2000: 45) summarized a more detailed definition by Mayer and Salovey (1997), which consisted of four constructs: 'the perception, appraisal and expression of emotion; emotion facilitation of thinking; understanding and analysing emotions, and employing emotional knowledge; and reflective regulation of emotions to promote emotional and intellectual growth'. This definition has also been described as having 'four branches: (a) perceiving emotions, (b) using emotions to facilitate thought, (c) understanding emotions, and (d) managing emotions' (Salovey and Pizarro, 2003: 263) and forms the framework for the Mayer–Salovey–Caruso Emotional Intelligence Test (MSCEIT) which has been used as a tool in this study. The Ability model of EI was first constructed by Salovey and Mayer (1990) and begins with the idea that emotions contain information about relationships and whether these relationships are actual, remembered, or imagined, they coexist with emotions - the felt signals of the relationship's status (Mayer, Salovey, Caruso, & Sitarenios, 2001). Salovey & Mayer's four branch Ability model of EI facilitates an ability to recognise the meanings of emotions and their relationships, and employ them to enhance cognitive activities (Mayer et al., 2001). The Ability model divides EI into four branches: (1) perceiving emotions, (2) using emotions to facilitate thought, (3) understanding emotions, and (4) managing emotions in a manner that enhances personal growth and social relations (Dulewicz & Higgs, 2000; Mayer et al., 2001; Salovey & Mayer, 1990). The model has undergone continual improvement since its construction and the most recent version is offered by Caruso, Mayer, and Salovey (Caruso et al., 2002), represented in Table 1.

Ability skills

The *Perceiving* branch addresses the perceptual skills of self-identification of emotions in thoughts, identifying emotions in other people, accurate expression of emotions, and the ability to differentiate and discriminate between accurate/real and inaccurate/phoney emotions (Caruso et al., 2002). The second branch, *Using Emotions*, advocates their use in prioritising thinking by directing attention to important events/factors, to generate emotions that assist judgement and facilitate decision making, to utilise self-mood swings to change perspective, and to use different emotional states to promote different means to problem solving (Caruso et al., 2002). The third branch, *Understanding Emotions*, is based on the ability to understand complex emotions and emotional 'chains', the transition of emotions through stages, the ability to understand relationships among emotions, and interpret the meanings emotions convey (Caruso et al., 2002). The fourth branch, *Managing Emotions*, encompasses the ability to reflectively monitor emotions and stay open to them, and the ability to engage or detach from emotions. The branch also advocates the ability to determine whether an emotion is clear or typical, and the ability to solve emotion-based problems without necessarily suppressing the negative emotions (Caruso et al., 2002).

Ability	Skills
Perceiving	Identify emotions in thoughts Identify emotions in other people Express emotions accurately Discriminate between accurate and inaccurate feelings
Using	Prioritise thinking by directing attention Generate emotions to assist judgement Mood swings change perspective Emotional states encourage problem solving
Understanding	Label and recognise relations among emotions Interpret meanings emotions convey Understanding complex feelings Recognise emotional transitions
Managing	Stay open to feelings Engage/detach from an emotion Reflectively monitor emotions

Table 1. The Ability Model of Emotional Intelligence (Caruso et al., 2002, p. 57)

Definitions of emotional intelligence tend to encompass long lists of personal attributes and it is perhaps inevitable that to fully understand emotional intelligence, there needs to be an understanding of emotion. Russell and Barchard (2002) commented that we are all able to recognize emotions when we see them but the distinction between emotions and non-emotions are less clear. In essence, emotions are either about something or directed at something with behaviour change depending on the emotion.

Goleman (1995) helped popularize emotional intelligence through his book of the same name. He emphasized its importance and cited Thorndike (1920), Sternberg (1985) and Salovey and Mayer (1990) as psychologists who have recognized that it has a part to play in life, indicating that if you are able to manage your emotions, you are more likely to be successful. Many have developed measurement tools to test for emotional intelligence, such as Bar-On's (2000) emotional quotient inventory (EQ-I) as previously noted, the 360-degree evaluation method (Jacobs, 2001), the EQ map (Cooper and Sawaf, 1997), the emotional competence inventory (ECI) (Boyatzis, Goleman and Hay/McBer, 1999) and the MSCEIT (Mayer, 2001) as previously referred.

2.3.1 Emotional intelligence and the leadership process

Leadership is a process of social interaction where the leader's ability to influence the behaviour of their followers can strongly influence performance outcomes (Humphrey, 2002; Pirola-Merlo et al., 2002). Leadership is intrinsically an emotional process, whereby leaders recognise followers' emotional states, attempt to evoke emotions in followers, and then seek to manage followers' emotional states accordingly (Humphrey, 2002). Pescosolido (2002) argues that leaders increase group solidarity and morale by creating shared emotional experiences. The ability of leaders to influence the emotional climate can strongly influence performance (Humphrey, 2002). EI is a key factor in an individual's ability to be socially effective (George, 2000; Mayer et al., 2000b) and is viewed in leadership literature as a key determinant of effective leadership (Ashkanasy and Tse, 2000; Boal and Hooijberg, 2000; George, 2000). George (2000) argues that emotionally intelligent leaders can promote effectiveness at all levels in organisations. The EI of the leader plays an important role in the quality and effectiveness of social interactions with other individuals (House and Aditya, 1996). Mayer et al. (2000a) hypothesized that employees who have high levels of EI may have smoother interactions with members of their work teams. Salovey et al. (1999), found that individuals who rated highly in the ability to perceive accurately, understand, and appraise others' emotions were better able to respond flexibly to changes in their social environments and build supportive networks. Mayer et al. (2000b) proposed that a high level of EI might enable a leader to be better able to monitor how work group members are feeling, and take the appropriate action.

2.3.2 Why do leaders need emotional intelligence?

The Ability model of EI provides a suitable medium for examining why leaders need emotional intelligence through asking why leaders need to be able to (1) identify, (2) use, (3) understand, and (4) manage emotions. Caruso, Mayer, and Salovey (2002) report that studies have found that the ability for a leader to identify emotions and feelings within themselves also allows them to accurately identify the emotions of peers and groups, to express emotions accurately, and to differentiate between honest and phoney emotional expressions. Empathy, the ability to understand and experience another person's feelings or emotions, is an important component of EI and facilitates a leader's social support and positive inter-personal relationships (George, 2000).

In their study comparing emotional and cognitive competencies as a basis of subordinate perceived effective leadership, Kellet, Humphrey and Sleeth (2002) report that empathy (a substantial EI component) bore the strongest correlation with perceived effective leadership. This suggests that perceiving others' feeling and empathizing with them may establish an affective bond that is beneficial for leadership. Leaders use of emotions can enhance cognitive processes and decision making (George, 2000), and allows leaders to understand and motivate others by making emotions available, engaging in multiple perspectives that facilitate more flexible planning, and more creative, open-minded, and broader thinking and perspectives (Caruso et al., 2002; George, 2000). George (2000) reports research findings that when people are in positive moods they tend to be more optimistic and have more positive perceptions and perspectives, compared with negative moods, that result in the converse of pessimism and negativism.

Understanding EI provides functional insights into human behaviour and perceptions. This understanding includes the ability to recognise relationships between emotions, determine emotions' underlying meaning, comprehend complex feelings and recognise and accept emotional fluctuation (Caruso et al., 2002). Identification, use and understanding of emotions facilitates effective management of emotions. In a longitudinal study of 382 team members comprising 48 self-managing teams, Wolff, Pescosolido, and Druskat (2002), found that empathy is the foundation for the cognitions and behaviours that support the emergence of leadership. Overall, they conclude their results suggest that emotional intelligence, particularly empathic competency, is a dominant factor of the leadership emergence in self managed teams. Managing emotions allows leaders to dissipate and alleviate the effects of negative events and provide redirection and focus towards more positive events and moods (Caruso et al., 2002; George, 2000), termed by Mayer and Salovey (1997, cited in George, 2000) as meta- regulation of mood. Lewis (2000) reports that her laboratory study found that the emotional tone of a CEO level leader has a significant effect on follower affect and perception of leader effectiveness. Indeed EI leadership prescribes not just the ability to manage self-feelings and moods, but ability to manage moods and emotions of others (George, 2000). In a field study on the emotional dynamics of 20 self-managed groups, Pescosolido (2002) reports that emergent leaders within groups adopt the role of managing the group's emotional state. They use their emotionally intelligent behaviour, (empathy, emotional perception of self and others, emotional management of self and others, emotional expression, emotional communication, inspirational leadership, role modelling) to communicate messages to group members regarding group performance and contextual events. Resultantly, group members read their leader's behaviour and crafted emotional interpretations of the situation, which then guided their own behaviour. This empirical evidence has demonstrated the strong relationships between emotional intelligence and performance, the existence of a relationship between emotional intelligence and leadership style, and the need to combine emotional intelligence abilities and competencies with leadership skill. Goleman et al. (2002) provide this linkage with the EI based model of leadership.

3. Quality in higher education

Quality of higher education and the need for effective quality assurance mechanisms beyond those of institutions themselves are becoming priority themes in national strategies for higher education. This is driven by the importance attached to higher education as a driver of growth and in achieving the MDGs, on one hand, and the emergence of new types of higher education providers (beyond public institutions), on the other. At the institutional level, increasing demand for accountability by governments, other funders and the public, coupled with the desire to be comparable with the best in-country and internationally is pushing HEIs to pay more attention to their QA systems. Structured QA processes in higher education at the national level are a very recent phenomenon in most African countries but the situation is changing rapidly. Existing QA agencies are young, the majority having been established within the last 10 years. Currently 16 countries have functioning national QA agencies. The emergence of private tertiary institutions and the need to regulate their activities appears to have been the main trigger for the establishment of formal QA agencies in most countries. Perhaps because of this historical fact, the main purpose of QA agencies in Africa has been regulation of the development of the sector rather than to enhance accountability and quality improvement. Several countries have now changed their laws to make accreditation of public institutions mandatory.

This positive step needs to be buttressed by an effective incentive system (currently absent) in order to encourage compliance and hence, quality improvement. Also needed is a stronger link between the results of QA processes and funding allocations, as well as learning outcomes (quality of graduates), in order to promote accountability. There is convergence in methodology across countries. At the national level, three different types of quality assurance practices can be observed: institutional audits, institutional accreditation, and program accreditation. But irrespective of the approach taken, a convergence among these methodologies is becoming apparent. Evidence from country case studies shows that all QA agencies follow the same basic approach — which is similar to that followed by QA agencies in developed countries. This approach entails an institutional (or program) self-assessment, followed by a peer review and transmission of findings to the institution, the government and even to stakeholders. This tends to be the norm regardless of whether it is an audit or accreditation. When conducted properly, this is a rigorous process which produces useful data that can be used for strategic planning and other purposes. However, experience from the case study countries shows that the methodology demands a high level of human and financial capacity. In a situation where the pool of qualified human resources is already strained, not all countries can afford to set up a full scale national agency. In fact, it is not justifiable for countries with small tertiary education systems.

The process is as important as the outcome. Experience from institutions within case study countries shows that the self-assessment process (at institutional or unit level) has positive effects on the culture of quality within an institution or unit. Because it is conducted within a collegial atmosphere without any pressure from an external body, the self-assessment fosters social cohesion and teamwork among staff and also enhances staff accountability of the results of the process. More concretely, self-assessment also helps institutions to identify their own strengths and weaknesses, while generating awareness of key performance indicators. The process of self-assessment is widely seen as the most valuable aspect of quality assurance reviews because it helps institutions to build capacity from within. This capacity-building function of self-assessment is valuable in any context, but it is particularly important in the countries of Sub-Saharan Africa where capacity remains very weak. Self-assessment is also less costly than accreditation and can be conveniently planned within an institution's annual calendar.   Thus, irrespective of whether a country has a full-scale national QA agency or not, regular self-assessments at the institutional and unit levels are the backbone of a viable quality assurance system.

This therefore calls for very effective quality assurance managers to be able to harness the human resource capacity of their directorates. This effectiveness will call for innovative approaches such as the application of emotional intelligence in the management of the directorate units in the various universities. The standards being applied by national QA agencies are mainly input-based with little attention being paid to process, outputs and outcomes. However, in almost all countries, no link between quality assurance results and funding allocations can be found. The most common QA standards in the case studies are mission and vision, academic programs, library resources, physical and technological resources, number and qualifications of staff, number of students and their entry qualifications, and financial resources (relative to number of students). The study found no evidence of output standards such as through-put ratio (percent of a cohort that graduates within a specified time) or volume and quality of research. There was also no evidence of any link between quality assurance results and funding allocations to institutions or units.

3.1 Why quality higher education is so important in Africa

Increasing importance of tertiary education to competitiveness and economic development cannot be overstated. Changes brought about by the transition to a knowledge economy have created a demand for higher skill levels in most occupations. A new range of competences such as adaptability, team work, communication skills and the motivation for continual learning have become critical. Thus, countries wishing to move towards the knowledge economy are challenged to undertake reforms to raise the quality of education and training through changes in content and pedagogy. Recent studies have demonstrated that for developing countries, higher education can play a key "catch-up" role in accelerating the rate of growth towards a county's productivity potential (Bloom, Canning, and Chan 2006). The international community is also paying increased attention to this new thinking. The World Bank's Africa Action Plan (2005) underscores the critical importance of post-primary education in building skills for growth and competitiveness in low- and medium-income countries. The Plan includes among its core actions during 2007–09, the monitoring and assessment of the quality of post-primary education and training, and the development and implementation of operational plans for IDA support to technical, tertiary and research institutions in at least eight African countries by FY08 (World Bank 2005).

Higher Education is critical to achieving the EFA and Millennium Development Goals (MDGs). Higher Education institutions educate people in a wide range of disciplines which are key to effective implementation of MDGs. These include the core areas of health, agriculture, science and technology, engineering, social sciences and research. In addition, through research and advisory services, they contribute to shaping national and international policies. Supporting other levels of education and buttressing other skill levels. Higher education plays a key role in supporting other levels of education (Hanushek and Wossmann 2007). This ranges from the production of teachers for secondary schools and other tertiary education institutions, to the training of managers of education and conducting research aimed at improving the performance of the sector. According to a recent study, low quality or

lack of a critical mass of graduates at the secondary school level reduces the productivity of tertiary-educated workers and dampens the overall incentives for education investments (Ramcharan 2004). The study also shows that the presence of tertiary-educated workers in the workplace raises the productivity of medium-skills workers. Increasing the value of investments to expand access. The challenge for Africa in creating knowledge economies is to improve the quality of tertiary education and at the same time increase the number of people trained at high quality levels in appropriate fields. The record to date in this area is not particularly good. Examples abound of rapid growth in the number of students in higher education while at the same time higher education quality drops substantially.

3.2 Quality assurance within higher education institutions

Within institutions of higher learning, use of external examiners, self-evaluation and academic audits are the most common forms of quality assurance processes. Institutions readily accept self-assessment because it empowers them and their staff to take charge of the quality of their performance without the pressure usually associated with an external review. Self-assessment also helps institutions to identify their own strengths and weaknesses, while generating awareness of key performance indicators. As noted above, it is the process of self-assessment that is widely seen as the most valuable aspect of quality assurance processes. The capacity-building function of self-assessment is particularly important in the countries of Sub-Saharan Africa where capacity remains very weak. In a few institutions (for example, the University of Dar es Salaam in Tanzania), these processes existed even before the stablishment of national QA agencies. At present, self-evaluation is increasingly being done as preparation for accreditation (for example, in Nigeria, South Africa and Tanzania). However, expertise in conducting self evaluation/academic audits is limited within Africa. Strengthening professional capacity (through initiatives involving capacity development in EI) in these areas is a major recommendation of this study.

The shortage of qualified personnel is one of the major constraints to developing widespread and effective quality assurance practices in the region. Some outputs of higher education are more easily measured than others. The challenge addressed in this study is to consider how to embed a quality culture within a university that is manifested by a university-wide commitment to a shared vision and a desire for continuous improvement (Ayiro,2011) and then identify indicators that show this has been achieved. Gauging this is far more problematic than, for example, assessing whether explicitly stated learning outcomes have been achieved or whether the occupancy rates of university buildings are increasing. In order to lay strategies that could lead to the successful embedding of a quality culture, issues related to quality assurance and quality enhancement will be examined and effective leadership provided beyond shear management. It will be argued that there should be a concentration on one of the core activities of universities, i.e. teaching and learning, in order to have greater success in achieving quality improvements and embedding a quality culture. The directors of quality assurance must therefore embrace innovative approaches of management in pursuit of quality in the universities. As Mayer et al. (2000b) proposes a high level of EI might enable a leader to be better able to monitor how work group members are feeling, and take the appropriate action. It is the argument of this paper that embracing emotional intelligence constructs will enhance leadership in this area of quality assurance.

4. Methodology

Participants

The study involved administering the Mayer Salovey Caruso emotional intelligence test (MSCEIT) EI test to 75 Quality Assurance Managers in Kenyan universities. There were 25 female and 50 male. Ratings of managerial leadership effectiveness were assessed via junior staff ratings on an attitude survey detailing questions relating to manager performance. Altogether data were collated from a total of 150 (with an average age of 42.7 years with 45 percent having earned a postgraduate degree) survey responses.

Measures

The MSCEIT measures an individual's overall level of EI and their ability levels in relation to the four branches of the model: perceiving emotions, using emotions, understanding emotions, and managing emotions.

The MSCEIT consists of 141 items that provide 15 scores: total EI score, two area scores, four branch scores and eight task scores. Research has suggested the MSCEIT has good reliability (Brackett and Mayer, 2003; Lopes et al., 2003; Mayer et al., 2004) and a supported factor structure (Day and Carroll, 2004; Mayer et al., 2000b). Altogether 75 quality assurance managers took the MSCEIT in a pencil and paper format. A total of 150 employee survey responses were accumulated for data analysis. The employee response per supervisor ranged from 1 to 2.

Procedures and Data Analysis

Part of the survey involved deploying attitude surveys to assess employee perceptions of among other things managerial performance of quality assurance officers. Validity and reliability evidence was provided by a pilot test before full-scale university wide implementation occurred. Each survey was identical and contained 12 questions under the section headings of "managerial leadership" "working conditions" and "training". High response rates were realized (over 79 per cent) and therefore reduced potential bias due to non-respondents. The attitudinal survey adopted a 5-point Likert-type scale ("1 = strongly disagree" to "5 = strongly agree"), and consisted of several questions relating to the perceived performance effectiveness of their respective Quality Assurance Managers.

5. Results

A stratification of the MSCEIT scores is necessary to allow for the hierarchical nature of the construct. For example, experiential EI comprises both the perceiving emotions and using emotions branches. Figure 1 shows the hierarchical levels of the MSCEIT factor structure.

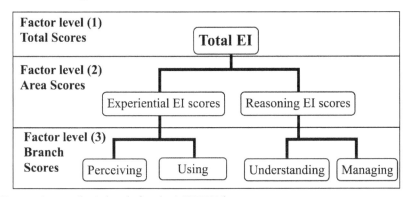

Fig. 1. Regression analysis levels for the MSCEIT factor structure.

MSCEIT scores	r	r2
Total EI	0.41 * **	0.168
Area scores		
Experiential EI	0.56 * * *	0.314
Reasoning EI	0.08 2	.0067
Branch scores		
Perceiving emotions	0.53 * *	0.281
Using emotions	0.57 * * *	0.325
Understanding emotions	0.34	0.116
Managing emotions	-0.11	-0.0121

Notes: *p, 0.05, * *p, 0.01, * * *p, 0.001

Table 2. Correlations of EI scores and Quality Assurance Manager Ratings.

The Pearson product-moment correlation coefficient is a measure of the linear relationship between two variables and is the most frequently used measure of association between variables. As expected a number of positive correlations were found between MSCEIT scores and manager ratings (e.g. perceiving emotions, r = 0.53, p, 0.01; using emotions branch, r = 0.57, p, 0.001). Of Interest was the fact that both the understanding and managing emotions branch scores, and their corresponding reasoning EI domain, did not reflect a significant relationship in so far as manager ratings by the employees was concerned.

6. Discussion

Data analysis found that the total EI score displayed a strong positive correlation with manager ratings (r = 0.41, p, 0.001). The results indicate that 16.8 per cent of the variation in supervisor ratings can be attributed to the supervisor's total emotional intelligence score. The American Psychological Association's (APA) taskforce on psychological testing asserted that psychologists studying highly complex human behaviour should be rather satisfied with correlations in the r = 0.10 to 0.20 range, and that these outcomes of correlations in the region 0.25-0.35 are indeed convincing (Meyer et al., 2001).

As far as the MSCEIT domain scores are concerned, the Experiential Emotional Intelligence (EEI) score was found to be highly correlated with manager ratings (r = 0.56, p, 0.001), whereas the Reasoning Emotional Intelligence (REI) score displayed no significant correlation (r = 0.082). These results indicate that the EEI limb of the MSCEIT accounts for almost all significance in the relationship between Total EI (TEI) and manager ratings. The r^2 value rises from 16.8 per cent for TEI at MSCEIT factor level 1, to 31.4 per cent for the EEI at MSCEIT factor level 2. This suggests that whereas the TEI score can predict 16.8 per cent of the variation in manager ratings the EEI score alone can predict 31.4 per cent of the variation. This increase, along with the lack of any significant statistical relationship found between REI scores and manager ratings (REI: r = 0. 08 2), indicates that the REI value does not possess any significant predictive power in regards to manager ratings. Indeed, these findings suggest that when the REI score is added to the EEI score (to create the overall TEI value) the REI score dilutes the overall level of correlation with the dependent variable, thus we witness a reduction in the value of r^2.

The perceiving emotions branch refers to the ability to recognize how an individual and those around the individual are feeling and this involves the capacity to perceive and to express feelings (Mayer et al., 2002, p. 19). Perceiving emotions branch scores displayed a high positive correlation with manager ratings (r = 0.53, p, 0.001). The r^2 value indicates that managers' respective perceiving emotions branch scores can account for 28.1 per cent of the variance in manager ratings. These findings indicate that the individuals they manage view managers who are adept at perceiving emotions as more effective in their managerial role. The using emotions branch of the MSCEIT involves using emotions to enhance reasoning (Mayer et al., 2001). The branch aims to measure how much a respondent's thoughts and other cognitive activities are informed by their experience of emotions. Using emotions branch scores displayed a highly significant positive correlation with manager ratings (r= 0.57, p, 0.001). Indeed, the regression coefficient for the using branch was more significant than all other branches (r^2 = 0.281; Table 1). Perceiving emotions and using emotions had the greatest overall impact on manager ratings. The understanding emotions branch assesses an individual's ability to understand emotions and to reason with emotional knowledge (Mayer and Salovey, 1997). High levels of emotional understanding enable superior comprehension of the advantages and disadvantages of future actions (Mayer et al., 2002), andmore effective self-management of emotions, particularly negative emotions (Mischel and DeSmet, 2000). Surprisingly, understanding emotions branch scores had a non-significant positive correlation with manager ratings (r = 0.34). These findings indicate that the level of managerial emotional understanding, as measured by the MSCEIT, has little bearing on employee perceptions of manager effectiveness. Matthews et al. (2002) propose that expert knowledge of appropriate emotional behaviour does not necessarily translate into the actual application of emotionally appropriate behaviour. They argue that an emotionally inept scholar of emotion is not an oxymoronic amalgam of expertise and action. This study suggests that an individual's greater understanding of how emotions may change over time and a greater emotional vocabulary does not necessarily translate into superior emotional behaviour. Swift (2002) found that an individual's increased awareness of the potentially negative impact of their behaviour had little impact on the actual behaviour they subsequently displayed. Therefore, it seems an individual may be able to identify the most socially effective behaviour to engage in but may be unwilling or unable to pursue such a course of action.

The managing emotions branch is viewed as the most advanced emotional ability within the ability-based model (Mayer et al., 2000), and therefore, has the potentially greatest impact on the management function (George, 2000). However, the actual results of the data analysis on the managing emotions branch scores are contrary to expectations. Correlation analysis identified no significant correlations between managing emotions branch scores and manager ratings (r = -0.11). The correlation, though non-significant, was also in an opposite direction than expected (negative instead of positive). The managing emotions branch and corresponding tasks were the only factorial components of the MSCEIT to display a negative relationship with manager ratings. Measuring an individual's ability to manage emotions is intrinsically more difficult than other branches of the ability model. Earlier branches of the MSCEIT are easier to assess as they have fewer parameters to consider (Mayer et al., 2004) and are accompanied by an established body of related knowledge, such as coding emotional expressions for perceiving emotions (Ekman and Davidson, 1994), how emotions impact on cognition for using emotions (Salovey and Birnbaum, 1989) and delineating emotional understanding for understanding emotions (Ortony et al., 1988). Mayer et al. (2004) believe that test items within theMSCEIT can be operationalised in such a fashion that there are more-or-less correct answers. However, Lopes et al. (2003) accede that ability tests of EI cannot encompass all the skills that contribute to people's capacity for emotional regulation. Emotional regulation includes both reactive and proactive coping requiring all sorts of skills, including analytical, creative, and practical competencies (Frijda, 1999). The managing emotions branch tasks are, in principal, closer to a self-reporting format than any other section of the MSCEIT. Whereas the other tasks focus on an individual determining what they thought was the "right" (i.e. correct) answer, the managing emotions tasks asked respondents to place themselves within a situation and identify which behaviour would be most socially effective to engage in. An individual's ability to regulate their emotions is not truly tested. The individual is to a large extent detached from the actual emotional stimulation the situation would invoke, allowing the individual to answer questions from an "emotional vacuum". Thus, the Managing Emotions branch seems vulnerable to similar criticisms applied to other self-report tests, that is, self-reported ability and actual ability are only minimally correlated in the realm of intelligence research (Davies et al., 1998; Mayer et al., 2000b). However, it must be noted that there is a lack of research supporting this proposition.

7. Implications of EI for Human Resource Development (HRD) research and practice in higher education

The implications of EI for HRD research and practice are captured under this section in addition to aspects of the effect of HRD and EI on individual and organizational productivity, EI and leadership development, and the relationship between EI and job performance. The need for organizations such as universities to invest in people through HRD programs, EI activities, and promotion of the development of social capital to remain competitive and succeed in the current knowledge-based economy characterized by uncertainty and inevitable change is critical. The research linking HRD and performance improvement is a relatively

new body of literature and has endeavoured to integrate economic theories, psychological theories, and systems thinking models (Nafukho, Hairston, & Brooks, 2004; Nafukho & Hinton, 2003; Pate, Martin, Beaumont, & McGoldrick, 2000; Swanson, 1999). The current literature specifically linking HRD, EI, social capital, and organizational productivity is limited at best (Brooks & Nafukho, 2006). Although a universally accepted definition of HRD is nonexistent, several scholars have attempted to identify its essential elements. For instance, McLagan and Suhadolink (1989) grouped organization development, training and development, and career development as the primary foci of HRD. Swanson and Holton (2001) define HRD as "a process for developing and unleashing human expertise through organization development and personnel training and development for the purpose of improving performance" (p. 4). This definition is more inclined toward individuals, organizations, and work groups or teams. An exploratory study of the definitions of HRD concluded that HRD's definitions were culturally influenced and varied internationally in scope of activities, intended audiences, and beneficiaries (McLean et al., 2003; McLean & McLean, 2001; Weinberger, 1998). Social capital theory has emerged from sociology as a potential influence on performance at the individual, process, and organizational levels. Social capital can be expressed as "the resources embedded in social networks accessed and used actors . . . and can also be envisioned as investment by individuals in interpersonal

relationships useful in the markets" (Lin, 2001, p. 25). Coleman (1990) explains that in social capital, the social relationships are relations with predictive capacity and can be used to create something of value. Unlike human capital and traditional organizational assets, social capital is unique in that it is developed by and is a result of meaningful social relationships that individuals invest in creating together over time (Storberg-Walker, 2002). In her excellent review of the evolution of social capital theory, Storberg-Walker (2002) indicates that like human capital theory and HRD, conflicting definitions and rationale for its measurement can be found in the management, sociology, and HRD literature. However, Lin (2001) suggested that although definitions may differ, most scholars agree that social capital "benefits both the collective and individuals of the collective" (pp. 11-13).

During the past 15 years, new technology has allowed breakthroughs in brain research that have increased our understanding about the mutual interaction between feelings (affect) and cognition (thought). Defining the nature and significance of this interplay between thought and emotion is at the heart of the emerging research on EI. HRD professionals continually grapple with the issues associated with organizing, motivating, enhancing, and evaluating human activity; EI research can inform HRD practices to this end within organizations. Fineman (2000) noted that "feelings shape and lubricate social transactions; hence emotional intelligence as an organizational development tool is widely accepted among managers, consultants, and practitioners as a means for solving problems and enhancing social capital" (pp. 1-24).

7.1 Utilization of EI in HRD issues

Organizations continue the search for innovative approaches to increase their competitive advantage in this knowledge-based economic era, which is defined by the utilization of people's talent. According to Appleby and Mavin (2000), "the unique positioning of each individual organization provides that difference through its culture and the human resources. It is human capability and commitment which distinguish successful organizations from the rest" (p. 555). They further suggest that people, and the way they are managed and deployed, are the single most sustainable source of competitive advantage (Appleby & Mavin, 2000). As noted, other advantages, such as technology, global reach, or IT systems, can all be copied and exceeded by competitors. The current drive for differentiation is to generate ideas and innovation through the organization's human resources (Appleby & Mavin, 2000). Appleby and Mavin lastly highlighted the fact that "ideas are now the DNA of organizations and therefore learning and development of people become crucial to economic survival" (p. 555). Statements like these reinforce the importance of HRD to the strategic initiatives of the enterprise. It is widely held that we live in a knowledge age. However, there is evidence that the ideas or innovation era has emerged. In an ideas or innovation era, individuals and organizations with the capacity to create and re-create themselves and their outputs are rewarded by developing and sustaining a competitive advantage in the marketplace, and HRD becomes the delivery system of individual and organizational development on which such organizations depend.

Furthermore, just as the human pulmonary system is affected by the type of inhalants to which it is exposed, the organizational climate is reactive to the emotions that are evident within the workplace. Organizations are illustrative of open-loop systems, those systems that depend on external sources to sustain themselves (Goleman et al., 2002). At the individual level, individuals rely on others for emotional stability while subsequently influencing the emotions of others. For example, displays of toxic emotions such as rage and unbridled coercion can contribute to negativity and impede collaboration, innovation, and good performance (Ayiro, 2010). Whereas positive emotions promote collaboration and feedback, these elements are essential too for innovation and productivity and improved performance in the workplace.

8. The relationship between EI and job performance

One of the largest areas of contention within the EI research community appears to relate to the impact of job performance. Some researchers have argued that the currently available data on EI as it relates to job performance may demonstrate a disconnect because it represents in fact emotional competencies that affect job performance. In this vein, Abraham (2004) wrote:

As emotional intelligence is the composite of 27 competencies, and as the competencies themselves never have been tested separately to determine their ability to predict superior performance, it is possible that the weak relationship between emotional intelligence and performance may result from the suppression of effects of some competencies with little or no impact on performance by others. (p. 121)

Arguments such as this focus on EI's overall representation of composite emotional competencies without addressing those specific competencies that may actually be the catalyst for success. However, there is an overwhelming amount of research that supports EI's ability to predict performance. Specific measurement tools such as the MSCEIT V.02 have been designed to incorporate emotional competency (abilitybased measurement) into reports of ability branches as well as the general EI measurement score. Researchers have found that an employee's ability to perceive his and other's emotions, to understand the implications of such emotions, and to regulate and manage emotion as described by EI has a direct impact on job performance. Furthermore, current research provides evidence that EI exists independently from other forms of intelligence (Carmeli, 2006; Lam & Kirby, 2002; Rosete & Ciarrochi, 2005). A study of 126 undergraduates who were placed in stressful situations were asked to accomplish mathematical problem solving and oratory presentations. It was found that the EI levels of these students positively predicted the performance of the assigned task ithin the stressful environment (Lyons & Scheneider, 2005). Research studies have even attempted to explore relationships between EI, an employee's sense of spirituality, and workplace performance (Tischler, Biberman, & McKeage, 2002). There is great interest in thinking out of the box to discover previously untapped areas for increased organizational performance. Research thus indicates that direct links between emotion and organizational performance have been established. In a study examining the relationship between a leader's mood and its impact on organizational productivity and performance, researchers determined that the employees working under a manager with a positive mood were likely to experience positive moods. These employees also demonstrated a more positive affective tone. It was ultimately discovered that leaders with positive moods supported a more cohesive work environment and expended a great deal less energy than did leaders with a negative mood, for similar results in productivity (Sy, Côté, S., Miners, & Saavedra, 2005). Further studies have even determined that EI predicts positive increased task performance in specific areas as cognitive levels of intelligence decrease (Côté & Miners, 2006).

In a study of the predictability of EI to sales outcomes, Rozell, Pettijohn, and Parker (2006) determined that positive or negative sales productivity was significantly related to EI. The effects of psychologically based intervention programs have been the subject of research for many years. The overwhelming consensus is that psychosocially based workplace training programs can significantly increase organizational effectiveness (Guzzo, Jette, & Katzell, 1985). It should come as no surprise then that with the increase in interest in the effects and predictive abilities of EI to increase organizational performance, many studies have focused their attention on the effect of EI on leader or follower performance outcomes (Wong & Law, 2002). The fact that EI demonstrates the ability to identify and manage both one's own emotions and the emotions of others allows for the use of such concepts as goal identification as a vital component of EI methodology in an effort to improve workplace performance levels (Brett & VandeWalle, 1999). This further strengthens the need for Quality Assurance Managers in the university to undergo capacity development in the area of EI.

9. Assumptions and limitations

This study sought to determine the degree of association between Quality Assurance Managers EI and the performance of the Quality Assurance Managers as rated by their immediate subordinates. It is assumed that the university councils whose mandate is to recruit university staff has ensured that any Quality Assurance Manager working in the university has satisfied the required academic and professional certifications and requirements to be placed in his or her current position as the Quality Assurance Managers. It was further assumed that the academic and training programs from which these Quality Assurance Managers received their administrative training were of even and global standards. There are multiple factors that may affect a quality directorate to do well (Ayiro, 2010). A Quality Assurance Manager's cognitive abilities would have an impact on university success with regard to quality imperatives. Specific aspects of a Quality Assurance Manager such as previous educational and training experiences will influence university success levels. Other factors may include variations in the macroeconomic context in the country/ university at any given time. This study did not address the Quality Assurance Managers' staff on issues such as experience, education, or interest, and/or motivation to be creative in helping the directorate achieve desirable quality attainments for the university.

Depending on the university's operational systems, Quality Assurance Managers do have varying degrees of interactions with students, management, and staff, which could have had an impact on the success of the quality function in the university. Issues of support for the Quality Assurance Managers were also not explored within this study. The final limitation of the study is the restricted scope of variables measured. There are several competencies not related to EI that are extremely important to leadership success that were not measured. Variables such as motivation, technical skills, experience, and extent of one's network can all lead to increased levels of success in leadership in various situations and these competencies were not accounted for in this study. The small size of the sample studied also limits the generalization of the findings of the study.

10. Conclusion

The aim of this investigation was to determine the relationship between managerial EI of personnel in the quality assurance directorates (as measured by the MSCEIT) and a rating of their effectiveness (by their subordinates). The overall results of the data analysis indicate that an individual's EI may indeed be a key determinant of effective leadership. Employee perceptions of manager effectiveness are strongly related to the EI of the manager. The results suggest that half of the MSCEIT scores may act as significantly large predictors of manager ratings (Mayer and Salovey, 1997; Mayer et al., 2000; Meyer et al., 2001). This being the case then the results supports the inclusion and consideration of a manager's level of EI within the recruitment and selection and the training and development process for managerial personnel for the quality assurance departments in the universities.

Even in the absence of external accreditation, institutional academic reviews (academic audits) are an effective way to introduce a culture of quality into an institution. A necessary pre-requisite is training of staff in self-evaluation and peer-reviewing. The need for investment in EI development in the quality assurance managers in the universities is therefore necessary. Involvement of peer reviewers from other institutions within or outside the country in self-assessment exercises can enrich the process, but selection must be done carefully to justify the high costs involved. Experience from the case studies shows that establishment of a dedicated quality assurance unit within an institution helps to ensure monitoring and evaluation of QA processes, maintains institutional memory and ensures implementation of recommended quality improvement measures.

11. References

Abraham, R. (2004). Emotional competence as antecedent to performance: A contingency framework. *Genetic, Social and General Psychology Monographs, 130*, 117-143.

Appleby, A., & Mavin, S. (2000).Innovation not imitation: Human resource strategy and the impact on world-class status. *Total Quality Management, 11*, 554-561.

Ashkanasy, N.M. & Tse, B. (2000). Transformational leadership as management of emotion: a conceptual review, in Ashkanasy, N., Hartel, C.E.J. and Zerbe, W.J. (Eds), Emotions in the Workplace: Research, Theory, and Practice, Quorum Books, Westport, CT, pp. 221-35.

Ayiro, P., L. & Sang, J., K. (2011).The award of the PhD degree in Kenyan universities: a quality assurance perspective. *Quality in Higher Education,* 17(2), 163–178

Ayiro, P., L. (2009). An Analysis of Emotional Intelligence and the Performance of Principals in Selected Schools in Kenya. *Advances in Developing Human Resources,* 11(6) 719–746.

Bar -On, R. (2004). The Bar-On Emotional Quotient Inventory (EQ-i): Rationale, description, and summary of psychometric properties. In Glenn Geher (Ed.), *Measuring emotional intelligence: Common ground and controversy.* Hauppauge, NY: Nova Science Publishers, pp. 111-142.

Bar-On, R. (2000). Emotional and social intelligence: insights from the Emotional Quotient Inventory, in Bar-On, R. and Parker, J. (Eds), *Handbook of Emotional Intelligence,* Jossey-Bass, San Francisco, CA, p. 385.

Bar-On, R. (1997a). *The Emotional Quotient Inventory (EQ-i): A test of emotional intelligence.* Toronto, Canada: Multi-Health Systems, Inc.

Bar-On, R. (1997b). *The Emotional Quotient Inventory (EQ-i): Technical manual.* Toronto, Canada: Multi-Health Systems, Inc.

Bar-On, R. (1997). *Bar-On Emotional Quotient Inventory: Technical Manual,* Multi Health Systems, Toronto.

Boal, K.B. & Hooijberg, R. (2000). Strategic leadership research: moving on. *The Leadership Quarterly Yearly Review of Leadership,* 11 (4), 515-50.

Boyatzis, R. E. and Sala, F. (2004) The emotional competence inventory (ECI), in: G. Geher (ed.) *Measuring Emotional Intelligence* (Hauppauge, NY: Nova Science), pp. 147–180.

Boyatzis, R. E., Goleman, D., & Rhee, K. (2000). Clustering Competence in Emotional Intelligence: Insights from the Emotional Competency Inventory. In J. D. A. Parker (Ed.), *Handbook of Emotional Intelligence* (pp. 343-362). San Francisco: Jossey- Bass.

Brackett, M.A. & Mayer, J.D. (2003). Convergent, discriminant, and incremental validity of competing measures of emotional intelligence, *Personality and Social Psychology Bulletin*, 29, 1147-58.

Brett, J., & VandeWalle, D. (1999). Goal orientation and goal content as predictors of performance in a training program. *Journal of Applied Psychology, 84*, 863-873.

Brooks, K., & Nafukho, F. M. (2006). Human resource development, social capital, and emotional intelligence: Any link to productivity? *Journal of European Industrial Training, 30*, 117-128.

Brown, F. W., Bryant, S. E. and Reilly, M. D. (2006) Does emotional intelligence – as measured by the EQI – influence transformational leadership and/or desirable outcomes? *Leadership and Organization Development Journal*, 27(5), 330–351.

Carmeli, A. J. Z. E. (2006). The relationship among emotional intelligence, task performance, and organizational citizenship behaviors. *Human Performance, 19*, 403-419.

Caruso, D.R., Mayer, J.D. & Salovey, P. (2002). Relation of a measure of emotional intelligence to personality, *Journal of Personality Assessment*, 79, 306-20.

Caruso, D.R. & Wolfe, C.J. (2001). *Emotional intelligence in the workplace.* In: Ciarrochi J, Forgas JP and Mayer JD (eds) Emotional Intelligence in Everyday Life: A Scientific Inquiry. Philadelphia, PA: Psychology Press.

Cherniss, C. (2000). Emotional intelligence: what is it and why it matters, paper presented at the Annual Meeting of the Society for Industrial and Organizational Psychology, New Orleans, LA.

Coleman, J. (1990). *Foundations of social theory.* Boston, MA: Harvard University Press.

Construct. *Journal of Personality and Social Psychology*,75, 989-1015.

Cooper, R.K. and Sawaf, A. (1997). *Executive EQ: Emotional Intelligence in Leadership and Organisations*, Grosset/Putman, New York, NY.

Côté, S., & Miners, C. (2006). Emotional intelligence, cognitive intelligence, and job performance. *Administrative Science Quarterly, 51*, 1-28.

Davies, M., Stankov, L. & Roberts, R.D. (1998). Emotional intelligence: in search of an elusive

Day, A.L. and Carroll, S. (2004). Using an ability-based measure of emotional intelligence to predict individual performance, group performance, and group citizenship behaviours, *Personality and Individual Differences*, 36, 1443-58.

Dulewicz, V& Higgs, M.J. (1999). Can emotional intelligence be measured and developed? *Leadership & Organization Development Journal*, 20 (5), 242-52.

Ekman, P. & Davidson, R.J. (1994). *The Nature of Emotion: Fundamental Questions*, Oxford University Press, New York, NY.

Fineman, S. (2000). Emotional arenas revisited. In S. Fineman (Ed.), *Emotion in organizations* (2nd ed., pp. 1-24). London, UK: Sage.

Frijda, N.H. (1999). "Emotions and hedonic experience", in Kahneman, D., Diener, E. and Schwarz, N. (Eds), Well-being: The Foundations of Hedonic Psychology, Russell Sage, New York, NY, pp. 190-210.

George, J.M. (2000). Emotions and leadership: the role of emotional intelligence, *Human Relations*, 53, 1027-55.

Goleman, D., Boyatzis, R. and Hay, G. (1999) *Emotional Competence Inventory.* Available online at: http://web.ebscohost.com/ehost/detail?vid=5&hid=109&sid=a33c2f92-954f-4118-b5a1-53ea1fe 9600d%40sessionmgr111&bdata=JnNpdGU9ZWhvc3Qtb GI2ZQ%3d%3d#db=loh&AN=1712 2851 (accessed 19 December 2009).

Goleman, D. (1998). *Working with Emotional Intelligence*, Bantam Books, New York, NY.

Goleman, D. (1996). *Emotional Intelligence*. London: Bloomsbury.

Goleman, D., Boyatzis, R., & McKee, A. (2002). *Primal leadership*. Boston, MA: Harvard Business School Press.

Guzzo, R., Jette, R., & Katzell, R. (1985). The effects of psychologically based intervention programs on worker productivity: A meta-analysis. *Personnel Psychology, 38*, 275-291.

Hanushek, E.A., and L. Wossmann. 2007. "The Role of Education Quality in Economic Growth." World Bank Policy Research Working Paper No. 4122, The World Bank, Washington, D.C.

Higgs M & Dulewicz V (1999). *Making Sense of Emotional Intelligence.* Windsor: NFERNELSON

Higgs, M.J. & Dulewicz, S.V.D. (1999). *Making Sense of Emotional Intelligence,* NFERNelson, Windsor.

House, R.J. & Aditya, R.N. (1996). The social scientific study of leadership: quo vadis. *Journal of Management, 23* (3), 409-43.

Humphrey, R.H. (2002). The many faces of emotional leadership. *The Leadership Quarterly, 13* (5), 493-504.

Jacobs, R.L. (2001). *Using human resource functions to enhance emotional intelligence.* In: Cherniss C and Goleman D (eds) The Emotionally Intelligent Workplace: How to Select for Measure, and Improve Emotional Intelligence in Individuals, Groups and Organisations. San Francisco, CA: Jossey-Bass.

Kellett, J. B., Humphrey, R. H., & Sleeth, R. G. (2002). Empathy and Complex Task Performance: Two Routes to Leadership. *The Leadership Quarterly, 13*, 523-544.

Lam, L., & Kirby, S. (2002). Is emotional intelligence an advantage? An exploration of the impact of emotional and general intelligence on individual performance. *Journal of Social Psychology, 142*, 133-143.

Lin, N. (2001). *Social capital: A theory of social structure and action.* New York, NY: Cambridge University Press.

Lopes, P.N., Salovey, P. & Straus, R. (2003). Emotional intelligence, personality, and the perceived quality of social relationships. *Personality and Individual Differences*, 35, 641-58.

Lyons, J. B., & Scheneider, T. R. (2005).The influence of emotional intelligence on performance. *Personality and Individual Differences, 39*, 693-703.

Materu, P. 2006. "Talking Notes." Conference on Knowledge for Africa's Development, Johannesburg, South Africa, May.

Matthews, G., Zeidner, M & Roberts, R.D. (2002). *Emotional Intelligence: Science and Myth*, MIT Press, Cambridge, MA.

Mayer, J.D., Salovey, P. & Caruso, D.R. (2004). Emotional intelligence: theory, findings, and implications. *Psychological Inquiry*, 15 (3), 197-215.

Mayer, J. D., Caruso, D., & Salovey, P. (2002). Meyer, Salovey, and Caruso Emotional Intelligence Test User's Manual. North Tonawanda, NY. Multi-Health Systems Inc.

Mayer, J.D., Salovey, P., Caruso, D.R., & Sitarenios, G. (2001). Emotional intelligence as a standard intelligence. *Emotion, 1*, 232-242.

Mayer, J.D., Caruso, D.R. and Salovey, P. (2000a), "Emotional intelligence as Zeitgeist, as personality, and as a mental ability", in Bar-On, R. and Parker, J.D.A. (Eds), The Handbook of Emotional Intelligence: Theory, Development, Assessment, and Application at Home, School and in the Workplace, Jossey-Bass/Wiley, New York, NY.

Mayer, J.D., Caruso, D.R. & Salovey, P. (2000b), Emotional intelligence meets traditional standards for intelligence. *Intelligence*, 27 (4) 267-98.

Mayer, J.D. and Salovey, P. (1997). What is emotional intelligence?, in Salovey, P. and Sluyter, D. (Eds), Emotional Development and Emotional Intelligence: Implications for Educators, Basic Books, New York, NY, pp. 3-31.

Mayer, J.D., Salovey, P. & Caruso, D.R. (2000*). Models of emotional intelligence*, in Sternberg, R.J. (Ed.), Handbook of Intelligence, Cambridge University Press, Cambridge, pp. 396-420.

Mayer, J.D., & Salovey, P. (1997). What is emotional intelligence? In P. Salovey & D. Sluyter (Eds). Emotional development and emotional intelligence: Implications for educators (pp. 3-31). New York: Basic Books.

McLagan, P., & Suhadolink, D. (1989). *Models for HRD practice: The research report.* American Society for Training and Development. Alexandria, VA: ASTD.

McLean, G. N., & McLean, L. (2001). If we can't define HRD in one country, how can we define it in an international context? *Human Resource Development International, 4,* 313-326.

Merlevede,P.E., Bridoux, D& Vandamme, R. (2001). *7 Steps to Emotional Intelligence.* Bancyfelin: Crown House.

Mischel, W. and DeSmet, A.L. (2000), "Self-regulation in the service of conflict resolution", in Deutsh, M. and Coleman, P.T. (Eds), The Handbook of Conflict Resolution: Theory and Practice, Jossey-Bass, San Francisco, CA, pp. 256-75.

Morris, E. (1999). Are you emotionally intelligent? *The British Journal of Administrative Management*, 6, 8–10

Nafukho, F. M., Hairston, N., & Brooks, K. (2004). Human capital theory: Implications for human resource development. *Human Resource Development International, 7,* 545-551.

Nafukho, F. M., & Hinton, E. B. (2003). Determining the relationship between drivers' level of education, training, and job performance in Kenya. *Human Resource Development Quarterly, 14,* 265-283.

Ortony, A., Clore, G.L. and Collins, A.M. (1988). *The Cognitive Structure of Emotions,* Cambridge University Press, Cambridge.

Pate, J., Martin, G., Beaumont, P., & McGoldrick, J. (2000). Company-based lifelong learning: What's the pay-off for employers? *Journal of European Industrial Training, 24,* 149-157.

Payne, W. L. (1985) A study of emotion: developing emotional intelligence; self-integration; relating to fear, pain and desire (theory, structure of reality, problem-solving, contraction/expansion, turning in/coming out/letting go). Unpublished PhD thesis, the Union for Experimenting Colleges and Universities.

Pescosolido, A.T. (2002). Emergent leaders as managers of group emotion, *The Leadership Quarterly*, 13, 583-99.

Pirola-Merlo, A., Hartel, C., Mann, L. and Hirst, G. (2002). How leaders influence the impact of affective events on team climate and performance in R&D teams, *The Leadership Quarterly*, 13, 561-81.

Plake, B. S., & Impara, J. C. (Eds.). (1999). *Supplement to the thirteenth mental measurement yearbook.* Lincoln, NE: Buros Institute for Mental Measurement.

Ramcharan, R. 2004. "Higher Education or Basic Education: The Composition of Human Capital and Economic Development." *IMF Staff Papers* 51(2). Washington, D.C.: International Monetary Fund.

Rosete, D., & Ciarrochi, J. (2005). Emotional intelligence and its relationship to workplace performance. *Leadership and Organization Development Journal, 26*, 388-399.

Rozell, E., Pettijohn, C., & Parker, R. (2006). Emotional intelligence and dispositional affectivity as predictors of performance in salespeople. *Journal of Marketing Theory and Practice, 14*, 113-124.

Russell, J.A., & Barchard, J.A. (2002). *Toward a shared language for emotion and emotional intelligence.* In: Feldman Barrett L and Salovey P (ed.) The Wisdom in Feeling: Psychological Processes in Emotional Intelligence. New York: Guilford Press.
Sala, F. (2002) *Emotional Competence Inventory (ECI): Technical Manual* (Boston: Hay/Mcber Group). Goleman, D. (1995) *Emotional Intelligence* (New York: Bantam).

Salovey, P., Bedell, B., Detweiler, J.B. &Mayer, J.D. (1999). Coping intelligently: emotional intelligence and the coping process, in Snyder, C.R. (Ed.), Coping: The Psychology of What Works, Oxford University press, New York, NY, pp. 141-64.

Salovey, P. and Birnbaum, D. (1989). Influence of mood on health-relevant cognitions, *Journal of Personality and Social Psychology*, 57, 539-51.

Salovey, P. & Mayer, J. (1990). Emotional intelligence, *Imagination, Cognition, and Personality*, 9 (3), 185-211.

Salovey, P., & Pizarro, D.A. (2003). *The value of emotional intelligence.* In: Sternberg RJ, Lautrey J and Lubart TI (eds) Models of Intelligence: International Perspectives. Washington, DC: American Psychological Association.

Sternberg,R.(1997). Managerial Intelligence: Why IQ isn't enough. *Journal of management*, 23,475-94.

Storberg-Walker, J. (2002). The evolution of capital theory: a critique of theory of social capital and implications for HRD. *Human Resource Development Review, 1*, 468-499.

Swanson, R. A. (1999). The foundations of performance improvement and implications for practice. *Advances in Developing Human Resources, 1*, 1-25.

Swift, D.G. (2002). *The Relationship of Emotional Intelligence, Hostility, and Anger to Heterosexual Male Intimate Partner Violence*, New York University, New York, NY.

Sy, T., Côté, S., Miners, C., & Saavedra, R. (2005). The contagious leader: Impact of the leader's mood on the mood of group members, group affective tone, and group processes. *Journal of Applied Psychology, 90*, 295-305.

Taylor, G.J., & Bagby, R.M (2000). An overview of the Alexithymia construct. In: Bar-On R and Parker JDA (eds) The Handbook of Emotional Intelligence: Theory, Development, Assessment, and Application at Home, School, and in the Workplace. San Francisco, CA: Jossey-Bass.

Thorndike, E.L. (1920). *Intelligence and its uses.* Harper's Magazine 140: 227–235. Sternberg (1985) Salovey P and Mayer JD (1990) Emotional intelligence. Imagination, Cognition and Personality 9: 185–211.

Tischler, L., Biberman, J., & McKeage, R. (2002). Linking emotional intelligence, spirituality and workplace performance: Definitions, models and ideas for research. *Journal of Managerial Psychology, 17*, 203-218.

Wolff, S. B., Pescosolido, A. T., & Druskat, V. U. (2002). Emotional Intelligence as the Basis of Leadership Emergence in Self-Managing Teams. *The Leadership Quarterly, 13*, 505-522.

Wong, C., & Law, K. (2002). The effects of leader and follower emotional intelligence on performance and attitude: An exploratory study. *Leadership Quarterly, 13*(3), 243.

8

Positive Human Tacit Signal Approach and Competence System Intelligence in Organization

Antti Syväjärvi and Marko Kesti
*University of Lapland, Rovaniemi,
Finland*

1. Introduction

Ghoshal et al. (2000) have showed that people's knowledge and competence will be increasingly critical for organizational success. The one who can recognize both human needs and emotional intelligence, but also is able to confront and lead people will probably be more successful with organization and work demands. However, the system complexity exists and human being such many-sided entity that organizational purpose may not be easily completed by traditional approaches and leadership (e.g. Stacey, 2001; Kets de Vries, 2006). In this context, thematic new approaches and designs are needed in order to tackle and develop the emotional intelligence in workplaces. In this chapter the positive human tacit signal approach and competence system intelligence are studied in order to recognize, develop and manage emotional intelligence in the workplaces. Also the importance of positive is studied to serve human leadership.

Our framework is organizational human capital development that is accomplished by leading positive human tacit signals and competencies in intelligent workplaces. The concept of positive has here major connotations like a focus on positively deviant performance, a focus on strength rather than weakness, a focus on virtuousness, and a focus on human experience and performance (Syväjärvi et al., 2005; Cameron, 2008; March, 2010). Human tacit signals approach and analyse are needed to identify organization development needs and to raise competence system intelligence. Tacit signals are based on employees' tacit knowledge and those will give guiding information for core competences improvement (Kesti & Syväjärvi, 2010). Positive human tacit signals and competence system intelligence are connected to the organizational development process in order to gain an effective organization change based on optimal workplace solutions.

Human tacit signals are rather well linked to system intelligence that consists of interrelated competencies or capacities (e.g. Luthans & Youssef, 2007). Thus it is possible to perceive and develop the "positive", but simultaneously to recognise the hidden human behaviour that might prevent the intelligence. As stated the current viewpoint is linked to both system intelligence and management in organization. System intelligence refers here to the sensitivity between competence environment and human. It shows human capabilities and experiences (incl. knowledge) but also invoke more positive performance. Now system intelligence is in accordance with emotional intelligence as the latter involves the ability to carry out reasoning about emotions and the ability to use emotions and knowledge (Mayer et al., 2008).

In addition, several years ago the centre of debate in both management and leadership studies was on what managers actually do and what is the nature of their work. However, nowadays workplaces and people are indeed under many changes and also the work itself is changing. Many of these instabilities also put a heavy stress on people and human capital centred management (Luthans & Youssef, 2009; Syväjärvi & Stenvall, 2009) and thus to emotional intelligence in workplaces. As organizational environments indeed are highly changing and turbulent there seems to be possibilities to well lead working societies to positive development. Therefore alongside the positive human tacit signals, we are after parallel leadership that may recognize affirmative strength, experience and performance and thus will be able to confront workplace situations with emotional intelligence (Spector & Fox, 2002; Cameron, 2008).

So is it possible to perceive and improve positivity, human-based well-being and system intelligence in order to gain sensitive and well performing workplaces? This has significant relevance for public policy, complex organizations, various knowledge-intensive workplaces and finally for humans (Stacey, 2009; Syväjärvi & Stenvall, 2010; Lewis, 2011). Given the weighty implications of abovementioned question, it is almost certain that one must move beyond cross-sectional and borderless research, and move towards approaches that account for extraordinary or new processes and methods. In our understanding when emotionally engaged to work, when giving the value for human experience and when executing the caring leadership one might be more likely to feel good and competent, and to have a sense of belonging and taken care. Also the emotional intelligence research has various concepts that are all valued here as overall study of the emotional intelligence (Salovey et al., 2009; Di Fabio & Palazzeschi, 2009). However, the tacit signal approach is now studied in order to see how organization detect, utilize and lead positive human tacit signals and how competence system intelligence with certain organization and government characters is specifically related to the emotional intelligence in workplaces.

2. Organization tacit knowledge utilizing approach

The organization is a complex and intelligent system that can be illustrated by applying various metaphors and models (e.g. Stacey, 2001). It has been shown with complexities and signal information that the spatial spread detection accompanied by knowledge collection is vital (Syväjärvi et al., 1999). Currently with human tacit signal and knowledge in organization it is important to pay attention to individual interaction and connectivity. Humans have learned to interact across space, time and many boundaries as such actions and connections create possibilities of cooperation and conflict (Stacey et al., 2000; Syväjärvi & Stenvall, 2009; Lewis, 2011).

Nagamachi (2008), as an example, has presented a model for developing industrial safety in which the innate reasoning of a person is illustrated with a model that has been divided into three sections. The lowest level is Akamiso, which comprises emotional experiences and subconsciously influences the actions of a person. In the middle of is the area of conscious management, while the highest level is Shiromiso to describe conscious practical activity.

Further, actions guided by the Akamiso level can be both impulsive without conscious management and neglectful to safety. In addition, it has been studied how emotional intelligence (Mayer et al., 2008) could be modelled or conceptualized in such way that it can be tackled more easily also to workplaces. For example, Di Fabio & Palazzeschi (2009) showed how emotional intelligence is related to career decision difficulties and they found the inclusive importance of emotional intelligence and how it is vital to construct relationships and to understand emotions. Salovey et al. (2009) have divided emotional intelligence to four branches, i.e. perceiving emotions, using emotions, understanding emotions and managing emotions.

Abovementioned approaches can be applied to describe the tacit knowledge interaction and connection processes of an organization. Those highlight emotional intelligence in organizational environment and describe quite well the challenges in detecting, recognizing, learning and managing competencies. Kesti (2010) recognize three levels which are separated with barriers that act as filters preventing interaction, connectivity and knowledge from one level to another. The tacit knowledge inventory, comprised of feelings and experiences, is situated at the lower level of the triangle, describing the large amount of tacit knowledge to be perceived. In the middle of the triangle is the level of rational thinking, using and understanding on which one's emotions and experiences are conceptualized for possible further needs. The highest level is the area of primary action where the on-going is processed, reflected and managed. The amount of primary actions is limited as we are incapable of doing or handling too much at once.

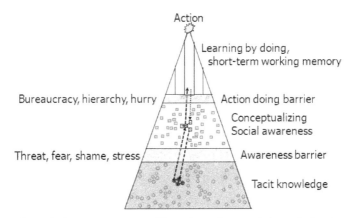

Fig. 1. The tacit knowledge interaction and learning where tacit knowledge is conceptualized into action.

The levels interact with each other over the filtering barriers. Therefore the filtering barrier between each of the levels of thinking creates a threshold for the flow of knowledge from one area to another, but might also hinder interaction and connectivity. There is an awareness barrier between tacit information and rational thinking. If the barrier is too opaque the tacit knowledge will not be able to ascend to the conceptualizing level. On the other hand, if the barrier is too transparent we will overanalyse or not identify our emotions and actions and thus, cause additional pressure to conceptualizing. The filtering barrier prevents becoming overloaded so that all emotional issues would not cause excess pressure. Finally when rational conceptualizing leads to action, the action doing barrier needs to be crossed. The action often requires sufficient motivation, creative tension and openness with pleasant and unpleasant experiences. The action doing barrier is lower in cases where the action is interesting and pleasant than in cases where the action is unpleasant and difficult.

The cognitive capability, collectiveness, behavioural self-management, shared experience and mutual appreciation are just few examples of the emotional intelligence that may either weaken barriers or create sufficient energy to facilitate the barrier crossing. Therefore inherent characters, external interventions, openness and human interaction, but also a group have great significance for complex adaptive work systems. When there is a healthy and happy work community then barriers are lower for positive outcomes and change. These can be innovative and unique, therefore creating new ideas and experiences that are recorded as tacit knowledge.

Kesti (2010) points out that the action doing barrier can be lowered by choosing a sufficiently concrete goals and actions that can be realized and indeed experienced in a workplace. Collective appreciation and agreement on an important issue will more probably motivate to take action. As an example, when a group succeeds in problem-solving then the amount of harmful stress is also reduced. This promotes the balance between negative and positive for human capital, which in turn highlight the awareness barrier. The interest of management and leaders towards the development is important because it lowers both the awareness barrier and the action doing barrier. In workplace the agreement on a schedule and follow-up procedures create an appropriate amount of positive tension.

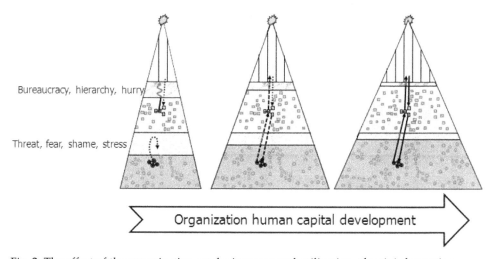

Bureaucracy, hierarchy, hurry

Threat, fear, shame, stress

Organization human capital development

Fig. 2. The effect of the organization on the increase and utilization of tacit information.

Several research studies indicate that organizations that are committed to their employees and promote the tacit knowledge base to increase are the most successful ones in a long term (Collins & Porras, 1994; de Geus, 1997; Liker, 2004). Tacit knowledge utilization model illustrate the meaning of sustainable positive organization development fostering workplace collaboration in development rather than defending and explaining the problems away. All this are in accordance with the idea of emotional intelligence and positive psychology appreciative inquiry and leadership (e.g. Cameron, 20008; Lewis, 2011; Haslam et al., 2011). Indeed appreciative inquiry principles value human tacit knowledge, contextual reality, dialogue, awareness and positivity in human collaboration (Fredrickson, 2001; Gergen & Gergen, 2004). In interactive and learning organization errors are prevented better and actions are continuously developed. These can be learnt and even achieved both systematic and efficient use of the positive tacit signal approach.

3. The positive, human tacit signals and intelligence

The background with "positive" is in both psychology and leadership studies. Leadership is grasped later on as one key theme, but indeed the positive psychology gives fundamentals for what makes life and also the working life significant. The term positive psychology has its' roots in 1950's. It was reintroduced as more attention needed to be paid to the good in human and changing workplaces (Seligman et al., 2005). Hence, the positive psychology has valuable impact on both humans and performance in organizations. Positive psychology has clear links to emotional intelligence in workplaces. Humans are after meanings in even more complex life situations. They care about the quality or nature of life and what will make, for example, a good working life for them. In workplaces, an individual as well even an organization needs to look after for holistic perspective in order to create meanings for them and for those they care (rf. Perttula, 2009).

According to Cameron (2008), the positive in organizational setting is keen about such deviant performance and successful performance that exceed standard. It has also an affirmative bias and thus strength, optimism and support overwhelm the opposite. Thirdly the tendency towards virtuousness (e.g. trust, optimism, love, care, forgiveness) is important as the good condition is possible with the positive and it might have an expectant influence to emotional intelligence in workplaces. All these are also essential in case of human tacit signals. These three connotations involve effective adoption to organizational environment. Nevertheless this does not mean that negative, disturbing or otherwise unwanted situations are neglected.

In organizational settings, however, some will rush to judgement on these important issues and offer oversimplified answers. Lewis (2011) indicates how positive psychology having elements of organizational life offers us an ethically viable choice with premises of organization and leader or manager. It is emphasized here that the experience plays a vital role for positive and human tacit signals when those are related to emotional intelligence in workplaces. The positive and human tacit signals give value to the human experience (incl. knowledge, intuition, beliefs, learning, etc.) as it shows interpretation of both life and working life. Human beings have desire to make sense of their experience and in complex workplace settings this means stability and change, but also positive and negative. Thus a certain kind of ambivalence is an important feature to explain the positive and human tacit signals in workplaces. In final, the concept of positive has a focus on positively deviant performance, a focus on strength and optimism rather than weakness and pessimism, a viewpoint towards virtuousness, and indeed a focus on human experience and performance (Syväjärvi et al., 2005; Cameron, 2008; March, 2010).

The importance of positive human tacit signal in the domain of emotional intelligence is quite profound. In short, the emotional intelligence indicates competence to identify, assess, and control the emotions of one and of others. The positive human tacit signals are connected to emotional intelligence as those refer to personal guiding abilities and experiences that can be used at improving the human competencies at working society (Stone, 2002; Kesti, 2005). Human competencies are needed for an individual to perform a work properly and thus a competency refers typically to abilities and behaviors. In working societies these employee opinions or experiences are related to competence development needs and to help solving problems which are important for the positive development, leadership and emotional intelligence. As emotional intelligence (Salovey et al., 2009) represents here the ability to perceive, appraise, and express emotions accurately and adaptively, thus aforementioned four connotations reflect the ability to understand, access, generate, control and process positive emotions in workplace. For example, the leader who wants to create an emotionally intelligent activity can start by helping the team raise its collective self-awareness (Goleman, 2007).

It seems that collective emotional intelligence is characteristic for top performing workplaces and positive energy (Wheelan, 2005). How to detect the positive and human tacit signal? By tacit signal approach it is possible to relate the human competence success factors with positive spiral and thus, for example, to minimize the risk of low human competence utilization. The mind set at tacit signals is to measure development needs so that the result will help hermeneutic improvement. Mind set is human positivism comparing to statistical Likert inquiries that find out the situation but do not help humans in improving it. Tacit signal approach is based on the dichotomy scale, consisting two interrelated guiding forces (Kesti & Syväjärvi, 2010).

When measuring the competence development needs, the positive performance is achieved when these forces are both optimally utilized and therefore in balance. This approach of two interrelated guiding forces is included at the the Yerkes-Dodson (1908) law of tension-performance relation (an inverted U-curve). The pressure – performance relation is recently studied and verified in several research studies (Abercrombie et al., 2003; Goleman, 2007; Putkonen, 2009). It is important basis of human performance and thus to emotional intelligence development. The principle of interrelated and opposing factors affecting at organization, and even multitude dichotomies, are affecting on organization's knowledge creation (e.g. Nonaka & Takeuchi, 1995; Losada & Heaphy, 2004). The competence system intelligence is further discussed in later parts.

3.1 The tacit signal inquiry connection to inverted U-curve

The Yerkes-Dodson law describes excellently this dichotomy in practice at the personal tension – performance correlation. Each human has personal best performance that correspond their 100 % performance at each measured competence area. Using this scale the focus is not to measure absolute competence against some fixed scale but rather relative and situation-based personal scale from 0 to 100 %. Each human is bodily and knowledgeable psychophysical being and tied at time and to own situation, context, identity and categorization (Haslam et al., 2011).

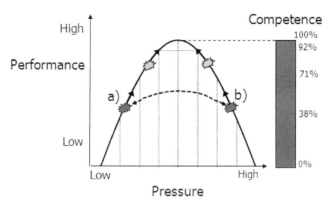

Fig. 3. Figure illustrates the principle of inverted U-curve in competence analyzing.

At figure 3 the point a) illustrates the situation where the person has not enough challenges and feels bored. Therefore self-esteem might be lower and it is linked to poorer performance. Person needs more challenges for increasing creative pressure to activate doing things, which typically increase performance. However, it is essential to proceed in balance so that the pressure does not exceed too much. If pressure gets too high the situation can turn to the opposite side of the inverted U-curve and quite often anxiety and stress might follow (point b). (Kesti 2007)

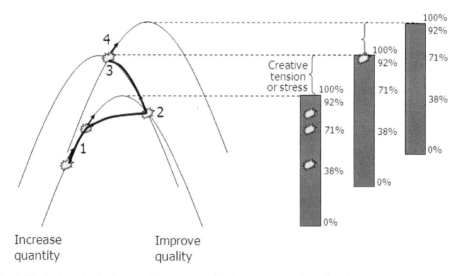

Fig. 4. Tacit signal relative performance scale phenomena when the challenges are increasing.

At figure 3 the point b) illustrates the situation where the person is under harmful stress and does not feel able to survive over situational challenges. Anxiety causes such stress that is harmful for mind and body. As a symptom the person tends to forget things and the body immunity resistance decreases. For example, one classical symptom is cynicism which might be destructive for happy working community (Wu et al., 2007). The situation can be improved by decreasing the stress by improving the quality of doing. This may mean new workload distribution in the group so that person is able to improve the quality of chosen tasks. New workload arrangement may also change the situation to the opposite side of the inverted U-curve which actually may be good way for persons' performance development.

The position at inverted U-curve is constantly changing. Also the altitude of personal curve changes depending on the competence area and situation. Because the performance is measured by asking the development need and being after positive, the analysis is relative which means that it can change in different situations. For example if organization implements new challenging strategy and targets, the situation is changed and more development needs may rise. This phenomenon was found empirically at our cases, and thus is under further studies.

The tacit signal approach can be described by using inverted U-curve. The situation at the inverted U-curve can be measured by asking the person's experience about the development need concerning the competence attribute. For example "working community meeting practices" are one competence attribute at the team culture competence. A person may feel that this competence is not positively utilized since there is need for further development and therefore the opinion or one's experience is at the right side of the inverted U-curve.

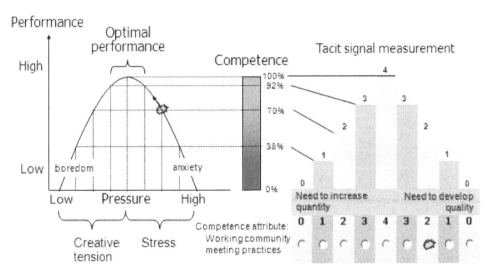

Fig. 5. The tacit signal method connection to inverted U-curve.

The guiding factors are chosen so that they follow the dichotomy principle. Hence, one guiding force is guiding to more straightforward actions (e.g. quantitative) and the other is more related to emotions (e.g. qualitative) thus guiding to dialog between the parties and individuals. The positive human tacit signal competence analysis use the sin-curve following the formula

$$C = \sin(\text{pii}/8 * x) \tag{1}$$

where x is tacit signal inquiry guiding opinion/experience. Kesti (2005)

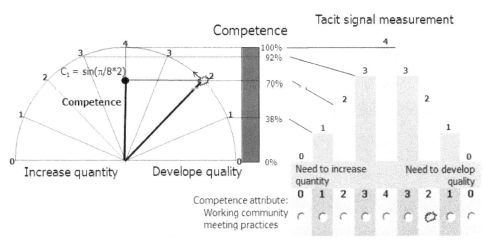

Fig. 6. The tacit signal inquiry analysing.

The tacit signal inquiry consist several competence attributes that are validated to be important for the organization and thus supporting the positive goals. Each person gives guiding opinion or experience about the possible development need on each item. There is possibility to choose only one guiding option in the dichotomy scale and thereby the inquiry triggers the tacit signal for retrieving the possible deviance in desired balance. In this context Nonaka and Takeuchi (1995) have pointed out this fundamental idea as:

"Written primarily for the academic reader, our discussion here revolves around our observation that organizational knowledge is created by transcending a multitude dichotomies presented throughout our book. "

and

"We maintain that any adequate theory of knowledge creation must contain elements of both".

These guiding factors are related to each other meaning that when the quantity is increased it affects to the quality and therefore the activating is done utilizing best practices. Correspondingly when quality is improved then it affects to the quantity. For example, the meeting practices quality development might first need more time to learn positive way and unlearn harmful habits. When new meeting practices are adapted it can decrease the time consumption. Besides the dichotomies related to positive improvement actions there is other balancing process to be considered and balanced. This other essential dichotomy is the interaction between self and other (e.g. Losada & Heaphy, 2004; Haslam et al., 2011).

3.2 Tacit signal inquiry and analysing

The current tacit signal approach is in accordance with the appreciative inquiry as it is an organizational development method that engages humans to detect, recognize, change and improve performance (Cooperrider & Srivastva, 1987). Each employee gives their tacit signal opinions or experiences (total feedback) which are combined to the working society collective knowledge of necessary development needs. People are reflecting their "self" in the group where the development is done together in constructive dialog between others. The tacit signal inquiry is needed to get the balancing feedback for starting the balancing process (see Senge, 2006) for working society and organization wide performance development. The balancing means also that both positive and negative feedbacks are valued. For example in case of leadership competence improvement, it needs the leader and each group member's collaboration for success.

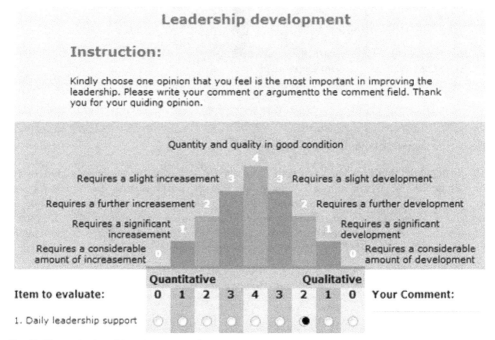

Fig. 7. The tacit signal inquiry example.

High performance organizations prevent possible problems in advance (Blanchart & Thacker, 2004; Fenwick, 2006; Mankin, 2009). This requires the organization culture where certain triggering events are enough for starting the improvement actions for preventing the performance problem. Blanchart and Thacker (2004) point out that performance problem may or may not actually exist; it is enough that one or more decision makers believe it does. Fenwick (2006) argue that the traditional assumption that observed problem, such as a task being carried out incorrectly, can be corrected simply by training is flawed. The performance problem – observed or suspected – can be due to wide range of factors and therefore it is difficult to isolate (Wexley & Latham, 2002; Gilley et al., 2002; McClernon, 2006).

Present approach has been found useful at the organization development purposes for it provides positive feedback about the human-based development needs. It seems that the tacit signal gives guiding information for improving the competencies (Kesti & Syväjärvi, 2010). However, analyse itself only guides to improvement, providing information for conceptualizing the problems to improvement actions. It should be noted how alongside measurements such collective and qualitative practices (i.e. meetings, discussions, and group forums) are performed that truly value human experiences and the importance of human interaction. The approach supports the idea of inverted U-curve, and practical cases have shown that measured competencies correlate with the organization performance.

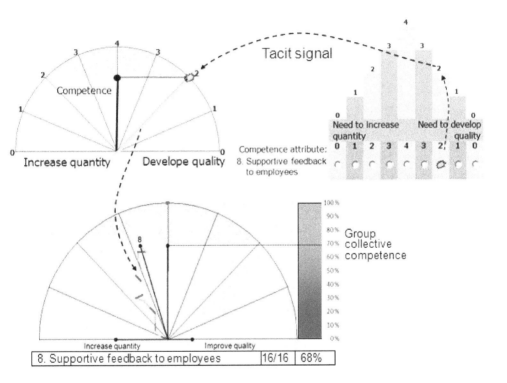

Fig. 8. Figure illustrates the tacit signal analysing principle in measuring working group collective competence. The 70% competence level is the alarm zone so that all competence attributes should be over it.

The analyse show if the group's collective development need is below the chosen alarm level (e.g. 70 %) which is the triggering level for urgent competence attribute development. The analyze result at the semicircle tells following essential information for the development purposes:

1. Competence level and development need
2. The homogeneity or heterogeneity of each opinion/experience compared to others
3. The direction of development need

Opinions or experiences are visualized by analyser. The inquiry and analysing is done by internet-based human resource information system (Kesti et al., 2008), where software is provided as a service (SaaS). In the analyzing the measured competences are shown at competence semicircular scale. Competence development semicircle radius is divided by number of individual answers. Therefore in bigger group one employee opinion has less meaning to group collective sum of opinions but always each person experiences have same importance weight. Tacit signals are gathered anonymous from each working society. The mathematical formula for balanced total competence for the entire group is illustrated in formula 1 as follows

$$C_{R1} = \sum_{i=1}^{N_x}(P_i * \sin(\frac{\pi}{8} * S_i)) = \sum_{i=1}^{N_x}(P_i * \sin(\alpha)) \tag{1}$$

where   C   = group competence

        P   = group member competence potential

        Si   = tacit signal guiding opinion from the inquiry, Si $\in$ (0 ... 8)

        п/8   = angle interval at the semicircle opinion scale

        α   = angle of the potential segment of a line (0 ≤ α ≤ п)

        Nx   = number of group member answers

Inquiry of this kind provides a reliable procedure and tool for measuring human competence, in relation to set goals and continuous interaction for optimizing the probability for attaining goals. Competence in this connection refers to the essential work capability of a person, work team or organization, in other words, human resources to attain the given goal. With the help of the tacit signal inquiry an organization can set goals that are in balance with the human competence of the team realizing those positive goals. As the tacit signals help finding the corrective actions towards desired direction, for example, the knowing –doing gap can be decreased (Pfeffer & Sutton, 2000). Performance improving comes from doing the right actions based on the data or information of the organization (Syväjärvi et al., 2005; Syväjärvi & Stenvall, 2010). As an example, if it is known that the leadership should be improved then one is able to activate the optimal improvement actions. The personnel can be brought to improve the working society competences and the management is informed of the probability for the realization of the goals and the possible needs to improve the organization competences in advance.

The inquiry is anonymous, providing mechanism where employees can inform possible non-compliances without fear of retribution. Before the tacit signal inquiry is launched the competence attributes are agreed with management and employee representatives. The tacit signals are measured concerning the organization performance drivers as positive human competencies. These competencies are management, leadership, culture, skills and processes, forming the organization system intelligence model. Thus tacit signal inquiries form a set of competences that are established as behavioral guidelines for effective organization performance. Therefore the inquiry is also important in order to give a more holistic and qualitative perspective for governance.

4. Human competence system intelligence

According to Schein (1985) the one of the most important tasks of the management is to support the culture in which the work communities are able to develop continuously and are able to react positively to the constant changes in the business. However it is common that leaders do not get adequate and honest information about the problems in the organization operations (Goleman, 1998). And when management knows what should be done to improve organization performance they usually have difficulties to implement the knowledge to practical improvements. Pfeffer and Sutton (2000) indeed describe the phenomenon so that there is knowing-doing-gap, which may lead to wrong decisions and thus prevent the optimal development of the organization.

The organization is build from the people who work together to achieve their objective. Goleman (1998) points out that only the group which wants and is able to operate together can be more efficient and more innovative than its individuals on their own. Thus even if the organization consisted of strong individuals, it can be weak as a system. Each organization group form a sort of microcosmos where defensive reasoning and other routines that are used to explain the problems are embedded. Senge (2006) and Argyris (1985) point out that the defensive routines are harmful because they tend to block the necessary development. Hence, it follows according to Senge (2006) that

"To understand how an organism works we must understand its balancing process – those that are explicit and implicit".

and

"In general, balancing loops are more difficult to see than reinforcing loops because it often looks like nothing is happening."

The tacit signals analyse help finding out the defensive routines that make the organization development difficult. For example the management culture may prevent team level improvements because the foremen have no real power for deciding the improvement actions. Teams may have adapted to this so that matters which require developing will not be brought out (awareness barrier).

When the organization system is in balance it is developing continuously and is easier to manage to the hoped direction. For example Senge (2006) has described the phenomen so that when the system is in balance, the power vectors inside the organization will be lined in the same direction towards the target. In the approach of system intelligence those internal power vectors can be seen as the tacit signal competence vectors from each individual working team as shown in Figure. This also shows the interactive and situational relationship between sensitive and mutual working groups.

Fig. 9. is illustrating the organization system intelligence phenomena where organization performance towards the target is composed from group individuals force vectors. Based on Yerkes-Dodson law of pressure-performance reverse U-curve, every worker has their individual capacity regarding every competence. Tacit signal approach indicates the utilized performance capacity and which direction it should be developed, in other words should be lined to achieve the target.

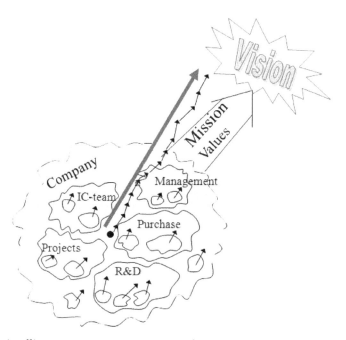

Fig. 9. System intelligence, competence vectors and vision.

Currently, and previously, we have counted on the study of complex adaptive systems (Stacey, 2001; Lewis, 2011). Thus the system intelligence approach considers how individual behaviour affects to competences which are both self-directed and interdependent. Human competence system intelligence means that human capacities, interaction and experience are central elements for performance. Dooley et al. (2004) argue that competencies establish the behavioral requirements needed to be successful in a given profession or task. Blanchard and Thacker (2004) describe that competences are relatively general in nature so they are applicable to a different jobs and hierarchical levels and they are adaptive to changing demands. According to Özcelig and Ferman (2006), the competencies are focused on organization goals and they incorporate feelings and emotions.

The organization is a complex adaptive system which also consists of organizational human success factors. These can be identified as key competencies in organization. The model of the system intelligence of the organization is based in the following optimal competencies (Kesti & Syväjärvi, 2010):

-   Management (management board and strategy capabilities)
-   Leadership (workplace and positive leadership capabilities)
-   Culture (situational and cultural workplace capabilities)
-   Skills (work abilities and know-how)
-   Processes (work methods, learning and interactions used for creating value)

The management should determine the vision and strategy of the organization, but also it should provide the necessary conditions for the development of the organization. The management is responsible that the structure of the organization is suitable to the situation and the abilities of the staff are in adequate balance with strategic objectives. Leaders organize operative work and responsibilities to the workers and should support working society's development in individual and group level. Culture refers in this context to the internal operational and situational settings in organization. In the work community everyone should be able to experience appreciation and collective competence. Skills refer to abilities and individual competencies that can be like the know-how either explicit or tacit. Processes are the work practices together which consist of methods interactions and learning possibilities at workplace. Usually these produce (like other elements) create value to benefiters (internal or external) and, for example, management should get high quality information from organizational processes for their decision making (Collins, 2001; Syväjärvi & Stenvall, 2009).

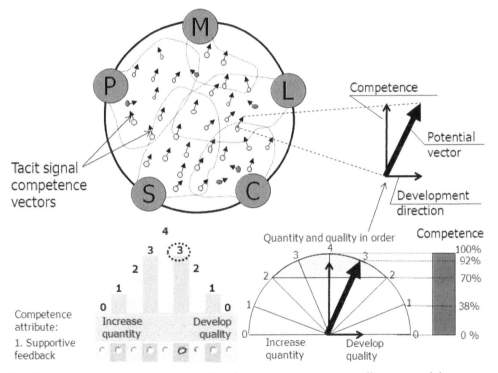

Fig. 10. Organization human tacit signal and competence system ingelligence model.

Thus system intelligence competencies are interrelated and affecting to each other. In positive spiral the management supports leadership and affect to culture. Leadership builds the culture and affects to humans. Team culture speeds up skills improvement and affect to processes. Good personal knowhow helps describing effective processes and gives initiatives to management. From effective processes the management gets high quality information for decision making and clear processes helps leadership. For example, knowhow is not always the problem as the interaction in utilizing the existing knowledge might need action. Furthermore in some organizations the process development is forced too much in case where development focus should be on leadership development.

It has been noticed that system intelligence model had both positive and negative interrelated competence connections (Mayer et al., 2008). In negative spiral, quite often the management does not support the leadership and thus neglected leadership support has an effect to team culture. Typically the humble interaction at the team does not support knowledge sharing and is negatively at processes and their development (Krone et al., 2009). Thus if knowhow is not shared but instead protected, the defensive mechanisms might disturb innovativeness which is important for organizational processes and management. If processes are not in order the management does not get high quality information for decision making. In final, the unclear processes cause mistakes and chaos affecting negatively to leadership which are often blamed.

Research has been done in many public and private sector organizations. These studies at several action research study cases support the competence system intelligence model practical benefits in understanding the phenomena of defensive routines and behavioral actions which otherwise would be difficult to see. For example, at one SME organization the tacit signal development process was carried out. Staff gave several written comments which support the tacit signal competence analysis like:

- *The managing director has too much management responsibilities over every department.*
- *There is no clear line at the management.*
- *For some the tasks and tittles are not in accordance with what is required.*
- *The independent deciding power of some departments is too small, the chief level person has not been appointed. Sometimes this lowers the motivation as the foreman's attitude is:"I'm not doing it, because it's not my task".*
- *More courage to the investments is needed.*
- *Do the foremen lead workers or the opposite?*
- *We have strong individuals at work, whose work dare not to comment. The counteractions can be so strong that rather leave not to say about improvement ideas, when there is possible conflict ahead.*
- *When there has not been the development discussion, there is no personal development plans either.*

Above qualitative examples show how competence analysis using system intelligence model indicate essential human related risks that otherwise could remain unnoticed. The system intelligence model provides method for identifying the probable risks so that management can communicate the optimal actions for mitigating the risks. Therefore system intelligence model can be linked to effective governance procedures of risk management and organization performance improvement. In our longitudinal study, we found positive interactions when the managing director showed interest at the team development by coming just to say hello to the development meeting. The management behaviour had once again positive effect on team members' motivation for innovating improvement actions, which was easy to observe (rf. Bezuijen et al., 2009). There are many similar cases showing that indeed there seem to be certain hermeneutic interaction between the competencies that is important to identify at organization improvement as an intelligent system. The mental model for the organization system intelligence utilizes the mental model of five elements interrelationship (Kesti, 2007).

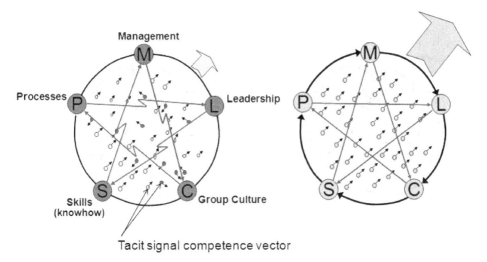

Tacit signal competence vector

Fig. 11. Mental model is illustrating the interaction of five competencies at the organization.

The competence relations need to be opened. At system intelligence model the competencies are interrelated and mutually interactive. There can be identified a positive spiral where management supports the leadership and has positive effect on the culture, the leadership builds the culture and promote personnel skills, good collaboration (culture) speeds up the skills improvement and affects positively to processes, and good personal skills help to describe effective processes and provide initiatives for the management, and finally from effective processes the management receives high quality information for decision-making, and good processes help leadership performance.

At competence system intelligence model negative spiral could go like this: the management does not support the leadership and may have negative influence on the team culture. Poor co-operation within the team does not activate knowledge sharing and this has negative effect on processes development. Once again if the know-how is not shared but protected, the defensive mechanism usually hinders innovativeness which hinges processes development and management possibilities to get necessary initiatives. If organizational processes are not in order, the management does not mine data or receive information for optimal governing (e.g. Syväjärvi & Stenvall, 2010). Furthermore, poorly performed processes will cause mistakes and waste labour which have a negative impact on the leadership.

We have approached the competence system intelligence that it is specifically linked to emotional intelligence with ability-based viewpoints. Thus competencies are seen as elements for emotionally intelligent workplaces and those help one to make sense of and navigate in organizational environment. Additionally the system intelligence method has been found useful in understand the complex organization system and seeing the development challenges especially among and between people (e.g. Lewis, 2011). Organization system intelligence model increase the social awareness in form of social cognition for understanding how social organization system works. So the competence system intelligence takes into account organization's environmental pressures and demands (Bar-On, 2001; Di Fabio & Palazzeschi, 2009) even though there is a stress on competencies. Especially at organization changes it is important to implement actions to support the organization emotional intelligence. Both strategic and working group level improvement needs can be detected using the positive tacit signal analysing. It is based on individuals' tacit knowledge concerning the competencies development in linkage to social and emotional intelligence.

To conclude, the current approach of positive human competence system intelligence is in good accordance with the positive initiative at workplaces, i.e. more precisely in line with the positive prospect and change, the positive psychology and experience, and with the positive leadership (e.g. Seligman et al., 2005; Syväjärvi et al., 2005; Cameron, 2008). The current approach has four major connotations that include the concept of positive: a focus on positively deviant performance, a focus on strengths rather than weaknesses, a focus on virtuousness, and finally a focus or value on human experience. Also in relation to emotional intelligence, it should be noted the importance of complex adaptive systems. Hence, the latter offer an analogy of how competencies are in touch with interaction between people and some competencies are overlapping or even redundant.

5. Positive tacit signal development and leadership

It was debated about the positive in earlier section three, but now it is considered how to develop and lead tacit signals. Goleman (2007) has studied the emotional intelligence of the working societies and found out that it seems to be one of the most significant factors affecting to the human performance. In an intelligent society members appreciate each other and want to improve the quality of the working life in constructive cooperation and thus utilizing emotion intelligence. According to Losada and Heaphy (2004), the group members' positive feelings increase the work community performance. When workers have positive feelings more than three times more than negative, the performance of the group increases strongly. Also it seems that working group that has good balance between dichotomies self-group and question-answer is able to create more positive feelings than negative.

In fact, there are many studies about positive behaviour and development that indicate how increasing contribution of positivity is touch with to desirable work-related outcomes (Luthans & Youssef, 2007). Hassard and Kelemen (2002) argue that knowledge can be seen as a set of cultural practices situated in and inextricably linked to the material and social circumstances in which it is produced and consumed. When a person is facing the new situation they evaluate the situation and start sense making process based on past experience and knowledge (Weick, 1995). In well-known study Argyris (1985) identified single and double loop learning where single loop learning could be seen as a process of correcting the fault using past experience and double loop learning as preventing the fault from happening again by creating new knowledge based on thorough reflection.

Communication is definitely one key factor in both organizational commitment and knowledge development. Elias (2009) found that positive and affective commitment together with the growth need strength is vital for the attitude toward organizational change. This highlights interactive relationship between leader and employee. Also group members should have positive mental attitude towards knowledge sharing and possibilities for open constructive discussion, which Nonaka and Konno (1998) describe with the knowledge creating concept of BA. Senge (2006) recognize three critical dimensions for team learning at the organization environment: 1) team members have motivation and ability to think insightfully about complex issues, 2) there is common need for innovative, coordinated action, and 3) there is ability to share practices and skills between the other teams at the organization. All this about attitudes, communications and the importance of balancing feedbacks at the organization are those that can give essential information for the start of balance process.

The social consciousness will be created when humans compare their own observations with the observations and ideas made by others (Festinger, 1954). Perttula (2009) has described a holistic perspective of psycho-social work that presumes human to exist and actualize as a whole. March (2010) indicate that intelligence normally entails two interrelated but different components, i.e. the effective adaptation to an environment and the elegance of interpretations of the experiences of life. These opinions are mostly based on experiences and therefore the interpretation of the human experience has a great influence on almost everything. This is the case with the growth need strength as when employees with strong needs for growth are given the opportunity to develop then such an opportunity is thought to be rewarding and increases affective organizational commitment (Elias, 2009). In addition to previous, the tacit knowledge is described as personal, context-specific, and therefore hard to formalize and communicate. The latter is supplemented Polanyi's (1967) action oriented concept of knowledge by assuming that knowledge is created through the interaction between tacit and explicit dimensions.

The current positive tacit signal process has following phases:

PHASE 1: Management and planning

Development process is planned and organized with management, leaders and employee representatives in order to guarantee good attitudes and commitments. Targets are set and the important human capabilities as essential competences are defined and agreed for tacit signal analysis. Only those competence attributes are included that are essential for organization performance. Management and HR specialists are coached for human capital development.

PHASE 2: The tacit signal collection

Tacit signals are collected from each working group of the organization. Signals are important collective balancing feedback that is needed for balancing process. Results are analyzed using the tacit signal development semicircle competence analysing method.

PHASE 3: Strategy development meeting

Strategic development focus is chosen according to organization tacit signals and mutual commitments.

PHASE 4: Development meetings at working communities

According to the group tacit signal analysis each organization group agree their own optimal improving actions with follow-up responsibility and time-schedule. Ideas and improvement actions are inquired and written down. These represent the group "BA", true workplace experiences and knowledge creation conversion process phases 1, 2 and 3.

PHASE 5 Follow-up and support

Actions implementation is followed up and supported by managers and leaders. Leadership forums are held where each leader presents their group improvement actions and possible problems or success. An internet based communication tool is used for action follow-up and best practices sharing. This phase correspond the knowledge creation process phase 4.

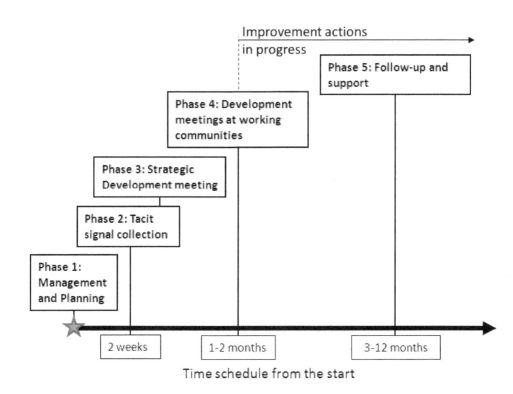

Fig. 12. The tacit signal development process schedule.

To make this development process effective for organization improvement there are four main factors to optimize. Firstly, all the improvement actions should be started as soon as possible from the beginning of the process. This motivates the participants and the improvement actions are able to affect to the organization performance as soon as possible. Secondly, the time consumption of the participants should be optimized so that the invested time for development gains more benefits than what it eats the organization capacity to make revenue and gross margin. Thirdly, people interact and share with their experiences as complex and demanding situations are managed by holistic perceptions and mutual understandings. Fourthly, the focus is on positive development as optimal improvement actions are valued. Development phases are shown in figure.

Some studies indicate that the difference between great and mediocre activity lies in the way how people face conflicts and complexities, and how they succeed with solving, interacting, responding and adapting those (e.g. Argyris, 1985; Stacey et al., 2000; Senge, 2006). Our experience from several cases where tacit signal process has been implemented supports finding that sensitivity to intervene in the matters which require attentions are learned behaviour models (Latane & Darley, 1969). The interference with the matters which require attention depends a lot from how humans have experienced or learned to be intervened. Therefore the successful implementation of positive tacit signal process can be seen as one implemented improvement action where the optimal improvement actions are agreed collectively. The development process creates certain mode of operation that stimulates, for example, opportunities for reflection, dialogue, creativity, learning and finally emotional intelligence throughout the workplace. However, in the core of positive tacit signal development is also the leadership.

The positive tacit signal development needs equal actions with leadership. At the same time it should be noted that the social construction of organizational realities might too easily or traditionally elevate the leadership to a lofty status and level of significance (rf. Meindl et al., 1985). It is not easy to build a comprehensive leadership approach in case of positive tacit signal development and emotional intelligence. It is not even our goal, but still the "great leadership" should note that human behavior, situation and organizational perception are not only about trying to fix what is wrong or dysfunctional in workplace and among employees. In fact preceding is recognized, but leadership should mean a more balanced perspective as it is more focusing on positive and the real nature of human experience.

In addition, the leadership quite typically linked to somewhat contingent and sensitive work situations. The contingency approach indicates that leadership is the product (and on the other hand produce itself) of a perfect match between particular and certain circumstance. Leadership is thus related to personality and situational factors that determine how humans experience and behave. Both contingency and situation are important to notice, but those are neither fixed nor beyond the realm of psychology (Haslam et al., 2011). Now a kind of caring leadership is presented alongside the positive tacit signal development. Caring leadership is a strength-based approach to workplace situation, human and overall management. The caring leadership is in line with the positive initiative at workplaces, i.e. more precisely in line with the complex adaptive system thinking, the positive prospect and change, the positive psychology and experience, and with the positive leadership (e.g. Stacey et al., 2000; Cameron, 2008; Kesti & Syväjärvi, 2010). This approach has four major connotations that include the concept of positive:

- a focus on complex situations together with human interaction,
- a focus on deviant human performance,
- a focus on human competencies,
- a focus on human experience and authenticity.

Emotional and intelligent workplaces do not necessarily need leadership to survive, but organizations with leadership are more likely to sustain or be successful. Current approach to leadership is needed in order to highlight the human bias, identity and development in workplace. It also has clear link to emotional intelligence in workplaces. Indeed the leadership is interested in what really goes on in organization and with human being. Leadership is not only for organizational performance and success but also strongly after and for human experience and intelligence. Thus the intelligence involves both the beauties of crafting understandings of experience and the efficiencies of adaptation (March, 2010). The positive leadership emphasizes organizational advantages and how to influence humans, but the current view even is more authentically and additionally keen about human and self, shared identity and human interaction. Nevertheless, any definition or approach to leadership ultimately rests on one's theoretical commitments. The positive tacit signal process seems to support emotional intelligence as in situations humans need to solve, adapt and to response multiple conceptual and behavioural complexities.

6. Conclusions

We have studied the positive human tacit signal approach and competence system intelligence. This is done in order to understand how positive human tacit signals are detected and used, but also in order to realise how competence system intelligence is related to emotional intelligence in workplaces. Experiences were seen in the core of human positive tacit signals and competence system intelligence. Additionally we found how positive human tactic signals and competence system intelligence are affecting and modifying the role of leadership in increasingly complex adaptive organizations and emotionally intelligent workplaces.

The positive human tacit signal approach works as an organizational development process that has gone through the evolution of systematic improvement (Kesti, Syväjärvi & Stenvall, 2008). This has been done by using massive and empirically grounded research data. At first there was an expectation that by method the guiding opinions or experiences can be measured for management since, for example, the tacit signal dichotomy scale seems to support the decision making. When essential capabilities can be recognized and improved then they form key competencies that are suitable for learning and growth scorecards and thus those are part of effective management and leadership. The tacit signal approach indeed gives guiding holistic information about human competencies and development.

According to current approach, it is possible to both detect and gain positive signals and performance (like optimism, hope, support, flexibility and interaction) that value human being as an individual and interactive subject. This does not mean that negative, disturbing or otherwise unwanted situations are neglected (Losada & Heaphy, 2004; Cameron, 2008). In knowledge-intensive and emotionally intelligent organizations and workplaces, the current approach enables positive meaning, positive climate, positive interaction and positive experiences. In human tacit signal approach it can be seen both individual and interactive development needs and also guiding values that will support in seeing and choosing the positive action in relation to emotional intelligence. All these are important viewpoints to manage with positive as organizational behaviour, psychology and leadership research has proposed that effective applications are needed to these purposes (Syväjärvi et al., 2005; Luthans & Youssef, 2007; Salovey et al., 2009).

The competence system intelligence was one key element in current study. We have seen that competence embraces various capabilities to perform needed tasks in organization. The competence-based approach was driven by factors that described and tackled organizational system intelligence in accordance to positive emotional intelligence in workplaces. Despite the central role of competence, there is such confusion surrounding the concept that it is almost impossible to impute a coherent theory in this context. However, the competence system intelligence can be related to the study that takes the organization as a complex adaptive system (e.g. Stacey, 2009). Additionally competence thus captures such positive elements that are related to personal and interpersonal intelligence, but are fundamentally behavioral and susceptible to learning and experience. At the end, the complex adaptive system offered a good analogy of how experience should be fundamental element to be added or weighted more heavily among, for example, the positive organizational scholar studies.

Human experience is thus stressed as it pays attention to social reality or awareness of an organization. This reality, like experience, means subjective guidance so that both individual and collective positive relations are valued. Subjective experience has been viewed as falling outside the sphere of human-based organizational study. At least to some degree this has been a reality also in positive organizational scholarship. Our viewpoints emphasize the meaning of experience as one determinant of social reality in organizations. The human experience has an emergent and adaptive nature, but it is shaped by both person and environment. Hence, now positive and subjective experience is seen as differentiated and integrated so that it originates from intuition, knowledge, belief, competence, etc. The tendency of the experience toward complexity means here that adaptation and response are like sources of positive as well as new competencies or abilities for optimal action in relation to existing goals. The abovementioned is thus related to emotional intelligence (see also Mayer et al., 2008).

Individual and group competencies increase social awareness and positive capabilities, which can be linked to various development actions. The current approach is in good accordance with some earlier studies (Luthans & Youssef, 2007; Haslam et al., 2011). Haslam et al. (2011) underline the importance of both social identity and self-categorization, when it is vital to experience that one belongs to certain social workgroup together with some emotional and value significance to him or her. Also the process of experiencing self as human being and an interchangeable person is highlighted. Luthans and Yuossef (2007) have indicated how positive state-like capacities are more flexible and thus open to change and development. For example, the social awareness increases motivation for solving the problems and might decrease the dissonance. Present approach followed the principle of inverted U-curve showing that both individual and group collective development competencies will guide to positive awareness's and improvements.

Quite much debate has been in leadership studies that concentrate on what and how leaders actually act or on the complex nature of leadership environment. These are still obvious and important viewpoints, but furthermore we put more pressure on leadership that cares about situational interaction, positive performance, human competencies and expediencies. Nowadays workplaces and people are under many changes and also the work itself is changing. Thus the caring leadership is able to facilitate emotional intelligence, meaningful work and happy work communities. Arnold et al. (2007), for example, have showed similar findings with leadership and psychological well-being as they found clear relationships among leadership, meaningful work and human well-being. Also leadership studies indicate that leader behavior with expectations (pygmalion effect) and people engagement have positive relation to human performance (Bezuijen et al., 2009).

Current approach seems to help the leaders to initiate the positive change process where problems can be turned to development needs and further to possibilities and optimal improvement actions. As problems are solved in constructive way, they will create positive feelings and so increase the group performance. This is in good accordance with findings about the growth need strength and the knowledge sharing in both change and knowledge intensive organizations (Elias, 2009; Krone et al., 2009). Current findings support the conclusion that the tacit signal process strengthens the group's emotional intelligence as the group members learn to solve problems constructively. Systematic development seems to create a certain mode of operation that stimulates opportunities for reflection, dialogue and sharing, creativity and workplace innovations throughout the organization. Thus tacit signal approach seems to be rather well in line with Appreciative Inquiry perspective that intention is to discover, understand, and foster innovations in social-organizational arrangements and processes (Cooperrider & Srivastva, 1987).

In final, the competence system intelligence illustrates how emotional intelligence might be perceived, but also how it can hinder or flourish workplace performance and experience. When existing complex human related outcomes can be conceptualized then one is able to develop corrective or supportive actions for situational demands. It seems that situational needs can be identified by using tacit signals approach, which instead seems to support hermeneutic positive problem solving but moreover human experience with the intelligence space. Many times organizational challenges are complex and thus sustainable solution or change requires such actions that give a great value to subjective and emotional human being. There are indeed many implications for organization and leadership research, but surely more research is needed in the fields of leadership psychology, positive organizational behavior and human experience-based organization. Future research should observe even more how various identities and human relations could be lead and how present type of or corresponding optimal interventions effect on multidimensional performance and employee wellbeing. More research is needed to explain optimal interventions that follow positive developments, competence system intelligences, and finally sensitive work communities.

7. References

Abercrombie, H.C., Kalin, N.H., Thurow, M.E., Rosenkranz, M.A. & Davidson, R.J. (2003). Cortisol Variation in Humans Affects Memory for Emotionally-laden and Neutral Information. *Behavioral Neuroscience*, 117(3), 505-516.

Argyris, C. (1985). *Strategy, Change and Defensive Routines*. Pitman, Boston.

Arnold, K., Turner, N., Barling, J., Kelloway, E.K. & McKee, M.C. (2007). Transformational Leadership and Psychological Well-Being: The Mediating Role of Meaningful Work. Journal of Occupational Health Psychology, 12(3), 193-203.

Bar-On, R. (2001). Emotional Intelligence and Self-actualization. In Ciarrochi, J., Forgas, J.P. & Mayer, J.D. (eds.), Emotional Intelligence in Every Day Life: A Scientific Inquiry. Philadelphia, PA: Psychology Press. pp. 82-97.

Bezuijen, X.M., van der Berg, P.T., van Dam, K. & Thierry, H. (2009). Pygmalion and Employee Learning: The Role of Leader Behaviors. *Journal of Management*, 35(5), 1248-1267.

Blanchard, P.N. & Thacker, J.W. (2004). *Effective Training: Systems, Strategies, and Practices.* Upper Saddle River, NJ: Prentice Hall.

Cameron, K. (2008*). Positive Leadership – Strategies for Extraordinary Performance.* USA: Berrett-Koehler.

Collins J. & Porras J. (1994). *Built to Last.* HarperCollins Publishers Inc. New York.

Collins, J. (2001). *Good to Great.* Harper Business, New York.

Cooperrider, D. & Srivastva, S. (1987). Appreciative Inquiry in Organizational Life. *Research in Organizational Change and Development*, 1, 129–169.

de Geus, A. (1997). *The Living Company.* Nicholas Brealy, London.

Di Fabio, A. & Palazzeschi, L. (2009). Emotional Intelligence, Personality Traits and Career Decision Difficulties. *International Journal for Educational and Vocational Guidance*, 9, 135-146.

Dooley, K.E., Lindner, J.R., Dooley, L.M. & Alagaraja, M. (2004). Behaviorally Anchored Competencies: Evaluation Tool for Training via Distance. *Human Resource Development International*, 7(3), 315-32.

Elias, S.M. (2009). Employee Commitment in Times of Change: Assessing the Importance of Attitudes Toward Organizational Change. *Journal of Management*, 35(1), 37-55.

Fenwick, T. (2006). Toward Enriched Conceptions of Work Learning: Participation, Expansion, and Translation Among Individuals Within Activity. *Human Resource Development Review*, 5(3), 285-302.

Festinger, L. (1954). A Theory of Social Comparison Process. *Human Relations*, 7, 117-140.

Fredrickson, B.L. (2001). The Role of Positive Emotions in Positive Psychology. *American Psychologist*, 56(3), 218-226.

Gergen, K. J. & Gergen, M. (2004). Social Construction: Entering the Dialogue. Chagrin Falls, OH: TaosInstitute Publishing, p. 20.

Ghoshal, S., Bartlett, C.A. & Moran, P. (2000). Value Creation: The New Millennium Management Manifesto. In Chowdhury, S. (ed.), *Management 21C*. London: Prentice-Hall. pp. 131-140.

Gilley, J.W., Eggland, S.A. & Maycunich, A. (2002). *Principles of Human Resource Development.* Cambridge, MA: Perseus Publishing.

Goleman, D. (1998). *Working with Emotional Intelligence.* A Bantam Book, USA.

Goleman, D. (2006). *Social Intelligence.* Arrow Books.

Hassard, J. & Kelemen, M. (2002). Production and Consumption in Organizational Knowledge: The Case of the 'Paradigms Debate'. *Organization*, 9(2), 331-155.

Haslam, S.A. Reicher, S.D. and Platow, M. (2011). *The New Psychology of Leadership. Identity, Influence and Power.* Psychology Press, USA.

Kesti, M. & Syväjärvi, A. (2010). Human Tacit Signals at Organization Performance Development. *Industrial Management & Data Systems,* 110(2), 211-229.

Kesti, M. (2005). *Tacit Signals – Key to Organization Development.* Edita Publishing, Helsinki.

Kesti, M. (2007). *High Performance Organization.* Edita Publishing, Helsinki.

Kesti, M. (2010). *Strategic Human Capital Management,* Talentum, Helsinki.

Kesti, M., Syväjärvi, A. & Stenvall, J. (2008). E-HRM in Competence Recognition and Management - The Tacit Signal HRIS. In Torres-Coronas, T. & Arias-Oliva, M. (eds.) *Encyclopedia of Human Resource Information Systems: Challenges in E-HRM.* Idea Group Publishing Inc, USA.

Kets de Vries, M. (2006).*The Leadership Mystique. Leading Behavior in the Human Enterprise.* Prentice Hall, UK.

Krone, O., Syväjärvi, A. & Stenvall, J. (2009). Knowledge Integration for Enterprise Resource Planning Application Design. *Knowledge and Process Management,* 16(1), 1-12.

Latane, B. & Darley, J.M. (1969). Bystander "Apathy". *American Scientist,* 57, 244-268.

Lewis, S. (2011). Positive Psychology at Work. How Positive Leadership and Appreciative Inquire Create Inspiring Organizations. Wiley-Blackwell, UK.

Liker, J.K. (2004). The Toyota Way, McGraw-Hill, New York.

Losada, M. & Heaphy, E. (2004). The Role of Positivity and Connectivity in the Performance of Business Teams: A Nonlinear Dynamics Model. *American Behavioral Science,* 2(1), 71-87.

Luthans, F. & Youssef, C.M. (2007). Emerging Positive Organizational Behavior. *Journal of Management,* 33(3), 321-349.

Luthans, F., & Youssef, C.M. (2009). Positive Workplaces. In Lopez, S.J. & Snyder, C.R. (eds.) *Oxford Handbook of Positive Psychology.* Oxford University Press, New York.

Mankin, D. (2009). *Human Resource Development.* Oxford University Press, USA.

March, J.G. (2010). *The Ambiguities of Experience.* Cornell University Press, USA.

Mayer, J.D., Roberts, R.D. & Barsade, S.G. (2008). Human Abilities: Emotional intelligence. *Annual Reviews in Psychology,* 59, 507–536.

McClernon, T. (2006). Rivals to Systematic Training. *Advances in Developing Human Resources,* 8(4): 442-59.

Meindl, J.R., Ehrlich, S.B. & Dukerich, J.M. (1985). The Romance of Leadership. *Administrative Science Quarterly,* 30(1), 78-102.

Nagamachi M. (2008). Shiromiso - Akamiso. Accident Prevention Management Based on Brain Theory. Hiroshima International University.

Nonaka, I. & Konno, N. (1998). 'The Concept of 'Ba': Building a Foundation for Knowledge Creation'. *California Management Review,* 40(3), 40-54.

Nonaka, I. & Takeuchi, H. (1995). *The Knowledge Creating Company.* Oxford University Press, New York.

Perttula, J. (2009). The Holistic Perspective to Psycho-Social Work. *Special Education,* 1(20), 55-63.

Pfeffer, J. & Sutton, R.I. (2000). *The Knowing-Doing Gap: How Smart Companies Turn Knowledge into Action*. Harvard Business School Press.

Polanyi, M. (1967). *The Tacit Dimension*. Doubleday, New York.

Putkonen, A. (2009). 'Predicting the Effects of Time Pressure on Design Work', *International Journal of Innovation and Learning*, 6(5), 477–492.

Salovey, P. Mayer, J.D., Caruso, D. & Yoo, S.H. (2009). The Positive Psychology of Emotional Intelligence. In Lopez. S.J. & Snyder, C.R. (eds.) *Oxford Handbook of Positive Psychology*. Second Edition. Oxford Univeristy Press, NY.

Schein, E.H. (1985). *Organizational Culture and Leadership: A Dynamic View*. Jossey-Bass, USA.

Seligman, M., Steen, T.A., Park, N. & Peterson, C. (2005). Positive Psychology Progress. Empirical Validation or Interventions. *.American Psychologist*, 60(5), 410-421.

Senge, P. M. (2006). *The Fifth Discipline*. Doubleday, USA.

Spector, P. E., & Fox, S. (2002). An Emotion-centered Model of Voluntary Work Behavior: Some Parallels between Counterproductive Work Behavior and Organizational Citizenship Behavior. *Human Resource Management Review, 12*, 269–292.

Stacey, R.D., Griffin, D. & Shaw, P.(2000). *Complexity and Management: Fad Or Radical Challenge to Systems Thinking?* Routledge, UK.

Stacey, R.D. (2001). *Complex Responsive Processes in Organizations. Learning and Knowledge Creation*. NY: Routledge

Stacey, R.D. (2009). *Complexity and Organizational Reality. Uncertainty and the Need to Rethink Management after the Collapse of Investment Capitalism*. Rotledge, USA and Canada.

Stone, R.J. (2002). *Human Resource Management*. Fourth edition. John Wiley & Sons Ltd., Australia.

Syväjärvi, A. Näsänen, R. & Rovamo, J. (1999). Spatial Integration of Signal Information in Gabor Stimuli. *Ophthal. Physiol. Opt.*, 19(3), 242-252.

Syväjärvi, A., & Stenvall, J. (2009). Core Governmental Perspectives of e-Health. In Tan, J. (ed.) *Medical informatics: concepts, methodologies, tools, and applications*. Information Science Reference. pp. 153-162.

Syväjärvi, A. & Stenvall, J. eds. (2010). *Data Mining in Public and Private Sectors; Organizational and Government Applications*. Information Science Reference, USA.

Syväjärvi, A., Stenvall, J., Harisalo, R., & Jurvansuu, H. (2005). The Impact of Information Technology on Human Capacity, Interprofessional Practice and Management. *Problems and Perspectives in Management*, 1(4), 82-95.

Weick, K. E. (1995). *Sensemaking in Organizations*. Sage Publications, Inc. USA.

Wexley, K.N. & Latham G.P. (2002). *Developing and Training Human Resources in Organizations*. Upper Saddle River, NJ: Prentice Hall.

Wheelan, S.A. (2005). *The Handbook of Group Research and Practice*. Sage Publications, Inc. USA.

Wu, C., Neubert. M.J. & Yi, X. (2007). Transformational Leadership, Cohesion Perceptions, and Employee Cynicism About Organizational Change. *The Journal of Applied Behavioral Science*, 43(3), 327-351.

Yerkes, R.M., & Dodson, J.D. (1908). The Relation of Strength of Stimulus to Rapidity of Habit-Formation. *Journal of Comparative Neurology and Psychology*, 18, 459-482.

Özcelig, G. & Ferman, M. (2006). Competency Approach to Human Resource Management: Outcomes and Contributions in a Turkish Cultural Context. *Human Resource Development Review*, 5 (1): 72-91.

9

Maternal Attitudes, Emotional Intelligence and Home Environment and Their Relations with Emotional Intelligence of Six Years Old Children

Ilkay Ulutas and Esra Omeroglu
Department of Early Childhood
Development and Education
Gazi University, Ankara
Turkey

1. Introduction

Mayer and Salovey have defined the emotional intelligence "perceiving emotions, using emotions in order to support ideas, understanding emotions and emotional information, adjusting emotions for emotional and mental development" (Mayer & Salovey 1997). Recently two conceptions of emotional intelligence (trait emotional intelligence and ability EI) have been indicated. Trait EI (or trait emotional self-efficacy) concerns emotion related dispositions and self-perceptions measured via self-report, whereas ability EI (or cognitive-emotional ability) concerns emotion-related cognitive abilities measured via performance-based tests (Petrides et all, 2007).

Emotional intelligence covers abilities like recognising, understanding and regulating emotions which are important for children to establish positive relationships with people (Mayer, Caruso, & Salovey, 2002, Goleman, 2001). It has come to light that children, who can understand emotions correctly avoid aggressive behaviours, establish more positive relations with their peers and other persons around them and they are accordant in their school and social life (Hughes, Dunn, & White, 1998, Fabes, et al. 2001).

Emotional intelligence also has a great importance in terms of ensuring social and universal unity. Today in many countries around the world it draw attention that social relationships have been declining and individualism has been arising in parallel with the rapid development of technology and increase in competition trend. Besides the necessity of emotional understanding and control has arisen in order to each individual accepts and works in cooperation with an individual from another culture. In recent years programs that increase emotional and social skills has been preparing and implementing at workplace and schools in many developed countries that acknowledge the importance of togetherness and cooperation Webster-Stratton, & Hammond, 2010, Elias, et al. 1997, Alegre, 2011). When we look at the results of these programs the decrease in violent behaviour among new generation revealed the importance of emotional intelligence.

Recent studies show that children interact with emotions before they born. During infancy child tries to recognize the emotions. As Piaget stated between the ages of two and four they display egocentric thinking. In these ages they can interact with adults and their peers freely but they are more focused on their selves and can't comprehend other's standpoints. However in following years with the increase of their need for association with friends egocentrism should decrease and emotional sharing and emotional control should increase (Berk, 2002). In this regard parents have very important responsibilities for children to turn towards to sharing from egocentric thinking.

Family is the first environment where child feels, observes and learns the emotional relationships (Warhol, 1998). Parenthood contains the skills like struggling against the various dangers that children may face and guiding them in a good way (Melmed, 1998). Children try to understand the emotions through the attachment and modelling with parents (Denham et al., 2000; Laible & Thompson, 1998; Ontai & Thompson, 2002; Raikes & Thomspon, 2006; Suess, Grossmann & Sroufe, 1992). How much child's attachments with his parents is strong his success increases in relationships with the people and he can establish social relationships without anxiety of acceptance, criticism and loneliness (Kerns, Klepac, & Cole, 1996).

The risk factors that lead unwanted behaviours of children who cannot attach securely like fighting, complaining appears in early childhood (Denham, 2007). Therefore it is important to examine the factors affecting the children and parents relationship.

1.1 Factors affecting children's emotional intelligence

Several factors affect the development of emotional intelligence in children. Child's character, neurophysiology and cognitive enhancement are the important factors (Eisenberg & Morris, 2002; Goldsmith & Davidson, 2004). However it has been seen that emotional intelligence may strengthen or dull with the effect of both these factors and social relationships like family and circle of friends. Family environment is especially the most important one among these (Cole, Martin, & Denis, 2004; Parke, 1994; Walden & Smith, 1997).

In Figure 1 family's effect on child's emotional intelligence has been shown.

According to Morris et al. (2007) family environment affects children's emotional intelligence in three aspects. Firstly children learn emotions by observing the people around them. Secondly their experiences and behaviours related to parent's emotions ensure children to become appropriate to society's expectations. Thirdly factors reflecting the emotional status of family such as the quality of emotional attachment between the child and the parents, attitude of parents, emotional and social openness, and marital relationship have impacts on emotional intelligence.

1.2 Emotional intelligence and parenting styles

Baumrind denotes ideal parents as "parents who manage child's activities in a rational way, promote verbal communication within the family, talk about their attitudes regarding child raising with the child, support child to overcome the obstacles that the child faces when he cannot adjusted" (Baumrind, 2005). As stated attitude of parents bring along with positive results as self control of child, self adjustment, adaptation and friendly relations (Jewell et. al., 2008).

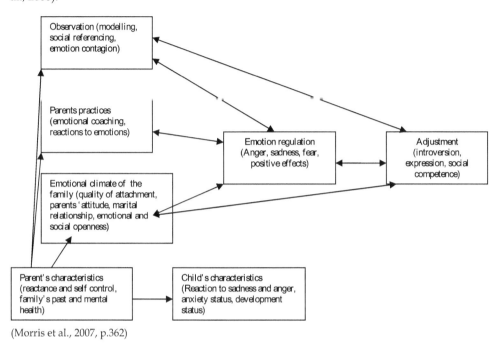

(Morris et al., 2007, p.362)

Fig. 1. Familial factors affecting emotional intelligence

Alegre (2011) reported four main dimensions of parenting are identified that are relevant to the study of emotional intelligence: parental responsiveness, parental positive demandingness, parental negative demandingness, and parental emotion-related coaching. Parental responsiveness, parental emotion-related coaching, and parental positive demandingness are related to children's higher emotional intelligence, while parental negative demandingness is related to children's lower emotional intelligence.

Thompson (1998) indicates that children, who have positive relations with parents and argue the emotions of others, have a better understanding of emotions when compared with others. Children learn emotions from their parents' speeches and enhance their emotional intelligence through the bond they attached with their parents (Raikes & Thompson 2006).

In a research by Chen et al. (2005) on attitudes of parents and children's social adaptation, it has appeared that supportive parenting attitude is influential on development of children's social adaptation.

Child raising attitudes of parents also affects the emotional environment of the family (Lopez, Bonenberger and Schneider; 2001), it was found that excessively authoritarian attitude of parents is associated with the low empathy level of child while inductive attitude is associated with high empathy level. It appears that authoritarian parents limit their child further (Marr & Ezeife, 2008).

Parenting styles associated with poor child emotion regulation, dismissive and disapproving responses to displays of emotions (Gottman et al., 1997; Ramsden & Hubbard, 2002). Ramsden and Hubbard (2002) found dismissive parenting was associated with poorer emotion regulation and increased aggressive behaviour in preschoolers. Denham and colleagues (2000) found a similar relationship, and concluded that dismissive parenting may be worse for children with more difficult temperaments. Also in several studies show that parents are influential on child's emotional reaction, motivation status, behaviours and emotional control (Eisenberg, Cumberland, & Spinrad, 1998; Gottman, Katz, & Hooven, 1997). Accordingly parents with warm and positive attitude will raise children who experience less anger and temper or who have fewer problems like aggressiveness stems from these emotions (Eisenberg et al., 2005).

1.3 Emotional intelligence and home environment

While parents' interaction with child and their form of attachment affect the emotional intelligence of child, home environment can be seen as a natural environment for the constitution of emotions and emotional attachments (Raikes, & Thompson, 2006). Parents' style of communication with the child, child's acceptance at home, the way they support the development and learning of child, signals they send to child, modelling, and physical environment are presumed as the indicator of sufficiency of home environment (Caldwel & Bradley, 1984).

Home environment is important in terms of ensuring the child to overcome the emotional barriers (Parke, et al., 1992; Thompson, 1994). It has appeared that negative impacts in home environment; especially mother's angry and furious communication style lowers preschool children's understanding of emotions. Nixon and Watson (2001) observed that children with positive home environment animate spousal relations positively in puppet plays while children who are subject to negative impacts animate it negatively. According to the study by Chen et al., (2005) parents with supportive attitude arrange home environment in such a way that is enhances emotional sufficiency of children. These parents organize home environment based on the thoughts and suggestions of children, choose and place the furniture and materials the way that this provide emotional comfort in order that children see themselves as a member of the family.

1.4 Aim of the present study

As stated by Eisenberg et al., (2005) mother's parenting attitudes and interactions with children have more powerful impact on their emotional and social development in the early years. It is also possible that the effects of positive parenting are especially strong in this period when children are more vulnerable and parents are highly salient emotional models compared with other models in their nearby. Therefore this study aimed to determine the relationship between maternal factors such as maternal attitudes, home environment and emotional intelligence and children's emotional intelligence. Mother negative parenting style was hypothesized to be negatively associated with child's emotional intelligence. Home environment was expected to be positively associated with child's emotional intelligence. Maternal emotional intelligence was hypothesized to be positively associated with child's emotional intelligence.

2. Method

2.1 Participants

144 sixth years old preschool children (78 boys and 66 girls) at two separate preschool sites, and their mothers, and teachers participated in the study. Sixth years old children were chosen because the early years were marked by the emergence of self regulatory capacities and an increase and diversification of emotional regulation abilities (Maughan & Cicchetti 2002; Cicchetti & Schneider-Rosen 1986). Children were recruited from the preparation classes of the primary schools at the centre of Ankara. All of them were Turkish and living in a household with both biological parents. The majority of the children had middle socio-economic status.

The mothers were aged from 20- 40 with a mean of 29 years (SD=3.42). The education level of the mothers ranged from less than 5 years of schooling to university graduates. 47.1 percent of mothers had less than high school education, 36.9 percent had a high school diploma, 16.0 percent had graduated from university. Most of them were from working-class families with a mean income of $1000 to $2000. The majority of the mothers had two children (62.7%, N = 153), the next largest group had one child (23.8%, N = 58). More than half of them were not working at the time of the study (61.9%, N = 151).

Classroom data were collected from ten teachers at two separate primary schools. Both schools were within public school districts, serving normal population. The teachers had bachelor's degree in early childhood teaching.

2.2 Measures

Demographic information obtained included sex, age, current living arrangements, participants' birth order and parents' age, educational status, job etc..

2.2.1 Children' emotional intelligence: The Sullivan Emotional Intelligence Scale for children, the Sullivan Brief Empathy Scale for children and the Sullivan Teacher Rating Scale of Emotional Intelligence for children were utilized

The Sullivan Emotional Intelligence Scale (Sullivan, 1999) consists of three main parts such as; Recognising emotions (with Faces and Stories subtest), Understanding emotions and Managing emotions. There are 19 faces in the faces subtest of Recognising section, 5 short stories in stories subtest of Recognising section, such as thunder, death of animal, 10 vignettes in the Understanding section and 7 interactive stories in the Managing section and 7 items in the managing section. The researcher read the each items to child and asks the questions following the item. The child is required to respond with "yes" or "no" or "I don't know".

The Sullivan Brief Empathy Scale for Children was designed to provide information about children's emphatic reactions. It contains ten items. The researcher read the each items to child, the child is required to respond with "yes" or "no" or "I don't know".

The Sullivan Teacher Rating Scale of Emotional Intelligence for Children is a scale of 11 items, from the lowest level perception of emotions to the highest level which is managing emotions. The teacher completes it for each child depending on classroom observations.

Items were first translated into Turkish and then back translated into English. Items with problematic back translations were thoroughly discussed and appropriately amended. Turkish adaptation of the scales proved adequate validity (α=0.68- 0.90) and reliability (.97-.99). Scales have two dimensions one from the researcher and other from the teacher to ensure a fairer assessment of each child's emotional intelligence (Ulutaş & Omeroglu, 2007).

2.2.2 Maternal emotional intelligence: Mothers' emotional intelligence was measured with the emotional intelligence self-evaluation test

This test was designed by Hall and adapted and translated into Turkish by Ergin (2000) and consists of 30 items. The scores received from the scale range between 30 and 180 and higher scores indicate higher emotional intelligence. When observed in terms of total score, a correlation coefficient at the level of 0.84 was found between the first and last application.

2.2.3 Maternal attitudes: Parental Attitudes Research Inventory (PARI)

The Parental Attitudes Research Inventory, developed by Schaefer and Bell, was used in this research to determine the attitudes of mothers towards their children. The test was adapted and translated into Turkish by LeCompte et al. (1978). There are 60 items and 5 subscales in the test. The subscales include overprotective mothering, democratic attitudes and recognition of equality, rejecting the role of housewife, marital conflicts, and strict discipline. A total score cannot be obtained from the scale; however, factor scores can be evaluated.

2.2.4 Home environment: Home observation for measurement of the environment (Home) inventory

This inventory was developed by Caldwell and Bradley (1984) in order to examine the facilities provided for children at home by the family and to observe the children's interaction with their mother. A validity and reliability study of the inventory on Turkish children was conducted by the researchers. The reliability coefficient emerged as .69. The inventory consists of eight subsections and a total of 55 items on the following aspects; "supporting learning", "supporting speaking", "physical environment", intimacy and acceptance", "academic stimulation", "modelling", "variety in experience" and "acceptance". The score received from the inventory are evaluated and higher scores point to a positive outcome in terms of home environment observation.

2.3 Procedure

Contact with most of the participants was made via a preschool teacher. The first 144 mothers and their children who expressed interest in participating were contacted to collect the data. A letter describing the study along with consent forms was sent to the parents of all the children in this study. Once consent from the parents was obtained, the surveys of demographic information, Emotional Intelligence Self-Evaluation Test and Parental Attitudes Research Inventory were sent home to mothers. The mothers were instructed to complete the measures independently, with these instructions provided in writing as well as verbally.

At the same time the researchers paid visits to mothers at home to fill the Home Observation for Measurement of The Environment (Home) Inventory. Home visits took approximately 40 minutes for per child. During this time mother's interaction with children and home environment of the child were observed and Home Observation Inventory completed by the researchers.

Children were assessed by the researchers using The Sullivan Emotional Intelligence and The Sullivan Brief Empathy Scale at the school in the interview room. It took 30-40 minutes per child. Additionally teachers completed The Sullivan Teacher Rating Scale of Emotional Intelligence for Children.

2.4 Data analysis

Firstly, gender differences in emotional intelligence were assessed performing Independent Sample T test. Secondly, relationship between the independent variables (mother emotional intelligence and parental styles, and home environment) and dependent variable (children emotional intelligence) was ascertained using the corresponding scores obtained from the variables and tested the same through bivariate correlation coefficient statistics. Finally simultaneous and multiple regression analyses were found out the predictors of children' emotional intelligence.

3. Results

3.1 Preliminary analyses

Because some researchers have found gender differences in emotional responding and managing (Goodvin, Carlo, Torquati, 2006) and to examine possible gender differences in the emotional intelligence Independent Sample t test was performed.

	Sex	N	Mean	Std. Deviation	
Recognising emotions					
Faces	Girl	66	14.23	2.12	
	Boy	78	14.71	2.01	$t_{(142)}$=-1.39
Stories	Girl	66	3.83	.83	
	Boy	78	3.49	1.07	$t_{(142)}$=2.14*
Understanding	Girl	66	7.50	1.69	
	Boy	78	7.31	1.64	$t_{(142)}$= .69
Managing emotions	Girl	66	4.61	1.51	
	Boy	78	4.80	1.59	$t_{(142)}$=-.73
Total EI	Girl	66	30.17	3.91	
	Boy	78	30.30	4.41	$t_{(142)}$=-.18
Empathy	Girl	66	9.38	1.05	
	Boy	78	9.28	1.15	$t_{(142)}$= .52
Teacher ratings	Girl	66	35.38	8.26	
	Boy	78	33.19	9.78	$t_{(142)}$=1.43

*p<.05

Table 1. Children's gender differences and emotional intelligence

An independent samples t-test revealed significant gender differences in "defining emotions" subtest of emotional intelligence (t=2,297 p<0.05) with girls scoring higher than boys (M (girls)=3, 89, SD = 0.84 ; M (boys) = 3.51, SD = 1.10). However, there were no significant differences in Understanding Emotions ($t_{(142)}$= ,693), Managing Emotions ($t_{(142)}$=--,727), Total EI ($t_{(142)}$=-,183), Empathy ($t_{(142)}$= ,524) and Teacher ratings ($t_{(142)}$=,1,434).

3.2 Correlations

Correlations among children emotional intelligence and maternal attitudes, home environment and maternal emotional intelligence are shown in table 2. Recognising emotions was negatively associated with overprotective attitudes of mothers (faces: r=-17, p<.05) and home environment (stories: r=-20, p<.05) on the other hand positively correlated with maternal emotional intelligence (r=24, p<.01). Understanding emotions was negatively associated with overprotective attitudes (r=-16, p<.05) but positively associated with democratic attitudes (r=20, p<.05). Overall there were negative relationship between children' total emotional intelligence and maternal overprotective behaviour (r=-20, p<.05) and positive and strong relationship with maternal emotional intelligence (r=20, p<.05).

	1.a	1b	2	3	4	5	6	7	8	9	10	11	12	13
1. Recognising emotions 1a.Faces		.27**	.29**	.11	.11	-.02	.71**	-.04	-.17*	.03	.09	.093	.06	.24**
1b. Stories			.17*	.14	.05	.10	.49**	-.20*	-.09	.05	.130	.15	.06	-.05
2.Understanding				.44**	.32**	.06	.74**	.04	-.17*	.20*	-.062	-.05	.04	.25**
3.Managing					.25**	.10	.63**	-.07	-.08	.01	.013	.01	.06	.04
4.Empathy						.05	.28**	.12	.02	.05	-.086	-.11	.02	.02
5.Teacher ratings							.08	.05	.09	.09	.200*	.09	-.01	.01
6.Total EI								-.07	-.20*	.11	.056	.07	.08	.22**
7.Home environment									-.15	.24**	-.136	-.10	-.15	.21*
8.Overprotective										-.05	.161	.16	-.07	-.27**
9.Democratic											-.029	.09	-.08	.39**
10.Rejecting Housewife role												.71**	-.15	.00
11.Marital conflicts													-.17*	.06
12.Strict discipline														-.09
13. Maternal EI														

*P<.05 **P<.01

Table 2. Correlations between children emotional intelligence and maternal characteristics

Maternal attitudes accounted for 7% of the variance in emotional intelligence ($F_{(5,138)}$ = 2.01 p<.05). As seen table 3 maternal attitudes results were significant only for the overprotective mothering (β=-.09, p<.05) indicating that overprotective attitudes had negative effect on children's emotional intelligence. Democratic mothering scores were not significant predictors in this analysis. Therefore, it appears that overprotecting attitudes in mothers would be a negative effect on emotional intelligence of children.

Independent variables	B	SEB	β
Maternal attitudes;			
Overprotective mothering	-.10	.04	-.21*
Democratic	.11	.09	.11
Rejecting the role of housewife	.03	.06	.07
Marital conflicts	.04	.09	.06
Strict discipline	.06	.06	.10
$R^2= .07$, $F_{(5,138)} = 2.01$*			
Maternal Emotional Intelligence	.02	.01	.22*
$R^2= .05$, $F_{(1,42)} = 7.45$*			
Home environment	-.06	.07	-.07
$R^2= .01$, $F_{(1,42)} = .75$			

*$p<.05$

Table 3. Summary of regression analysis predicting children's emotional intelligence from maternal and home characteristics

Beside this negative predictor, maternal emotional intelligence was found a positive predictor of children's emotional intelligence ($R^2= .05$, $F_{(1,42)} = 7.45$, $\beta=.02$ p<.05). High maternal emotional intelligence predicted high emotional intelligence in children.

Final result from Table 3, revealed that home environment failed to predict the emotional intelligence in children ($R^2= .01$, $F_{(1,42)} = .75$, $\beta =-.06$ p>.05). In sum, in the light of the analyses it can be seen that maternal protecting and emotional intelligence estimated the children's emotional intelligence stronger than home environment.

4. Discussion

This study aimed to evaluate and compare the relationship among children's emotional intelligence and maternal parenting style, emotional intelligence and home environment. The study findings suggest that gender differences partially had effect children's emotional intelligence. Consistent with results of many other studies (Bruno, England, & Chambliss 2002; Bosacki & Moore 2004) girls were recognising emotions more than boys.

Compared with the many prior research (Parke, et al., 1992; Thompson, 1994, Nixon and Watson 2001, Chen et al., 2005, McLaughlin, et al. 2007, Scheroeder & Kelley 2009) the home environment was not found as a significant predictor of children's emotional intelligence in the study. Consistent with this result Schimitz (2006) indicated that home environment was not predictive of child global self-esteem.

Negative associations found between emotional intelligence of children's and mothers' attitudes also. The overprotective attitudes revealed negatively with children's emotional intelligence. In Turkish mothers depending on the cultural characteristics and strict family interactions overprotective mothering has been frequently appeared. For instance Arı &

Secer (2003) also stated when the Turkish mothers were less protective their children had higher social problem solving capability.

Children's emotional intelligence can be supported with the positive or moderate parental behaviours rather than overprotective and harsh discipline parenting style (Alegre, & Benson, 2010). Moderate parents appreciate emotions of children and try to understand them through empathy. It has observed that children of this parents are usually conscious about their own selves and their environment, have developed social skills and self esteem, in other words they have high emotional intelligence (Shapiro, 2000, Eisenberg, et al., 2003, Alegre, 2011). Moreover overprotective behaviours of mothers restrict child behaviours, discourage child independence and lead the shyness and internalizing problems in childhood (Rubin & Burgess, 2002, Coplan, Reichel, & Rowan, 2009).

The results in this study provide perhaps the strongest support for the hypothesis that how maternal emotional intelligence predicts children's emotional intelligence. Results showed that as mother's emotional intelligence increases, children's emotional intelligence also increases. Parent's internal control, warm and positive family atmosphere also affect children positively (Ozabaci, 2006). Parents which are qualified emotionally seem to place emphasis on emotions within the family, develop empathy, display consistent attitudes and try to solve children's negative behaviours through empathy (Bradley et al., 2008).

In sum outcomes emphasize that mother' attitudes and emotional intelligence has a critical impact on emotional intelligence of children. A progress mother's attitude or emotional skills will lead a progress in emotional intelligence in children. If a child is raised to have poor emotional intelligence, that child is more likely to have difficulty, to make choices that are to his/her own detriment, to have problems dealing with stress and to be an unhappy and angry person (Sung, 2011).

Due to the attitudes of parents have direct effect on children's emotional intelligence, it should be accepted that the enhancement of the parents' attitudes would be the first step to support emotional intelligence of children (Alegre, 2011). While parents' attitudes are supported, children's emotional intelligence and home atmosphere are supported as well. Especially in early childhood it will be more effective to support parents' attitude to improve emotional intelligence of children.

Although there were many studies focus on emotional understanding and regulation and parental factors in school age children very little research aimed to focus on the emotional intelligence in the early years. Despite the potential limitations of survey data, the present study has theoretical and methodological significance. Motherhood is especially centre in emotional intelligence in the early years because child lacks many of the emotional understanding and managing considered necessary for emotional intelligence. Our expectation for the future is to improve all parents and children with emotional abilities.

There are several limitations in the study that should be mentioned. We were interested to study with children and their mothers. The results cannot generalise to fathers. We included children emotional intelligence and maternal factors. It will also be important to explore the role of the peer group in emotional intelligence such as the provision of emotional support and the enhancement of self-regard. Future research could also investigate the emotional intelligence of children who come from different home environments. Finally there is still need to further understanding with studies based experimental and longitudinal methods in the area.

5. References

Alegre, A. & Benson, M. J. (2010). Parental Behaviours and Adolescent Adjustment: Mediation via Adolescent Trait Emotional Intelligence. *Individual Differences Research* 8 (2), 83-96

Alegre, A. (2011). Parenting Styles and Children's Emotional Intelligence: What Do We Know?. *The Family Journal: Counselling and Therapy for Couples and Families*, 19(1) 56-62.

Arı, R. & Secer, Z. Ş. (2003). The Effects of The Parents' Attitudes on Children's Psychosocial Based Problem Solving Capabilities. *Selcuk University Journal of Social Science*, 10, 451-464.

Baumrind, D. (2005). Patterns of Parental Authority and Adolescent Autonomy. *New Directions for Child and Adoiescent Development, 108,* 61-69.

Berk, L. E. (2002). Infants and Children: Prenatal Trough Middle Childhood. U.S.A.; Allyn and Bacon Publishing.

Bosacki, S. L., & Moore, C. (2004). Preschoolers' Understanding of Simple and Complex Emotions: Links with Gender and Language. *Sex Roles*, 50, 659-675.

Bradley, R.G.; Binder, E.B.; Epstein,M.P.; Tang, Y.; Nair, H.P.; Liu,W.; Gillespie, C.F.; Berg, T.; Evces, M.; Newport, D.J.; Stowe, Z.N.; Heim, C.M.; Nemeroff, C.B., Schwartz,A.; Cubells, J.F.& Ressler, K.J. (2008). Influence of Child Abuse on Adult Depression. Archives of General Psychiatry 65, 190–200.

Bruno, K.; England, E. & Chambliss, C. (2002). Social and Emotional Learning Programs for Elementary School Students. available from http://search ERIC.Org/ericde/ED463097. htm

Caldwell, B. M., & Bradley, R. H. (1984). *Home Observation for Measurement of the Environment.* Revised edition. Little Rock: University of Arkansas at Little Rock.

Chen, X.; Chang, L;, He, Y.& Liu, H. (2005). The Peer Group as a Context: Moderating Effects on Relations between Maternal Parenting and Social and School Adjustment in Chinese Children. *Child Development*, 76(2), 417 – 434.

Cicchetti, D., & Schneider-Rosen, K. (1986). *An Organizational Approach to Childhood Depression.* in M. Rutter, C. E. Izard, & P. E. Read (Eds.), Depression in Young People (pp. 71-134). New York: Guilford Press.

Cole, P. M.; Martin, S. E., & Dennis, T. A. (2004). Emotion Regulation as a Scientific Construct: Methodological Challenges and Directions for Child Development Research. *Child Development*, 75, 317-333.

Coplan, R. J.; Reichel, M. & Rowan, K. (2009). Exploring the Associations between Maternal Personality, Child Temperament, and Parenting: A Focus On Emotions. *Personality and Individual Differences* 46, 241–246.

Denham, S. (2007). Dealing with Feelings: How Children Negotiate The Worlds of Emotions and Social Relationships. *Cogniţie, Creier, Comportament / Cognition, Brain, Behavior*, 11 (1)), 1 – 48.

Denham, S. A.; Workman, E.; Cole, P. M.; Weissbrod, C.; Kendziora, K. T., & Zahn- Waxler, C. (2000). Prediction Of Externalizing Behavior Problems from Early to Middle

Childhood: The Role of Parental Socialization and Emotion Expression. *Development and Psychopathology, 12,* 23-45.

Eisenberg, N., & Morris, A. S. (2002). *Children's emotion-related regulation.* In H. Reese, & R. Kail (Eds.), *Advances In Child Development And Behavior* (Vol. 30, pp. 189–229). San Diego, CA: Academic Press.

Eisenberg, N.; Cumberland, A., & Spinrad, T. L. (1998). Parental Socialization of Emotion. *Psychological Inquiry, 9,* 241 – 273.

Eisenberg, N.; Valiente, C.; Morris, A. S.; Fabes, R. A.; Cumberland, A.; Reiser, M., et al. (2003). Longitudinal Relations Among Parental Emotional Expressivity, Children's Regulation, And Quality of Socioemotional Functioning. *Developmental Psychology, 39,* 2 – 19.

Eisenberg, N.; Zhou, Q.; Spinrad, T.L.; Valiente, C.; Fabes, R. A. & Liew, J. (2005). Relations among Positive Parenting, Children's Effortful Control, and Externalizing Problems: A Three-Wave Longitudinal Study. *Child Development,* 76,(5), 1055 – 1071.

Elias, M., J.; Zins, J. E.; Weissberg, R. P.; Frey, K. S; Greenberg, M. T.; Haynes, N. M., Kessler, R.; Schwab-Stone, M, E. & Shriver, T. P. (1997). *Promoting Social and Emotional Learning, Association for Supervision and Curriculum Development.* U.S.A.

Ergin, F. E. (2000). A Study on the Relationship Between Emotional Intelligence Levels and Sixteen Personality Characteristics of The University Students. (master thesis). Turkey; Selçuk University.

Fabes, R.; Eisenberg, N.; Hanish, L. & Spinrad, T. (2001). Preschoolers' Spontaneous Emotion Vocabulary: Links to Likability. *Early Education and Development, 12,* 11–27.

Goldsmith, H. H., & Davidson, R. J. (2004). Disambiguating the Components of Emotion Regulation. *Child Development, 75,* 361–365.

Goleman, D. (2001). *Emotional Intelligence.* (Translator: Banu Seçkin Yüksel), İstanbul: Varlık Publication.

Goodvin, R.; Carlo, G.; Torquati, J. (2006). The Role of Child Emotional Responsiveness and Maternal Negative Emotion Expression in Children's Coping Strategy Use. *Social Development,* 15(4), 591-611.

Gottman, J. M.; Katz, L. F. & Hooven, C. (1997). Metaemotion: How Families Communicate Emotionally. Mahwah, NJ: Erlbaum.

Hughes, C.; Dunn, J., & White, A. (1998). Trick or Treat? Uneven Understanding of Mind And Emotion And Executive Dysfunction In Hard-To-Manage Preschoolers. *Journal of Child Psychology and Psychiatry, 39,* 981–994.

Jewell, J. D.; Krohn, E. J.; Scott, V. G.; Carlton, M. & Meinz, E. (2008). The Differential Impact of Mothers' And Fathers' Discipline on Preschool Children's Home And Classroom Behavior. *North American Journal of Psychology,* 10 (1), 173-188.

Kerns, K.; Klepac, L., & Cole, A. K. (1996). Peer Relationships and Preadolescents' Perceptions of Security in The Child-Mother Relationship. *Developmental Psychology, 32,* 457-466.

Laible, D. J., & Thompson, R. A. (1998). Attachment and Emotional Understanding in Preschool Children. *Developmental Psychology,* 34, 1038 – 1045.

LeCompte G.; LeCompte A.& Özer , S. et. al. (1978). Child-rearing Attitudes of Mothers in Three Socio-Economic Level, the Adaptation of Parental Attitudes Research Inventory. *Journal of Turkish Psychology,* 1:5-8.

Lopez, N.L.& Bonenberger, J.L., & Schneider, H.G. (2001). Parental Disciplinary History
Current Levels of Empathy, and Moral Reasoning In Young Adults. *North American
Journal of Psychology, 3(1),* 193-204.

Marr, K. & Ezeife, A . (2008). Empathy, Authoritarianism, and Recalled Parental Attitudes in
Child and Youth Workers. *Relational Child and Youth Care Practice,* 21(1), 26-

Maughan, A. & Cicchetti, D. (2002). Impact of Child Maltreatment and Interadult Violence
on Children's Emotion Regulation Abilities And Socioemotional Adjustment. *Child
Development,* 73(5), 1525;1542.

Mayer, J. D. & Caruso, D. R. and Salovey, P. (2002) 'Selecting a Measure of Emotional
Intelligence', in R. Bar-On and J. D. Parker (eds) The Handbook of Emotional
Intelligence, pp. 320-42. San Francisco, CA: Jossey-Bass.

Mayer, J. D. & Salovey. M. (1997). *What İs Emotional İntelligence?. Emotional Development And
Emotional İntelligence.* Edited By: Peter Salovey And David J. Sluyter, U.S.A.

McLaughlin, A. E.; Campbell, F. A.; Pungello, E. P. & Skinner, M. (2007). Depressive
Symptoms In Young Adults: The Influences of The Early Home Environment and
Early Educational Child Care. *Child Development,* 78, (3), 746 – 756.

Melmed, M. E. (1998). Talking with parents about emotional development. *Pediatrics,* 102 (5);
1317-1326.

Morris, A. S.; Silk, J. S.; Steinberg, L.; Myers, S. S.& Robinson, L. R. (2007). The Role of the
Family Context in the Development of Emotion Regulation. *Social Development,* 16,
2, 361-368.

Nixon, C., & Watson, A. (2001). Family Experiences and Early Emotion Understanding.
Merrill-Palmer Quarterly, 47, 300–322.

Ontai, L. L., & Thompson, R. A. (2002). Patterns of Attachment and Maternal Discourse
Effects On Children's Emotion Understanding From 3 To 5 Years of Age. *Social
Development,* 11, 433–450.

Ozabacı, N. (2006). "Emotional Intelligence and Family Environment". *Kyrgyzstan-Turkey
Manas University The Journal of Social Sciences* 16 (6), 169-177.

Parke, R. D. (1994). Progress, Paradigms, and Unresolved Problems: A Commentary On
Recent Advances In Our Understanding of Children's Emotions. *Merrill-Palmer
Quarterly, 40,* 157-169.

Parke, R. D.; Cassidy, J.; Burks, V. M.; Carson, J. L.& Boyum, L. (1992). Familial Contribution
to Peer Competence Among Young Children: the Role of Interactive and Affective
Processes. in R. D. P. G. W. Ladd (Ed.), *Family-peer relationships Modes of linkage* (pp.
107-134). Hillsdale, NJ: Erlbaum.

Petrides, K. V.; Pita, R. & Kokkinaki, F.(2007). The Location of Trait Emotional Intelligence in
Personality Factor Space. *British Journal of Psychology,* 98, 273-289

Raikes, H. A., & Thompson, R. A. (2006). Family Emotional Climate, Attachment Security
and Young Children's Emotion Knowledge In A High Risk Sample. *British Journal
of Developmental Psychology,* 24(1), 89-104.

Ramsden, S. R., & Hubbard, J. A. (2002). Family Expressiveness and Parental Emotion
Coach-Ing: Their Role in Children's Emotion Regulation and Aggression. *Journal of
Abnormal Child Psychology,* 30, 657–667.

Rubin, K. H., & Burgess, K. (2002). Parents Of Aggressive and Withdrawn Children (2nd ed..
In M. Bornstein Ed.). *Handbook of Parenting* (Vol. 1, pp. 383–418). Hillsdale, NJ: Sage.

Scheroeder, V. M. & Kelley M. L. (2009). Associations between Family Environment, Parenting Practices, and Executive Functioning Of Children with and without Adhd. *Journal of Child & Family Studies*, 18:227–235.

Schmitz, M. F. (2006) Influence of Social and Family Contexts on Self-Esteem of Latino Youth. *Hispanic Journal of Behavioral Sciences*, 28, 516-530.

Shapiro, L. E. (2000). *How To Rise A Child with High Emotional Intelligenc.* (translator: Ümran Kartal), İstanbul: Varlık publications.

Suess, G.J.; Grossmann, K.E. & Sroufe, L.A. (1992). Effects of Infant Attachment to Mother on Quality of Adaptation in Preschool. From Dyadic To Individual Organization of Self. *International Journal of Behavioral Development, 15*, 43-65.

Sullivan, A. K. (1999). *The Emotional Intelligence Scale For Children*. U.S.A.: The Faculty Of The Curry School Of Education., Univesity Of Virginia. (PhD Thesis).

Sung, H. Y. (2011). The Influence of Culture on Parenting Practices of East Asian Families and Emotional Intelligence of Older Adolescents a Qualitative Study. *School Psychology International*, 31(2): 199–214.

Thompson, R. A. (1994). *Emotion Regulation: A Theme In Search Of Definition. In N. A. Fox (Ed.),* The Development of Emotion Regulation: Biological and Behavioural Considerations. *Monographs of the Society for Research in Child Development*, Serial No. 240, 259 (242-243), 225-252.

Thompson, R. A. (1998). Early Socio-Personality Development. In W. Damon (Series Ed.) & N. Eisenberg (Vol. Ed.), Handbook of child psychology: *Social and personality development* (Vol. 3, pp. 25–104). New York: Wiley.

Walden, T. A., & Smith, M. C. (1997). Emotion Regulation. *Motivation and Emotion, 21*, 7–25.

Ulutas, I. & Omeroglu, (2007). The Effects of An Emotional Intelligence Education Program on the Emotional Intelligence of Children. *Social Behavior And Personality*, 35 (10), 1365-1372, ISSN: 0301-2212

Warhol, J. G. (1998). Facilitating and Encouraging Healthy Emotional Development. *Pediatrics*, 102(5), 1330-1331.

Webster-Stratton, C. & Herman, K. C. (2010). Disseminating Incredible Years Series Early-Intervention Programs: Integrating and Sustaining Services between School And Home. *Psychology in the Schools, 47*, 36-54.

Part 2

Emotional Intelligence:
Assessment and Training

10

The Equivalence of Online and Paper-Pencil Measures of Emotional Intelligence

Barbara B. Meyer, Susan E. Cashin and William V. Massey
University of Wisconsin, Milwaukee
USA

1. Introduction

Improved access to the Internet along with technological advances in hardware and software are prompting social scientists to move their research pursuits from the laboratory into cyberspace. While evidence suggests that online research is equivalent if not superior to traditional offline (i.e., paper-pencil [PP]) methods (Buchanan & Smith, 1999; Campos et al., 2011; Lonsdale et al., 2006; Meyerson & Tryon, 2003; Naus et al., 2009; Preckel & Thiemann, 2003), caution is urged in summarily generalizing research methods and results from one format to another. To address one of the key limitations of Internet research (i.e., measurement error), scholars have begun to examine the reliability and validity of online test formats. In studies of matched or paired samples who completed electronic and PP measures of various psychological constructs (e.g., personality, burnout, intellectual giftedness), results suggest comparable psychometric properties, factor structure, and outcomes across the data collection methods (Buchanan & Smith, 1999; Campos et al., 2011; Lonsdale et al., 2006; Meyerson & Tryon, 2003; Naus et al., 2009; Preckel & Thiemann, 2003).

While the literature reviewed above supports the general reliability and validity of Internet data collection in psychological research, it cannot be assumed that all psychological tests are equivalent across methods. Before we can consider online data collection as standard operating procedure and confidently combine the results of data collected from mixed formats, the influence of survey format on responses to specific assessment inventories must be evaluated. Little is known, for example, about the online assessment of the popular psychological construct emotional intelligence (EI).

2. Emotional intelligence

Since its introduction (Salovey & Mayer, 1990), EI, or the ability to perceive, utilize, understand, and manage emotions, has received consistent attention in both the scholarly and popular press. Despite ongoing debate over theoretical underpinnings and assessment techniques, scholars and practitioners alike have remained steadfast in their quest to use EI to describe, predict, and explain various outcomes (e.g., depression and anxiety, problem behavior, substance use, employee and customer satisfaction, etc.) across domains (Kafetsoios & Zampetakis, 2008; Martins et al., 2010; Siu, 2009; Trinidad & Johnson, 2002). Lack of agreement among applied researchers as to the conceptualization and assessment of

EI can result in, among other things, different EI profiles or recommendations for the same person (Brackett & Mayer, 2003). In an effort to better understand the need for a consistent approach to EI assessment in the applied context, we review below the theoretical models and corresponding assessment inventories typically used in EI research.

2.1 Conceptualization and assessment of emotional intelligence

Most of the research on the application of EI is informed by one of two models: the mixed model or the ability model. Mixed models suggest that EI encompasses both mental abilities (i.e., emotional self-awareness, empathy, problem-solving, impulse control) and self-reported personality characteristics (i.e., mood, genuineness, warmth) (Sternberg et al., 2000). Conversely, the ability model of EI represents an intelligence involving emotion, and the ability to use the information encoded in emotion to direct cognition and motivate behavior. The most commonly utilized mixed models and ability approaches, along with their associated assessment tools, are reviewed below.

2.1.1 Goleman's mixed model of emotional intelligence

According to Goleman (1995), EI includes "abilities such as being able to motivate oneself and persist in the face of frustrations; to control impulse and delay gratification; to regulate one's moods and keep distress from swamping the ability to think; to empathize and to hope" (Goleman, 1995, p.34). These capabilities are present in 20 competencies that fall within four separate domains: self-awareness, self-management, social awareness, and relationship management. Although Goleman's work is popular among laypersons and scholars who are new to the study of EI, comprehensive evaluation is made difficult because to date, little if any peer-reviewed research has been informed by Goleman's model or related measurement tool (Landy, 2005; Matthews et al., 2004).

The aforementioned assessment tool, the Emotional Competence Inventory (ECI) – Version 2, is a 110-item self-report measure of 20 behavioral competencies within four domains. Both the validity and reliability of the instrument have been called into question (Conte, 2005; Matthews et al., 2004), including the identification of considerable overlap between the ECI and measures of the Big Five personality factors (i.e., neuroticism, extraversion, openness, agreeableness, conscientiousness) (Conte, 2005; Matthews et al., 2004; Van Rooy & Viswesvaran, 2004). Since few *independent* peer-reviewed critiques of the ECI have been published, it is difficult to refute or confirm these concerns (Conte, 2005).

2.1.2 Bar-On's mixed model of emotional intelligence

Consistent with Goleman, Bar-On's mixed model approach suggests that EI is comprised of an array of trait and state characteristics, both of which influence an individual's probability of success. In his model, Bar-On (1997) identifies five areas of functioning related to success: (a) intrapersonal (i.e., emotional self-awareness, assertiveness, self-regard, self-actualization, independence); (b) interpersonal (i.e., interpersonal relationships, social responsibility, empathy); (c) adaptability (i.e., problem solving, reality testing, flexibility); (d) stress-management (i.e., stress tolerance, impulse control); and (e) general mood (i.e., happiness, optimism).

Bar-On uses the Emotional Quotient Inventory (EQ-i: Bar-On, 1997) to measure EI. The EQ-i is a 133-item self-report measure grouped into five higher-order dimensions. Although adequate test-retest reliability (r = .73) (Bar-On, 1997) and acceptable predictive validity (p = .20) (Van Rooy & Viswesvaran, 2004) have been established for the instrument, studies of concurrent validity suggest considerable overlap between the EQ-i and other psychological measures. Review of these convergent and discriminant validity data suggest that many items on the EQ-i pertain to personality attributes (e.g., optimism, emotional stability) (Bracket & Mayer, 2001; Conte, 2005; Dawda & Hart, 2000), so much so that it has been suggested that EI as conceptualized by Bar-On "may be a lower-level primary trait that could be placed below the Big Five in a multistratum model" (Matthews et al., 2004, p. 213).

2.1.3 Mayer and Salovey's ability model

In contrast to the mixed models explained above, the ability model describes EI as an ability to recognize the meanings of emotions and their relationships, as well as the ability to use emotions to inform cognitive activities (e.g., reasoning, problem-solving) (Mayer et al., 2001). Informed by the aforementioned description, Mayer and Salovey (1997) conceptualized an ability model consisting of the four following skills or *branches*: (a) Branch 1 (i.e., perception and expression of emotion), which encompasses the ability to identify and express one's physical states, feelings, and thoughts; (b) Branch 2 (i.e., assimilating emotion in thought), which consists of the ability to use one's emotions to prioritize thinking in productive ways; (c) Branch 3 (i.e., understanding and analyzing emotion), which encompasses the ability to label emotions and simultaneous feelings, and understand cognitions associated with shifts of emotion; and (d) Branch 4 (i.e., regulation of emotion), which consists of the ability to stay open to regulate emotions reflectively so as to promote emotional and intellectual growth. These branches represent a hierarchical structure whereby it is difficult to manage emotions (Branch 4) if you cannot first understand how your emotions influence your thoughts (Branch 3). Conceptualized in this way, EI is a mental skill or ability that develops over time with training and/or experience.

At the time of writing, two assessment inventories frequently associated with the ability model are the performance-based Mayer-Salovey-Caruso Emotional Intelligence Test, Version 2.0 (MSCEIT V2.0: Mayer et al., 2002) and the perception-based Emotional Intelligence Scale (EIS: Schutte et al., 1998). Early factor analysis calculations for both inventories suggest a factor structure consistent with the ability model of EI, yielding a score for total EI and each of the four branches (i.e., perceiving emotion, assimilating emotion in thought, understanding emotion, managing emotion) (Brackett & Mayer, 2003; Mayer et al., 2003; Schutte et al., 1998). More recently, however, Schutte and colleagues (Riley & Schutte, 2003; Schutte et al., 2002) have suggested that EI is a unidimensional construct with the EIS providing only an overall score of EI.

While research consistently suggests distinction between the MSCEIT and other psychological constructs, discriminant validity of the EIS has been called into question. For example, correlations between the MSCEIT and personality are weak, ranging from r = .03 to r = .28 for the Big Five (Brackett & Mayer, 2003; Brackett et al., 2006) and r = .04 to r = .24 for the 16PF (O'Connor & Little, 2003). Although the research of Schutte et al.

(1998) suggests nonsignificant correlations between the EIS and four of the Big Five personality constructs, the research of others (Brackett & Mayer, 2003; Brackett et al., 2006) suggests the EIS is not easily distinguishable from either personality or psychological well-being.

2.2 Perceived versus performance measures of emotional intelligence

Alluded to above, the MSCEIT and the EIS represent different types of EI measures, therefore potentially different EI constructs. A performance test like the MSCEIT evaluates individuals' item responses against objective or predetermined scoring criteria, whereas a self-report or subjective measure such as the EIS asks individuals to judge how good they themselves are at recognizing emotions. In utilizing and/or interpreting measures of EI, five major differences between performance and self-report measures should be considered: (a) performance tests assess actual EI (i.e., maximal attainment), while self-report measures assess perceived EI (i.e., personality traits); (b) performance measures typically require more time to complete, score, and evaluate than self-report measures; (c) self-report measures require respondents to have insight into their own level of EI; (d) self-report measures are susceptible to response and social desirability bias; and (e) self-report measures are more strongly related to personality traits and psychological well-being than performance measures (Matthews et al., 2002; Wilhelm, 2005). It appears then that performance measures of EI are less likely than self-report measures to be influenced by personality and other psychological constructs, thereby providing a more true representation of EI ability.

That said, there is a need to carefully consider not only the interpretation of results emanating from data collected by these diverse approaches, but also the instruments used to collect the data. Specifically, it has been suggested (Austin et al., 2004; Perez et al., 2005; Petrides & Furnham, 2000) that different types of measures assess two different constructs: self-report measures assess trait EI while performance measures assess state EI (i.e., EI ability). These discrepancies between trait and state EI have implications for the utility of the construct in professional practice, and may contribute to the contradictory profiles obtained for the same individuals (Brackett & Mayer, 2003).

The disparities in EI assessment outlined above have implications for future research and application, yet say nothing about the use of electronic data collection. The relative ease and cost effectiveness of online EI data collection may facilitate research, thereby expediting standardization of theoretical and empirical approaches to the study of the construct. While the correlation between PP and online administration of the MSCEIT has been reported at $r = .99$ by creators of the instrument (Mayer et al., 2003), independent confirmation is warranted. Furthermore, examination of the validity of the online version of the self-report instrument (i.e., EIS), and comparison between the self-report and performance measures will inform future EI research. By exploring further the relationship between psychometric equivalence of online and offline EI assessment, the current research contributes to the theoretical and empirical foundation upon which Internet research and EI application can be advanced. The purposes of the current study, therefore, were to: (a) examine the equivalence of online and PP measures of EI, and; (b) provide independent confirmation that the MSCEIT is a more accurate assessment of the ability model of EI, a conclusion that holds true in online format.

3. Methods

3.1 Participants

The sample of participants in the current study consisted of 157 individuals (109 women; 48 men), ranging in age from 19 to 69. For the purposes of this study, online data collected from these individuals were compared to offline data collected from individuals in previous research (Brackett & Mayer, 2003; Schutte et al., 1998). Participants in all three samples were predominantly female and Caucasian. Average age in the current online sample was 31.73 $\pm$11.65, while average age in the two offline samples were 18.93$\pm$1.51(F)/19.51$\pm$1.17(M) and 29.27$\pm$10.23, respectively (Brackett & Mayer, 2003; Schutte et al., 1998).

3.2 Measures

Two EI inventories, both informed by the ability model of Mayer and colleagues, were used to measure the construct. One inventory was used to measure the personality construct.

3.2.1 The MSCEIT

The MSCEIT Version 2.0 (Mayer et al., 2002), a 141-item performance inventory, was used to record scores for total EI as well as each of the four branches (i.e., perceiving emotion, assimilating emotion in thought, understanding emotion, managing emotion). Factor analysis calculations suggest that the MSCEIT has a factor structure consistent with the four-factor model of EI (Brackett & Mayer, 20001). Further analysis suggests a two-week test-retest reliability of $r = .86$. Similarly, results suggest a lack of convergence between the MSCEIT and self-report (i.e., mixed model) EI measures, and discrimination between the MSCEIT and well-being scales as well as Big Five personality measures (Brackett & Mayer, 2001; Conte, 2005). That is, EI as measured by the MSCEIT exists as a mental ability that is distinct from personality variables as well as other mixed measures of EI.

Because the test publisher scores the MSCEIT, we were unable to calculate internal consistencies for our sample (Day & Carroll, 2004). It should be noted, however, that branch score reliability coefficients for consensus scoring have been shown to range from $\alpha = .79$ to $\alpha = .91$ (Mayer et al., 2004).

3.2.2 The EIS

The EIS (Schutte et al., 1998) is a 33-item self-report inventory that assesses the extent to which an individual can identify, understand, harness, and regulate emotions in self and others. Using a unidimensional conceptualization, adequate internal reliability ($r = .87$ to $r = .90$) and test-retest reliability ($r = .78$) have been reported (Schutte et al., 1998). Similarly, meta-analysis results (Van Rooy & Viswesvaran, 2004) indicate that the EIS had higher predictive validity than other EI measures (i.e., EQ-i, ECI). Studies of concurrent validity suggest moderate to strong correlations between the EIS and other personality measures (Brackett & Mayer, 2003; Schutte et al., 1998; Schutte et al., 2002). Examination of discriminant validity data yields contradictory results (Brackett & Mayer, 2003; Ciarrochi et al., 2001; Schutte et al., 1998). For example, the research of Schutte et al. (1998) suggests nonsignificant correlations between the EIS and four of the Big Five constructs while the research of Bracket & Mayer (2003) suggests that the EIS is not easily distinguishable from either personality or well-being.

Internal consistency reliability for the EIS in the current study was calculated as α =.89.

3.2.3 Personality

The Mini-Modular Markers (3M40: Saucier, 2002), a 40-item self-report inventory, was used to measure Big Five Personality factors (i.e., extraversion, agreeableness, conscientiousness, emotional stability, openness). For the current sample, internal consistency reliabilities for the five scales of the 3M40 ranged from α = .74 to α = .86.

3.3 Procedure and data analysis

Online data collected in the current study were compared to PP data collected in previous studies.

4. Results

4.1 Online versus paper-pencil measures

Calculations of z-scores were used to examine differences in correlation coefficients between measures of EI and personality collected via online format in the current study and via PP format in previous research (see Table 1). No statistical differences were detected between electronic and PP data when the MSCEIT was used to assess EI. These results suggest that the relationships between EI (as assessed by the MSCEIT) and personality hold steady when using either electronic or PP data collection.

3M40	EIS			MSCEIT
	Current Study to Brackett & Mayer (2003)	Current Study to Schutte et al. (1998)	Brackett & Mayer (2003) to Schutte et al. (1998)	Current Study to Brackett & Mayer (2003)
Extraversion	.52	.42	.19	-.18
Agreeableness	3.47***	.86	-.75	-.10
Conscientiousness	.00	.18	.18	.18
Emotional Stability	5.60***	2.98**	.41	.46
Openness	-1.37	-1.23	-.61	-.57

Note: Current study utilized online data collection while previous studies used paper-pencil collection. 3M40 = Mini Module Markers; EIS = Emotional Intelligence Survey; MSCEIT = Mayer-Salovey-Caruso Emotional Intelligence Test.
**p<.01, ***p<.001

Table 1. z-Score Differences in Correlation Coefficients between Measures of Personality and Emotional Intelligence in Present and Previous Studies.

4.2 MSCEIT vs. EIS

In an effort to compare the psychometric properties of the two disparate online measures of EI, correlation coefficients were calculated (see Table 2). Correlations show a statistically significant yet relatively weak relationship between the MSCEIT and EIS total scores. Correlations also suggest that the EIS has greater convergence with measures of personality than does the MSCEIT. Concomitantly, the MSCEIT displayed divergence from measures of personality, with significant yet weak relationships identified for only the Agreeableness and Openness scales ($r = .27$, $p < .01$; $r = .19$, $p < .05$, respectively). In both cases, as illustrated in Table 1, the EIS had a significantly stronger relationship with those two personality scales. Additionally, when using the EIS three statistically significant differences were identified between electronic data collected in the current study and PP data collected previously. Taken together, these results suggest that the MSCEIT is a more accurate measure of EI ability, a finding which holds true regardless of data collection format.

| Measure | MSCEIT | EIS | 3M40 | | | | |
			Extraversion	Agreeableness	Conscientiousness	Emotional Stability	Openness
MSCEIT	1.00**	.25**	.09	.27**	.05	-.03	.19*
EIS		1.00**	.37**	.44**	.25**	.40**	.30**
Extraversion				.09	.08	.22**	.20*
Agreeableness					.38**	.46**	.19*
Conscientiousness						.26**	.11
Emotional Stability							.11

Note: 3M40 = Mini Module Markers; EIS = Emotional Intelligence Survey;
MSCEIT = Mayer-Salovey-Caruso Emotional Intelligence Test.
* $p<.05$, **$p<.01$, ***$p<.001$

Table 2. Intercorrelations for Scores on Two Emotional Intelligence Measures and Personality

5. Discussion

The primary purpose of the current study was to examine the equivalence of online and PP measures of EI. No statistical differences were detected between correlations of online and PP administrations of the MSCEIT. Correlations between the MSCEIT and personality also held constant when using online or PP data collection. These results are consistent with previous research conducted by inventory creators who identified uniformity between online and PP administrations of the MSCEIT (Mayer et al., 2003). The finding of psychometric equivalence in the current study is also consistent with studies of other psychological variables (Campos et al., 2011; Lonsdale et al., 2006; Meyerson & Tryon, 2003; Naus et al., 2009; Preckel & Thiemann, 2003), most notably those of Buchanan and Smith (1999) who utilized two different study samples. Taken together, these results support the use of online administration of the MSCEIT to assess EI ability.

A secondary purpose of the current study was to compare the psychometric properties of two disparate online ability-based measures of EI. Tests of convergent and discriminant validity suggest that the EIS conceptualization of EI lacks discriminant validity and is largely indistinguishable from personality constructs (Brackett & Mayer, 2003). It appears, then, that assessment inventories based upon the self-report and trait approaches fail to provide new information about this discrete concept, making it difficult to differentiate between EI and various personality constructs. Similarly, this strong grounding in personality traits contradicts claims that EI is a group of skills that can be learned and developed over time (Goleman, 1995). As such, it may be appropriate to consider the ability model (i.e., MSCEIT) of EI for identifying emotion-based contributions to behavior. Additionally, the self-report nature of the EIS makes it susceptible to social desirability bias (Austin et al., 2004; Schutte et al., 1998), a fact which is exacerbated by a lack of reverse-keyed items (i.e., lie-scale). These findings are consistent with those of other studies using traditional PP administration of the respective assessment inventories (Brackett & Mayer, 2003; Brackett et al., 2006).

5.1 Limitations and suggestions for future research conclusion

Results of the current study support the use of online data collection to assess EI performance. That said, several limitations exist in the current study which should be considered in future research. While tests of convergent and discriminant validity demonstrate the psychometric equivalence of data obtained from electronic and PP administration of the MSCEIT, different samples were utilized. Specifically, online data collected in conjunction with the current study were compared to PP data collected by other researchers on different samples. Although similar methods were used in several studies (Fouladi et al., 2002; Gosling et al., 2004; Meyerson & Tryon, 2003) to validate Internet-based psychological research, these threats to internal validity could be reduced by employing random assignment to online and PP groups or counterbalanced repeated measures designs (Lonsdale et al., 2006).

Similarly, various inventories were utilized to collect the personality data used in this study. Saucier's (2002) 3M40 was used to measure Big Five Personality factors in the current study, while the Revised NEO Personality Inventory was used to measure the Big Five Personality factors in previously conducted studies (Brackett et al., 2006; Brackett & Mayer, 2003). It should be noted that still other measures of personality (i.e., 16 PF, original NEO Personality Inventory) have been used in studies (Caruso et al., 2002; Day & Carroll, 2004; Roberts et al., 2001) examining the psychometric properties of various measures of EI. These disparate methods of assessing personality make it difficult to effectively assess the relationship between EI and personality. As such, researchers should consider coming to an agreement on the most acceptable measure for assessing personality.

6. Conclusion

Research in the area of EI continues to move forward, yet a lack of consistency in the assessment of the construct has slowed progress in the field from both an applied and an empirical standpoint. Given the interest in EI and its implications for performance in a variety of domains (e.g., sport, health, business; Meyer & Fletcher, 2007), the use of an ability model to define and measure EI is deemed most appropriate. In an effort to facilitate evidence-based practice and to advance this line of research (i.e., share and compare results across studies and populations), there is a need to standardize the measurement of EI (Brackett & Mayer, 2003; Meyer & Fletcher, 2007). The discriminant validity of other EI measures (e.g., overlap with personality) and the need for a performance-based evaluation, support the results of the current study which suggest that the MSCEIT V2.0 be used as the criterion for assessment of EI. That said, the financial costs associated with delivery and scoring of PP versions of the MSCEIT V2.0 may have hindered past efforts to standardize assessment of EI. The results of the current study, in conjunction with the relative ease and cost-effectiveness of online data collection, should make it possible for EI researchers to standardize their collection of EI data through use of the MSCEIT V2.0.

7. Acknowledgement

We would like to thank Blake Pindyck for his help in the preparation of this manuscript.

8. References

Ashkanasy, N. M., Hartel, C. E. J., & Daus, C. S. (2002). Diversity and emotion: The new frontiers in organizational behavior research, *Journal of Management,* VOL 28, NO 3 (June, 2002), pp. (307-338), ISSN 01492063

Austin, E.J., Saklofske, D.H., Huang, S.H.S., & McKinney, D. (2004). Measurement of trait emotional intelligence: Testing and cross-validating a modified version of Schutte et al.'s (1998) measure. *Personality and Individual Differences,* VOL 36, NO 3 (February, 2004), pp. (555-562), ISSN 01918869

Bar-On, R. (1997). *The emotional Quotient Inventory (EQ-i): Technical Manual.* Multi-Health Systems, Toronto, Ontario

Brackett, M., & Mayer, J.D. (2001). Comparing measures of emotional intelligence. *Proceedings of Third Positive Psychology Summit*, Washington, DC, October, 2001

Brackett, M., & Mayer, J.D. (2003). Convergent, discriminant, and incremental validity of competing measures of emotional intelligence. *Personality and Social Psychology Bulletin,* VOL 29, NO 9 (September, 2003), pp. (1147-1158), ISSN 01461672

Brackett, M.A., Rivers, S.E., Shiffman, S., Lerner, N., & Salovey, P. (2006). Relating emotional abilities to social functioning: A comparison of self-report and performance measures of emotional intelligence. *Journal of Personality and Social Psychology,* VOL 91, NO 4 (October, 2006), pp. (780-795) ISSN 00223514

Buchanan, T., & Smith, J.L. (1999). Using the Internet for psychological research: Personality testing on the World Wide Web, *British Journal of Psychology,* VOL 90, NO 1 (February, 1999), pp. (125-144) ISSN 00071269

Caruso, D.R., Mayer, J.D., & Salovey, P. (2002). Emotional intelligence and emotional leadership. In, *Multiple intelligences and leadership: LEA's organization and management series*, M. Riggio (Ed), pp. (55-74), Lawrence Earlbaum, ISBN 978-0805834666, Mahwah, NJ

Conte, J.M., (2005). A review and critique of emotional intelligence measures. *Journal of Organizational Behavior,* VOL 26, NO 4 (April, 2005), pp. (433-440), ISSN 08943796

Day, A.L., & Carroll, S.A. (2004). Using an ability-based measure of emotional intelligence to predict individual performance, group performance, and group citizenship behaviors. *Personality & Individual Differences*, VOL 36, NO 6 (April 2004), pp. (1443-1458) ISSN 01918869

Dawda, D., & Hart, S. D. (2000). Assessing emotional intelligence: Reliability and validity of the Bar-On Emotional Quotient Inventory (EQ-I) in university students. *Personality and Individual Differences*, VOL 28, NO 4 (April, 2000), pp. (797-812), ISSN 01918869

Fouladi, R.T., McCarthy, C.J., & Moller, N.P. (2002). Paper-and pencil or online? Evaluating mode effects of measures of emotional functioning and attachment. *Assessment*, VOL 9, NO 2 (June, 2002), pp. (204-215) ISSN 12066835

Goleman, D. (1995). *Emotional intelligence*. Bantam Books, ISBN 055309503X, New York

Gosling, S.D., Vazire, S., Srvastava, S., & John, O.P. (2004). Should we trust web-based studies? A comparative analysis of six preconceptions about internet questionnaires. *American Psychologist*, VOL 59, NO 2 (February, 2004) pp. (93-104), ISSN 14992636

Landy, F.J. (2005). Some historical and scientific issues related to research on emotional intelligence. *Journal of Organizational Behavior*, VOL 26, NO 4 (June, 2005), pp. (411-424), ISSN 10991379

Lonsdale, C., Hodge, K., & Rose, E.A. (2006). Pixels vs. paper: Comparing online and traditional survey methods in sport psychology. *Journal of Sport & Exercise Psychology*, VOL 28, NO 1 (March, 2006), pp. (100-108), ISSN 08952779

Matthews, G., Zeidner, M., & Roberts, R.D. (2002). *Emotional intelligence: Science and myth*. MIT Press, ISBN 978-0262134187, Cambridge, MA

Mayer, J. D. (2001). A field guide to emotional intelligence. In, *Emotional intelligence in everyday life: A scientific inquiry*. J. Ciarrochi, J.P. Forgas, and J.D. Mayer (Eds.), pp. (3-24) Psychology Press, ISBN 978-1841690285, New York

Mayer, J. D., & Salovey, P. (1997). What is emotional intelligence? In, *Emotional development and emotional intelligence: Implications for educators*, P. Salovey and D. Sluyter (Eds.), pp. (3-31), Basic Books, ISBN 978-0465095872, New York

Mayer J.D., Salovey P., & Caruso, D.R. (2002). *Mayer-Salovey-Caruso Emotional Intelligence Test (MSCEIT): User's manual*. Multi-Health Systems, Toronto, Ontario

Mayer, J.D., Salovey, P., & Caruso, D.R. (2004). Emotional intelligence: Theory, findings, and implications. *Psychological Inquiry*, VOL 15, NO 3 (November, 2004) pp. (197-215), ISSN 15327965

Mayer, J.D., Salovey, P., Caruso, D.R., & Sitarenios, G. (2003). Measuring emotional intelligence with the MSCEIT v2.0. *Emotion*, VOL 3, NO 1 (March, 2003), pp. (97-105), ISSN 12899231

Meyer, B.B., & Fletcher, T.B. (2007). Emotional intelligence: A theoretical overview and implications for research and professional practice in sport psychology. *Journal of Applied Sport Psychology*, VOL 19, NO 1 (January, 2007), pp. (1-15), ISSN 10413200

Meyer, B.B., & Zizzi, S. (2007). Emotional intelligence in sport: Conceptual, methodological, and applied issues. In, *Mood and human performance: Conceptual, measurement, and applied issues*, A. Lane (Ed.), pp. (131-154), Nova Science Publishers, ISBN 978-1600212697, Hauppauge, NY

Meyerson, P., & Tryon, W.W. (2003). Validating Internet research: A test of the psychometric equivalence of Internet and in-person samples. *Behavior Research Methods, Instruments, & Computers,* VOL 35, NO 4 (November, 2003), pp. (614-620), ISSN 03195541

O'Connor, R.M., & Little, I.S. (2003). Revisiting the predictive validity of emotional intelligence: Self-report versus ability measures. *Personality and Individual Differences,* VOL 35, NO 8 (December, 2003), pp. (1893-1902), ISSN 01918869

Perez, J.C., Petrides, K.V., & Furnham, A. (2005). Measuring trait emotional intelligence. In, *Emotional intelligence: An international handbook,* R. Schulze & R.D. Roberts (Eds.), pp. (181-201), Hogrefe & Huber, ISBN 978-0889372832, Cambridge, MA

Petrides, K. V., & Furnham, A. (2000). On the dimensional structure of emotional intelligence. *Personality and Individual Differences,* VOL 29, NO 2 (August, 2005), pp. (313-320), ISSN 01918869

Preckel, F., & Thiemann, H. (2003). Online- versus paper-pencil-version of a high potential intelligence test. *Swiss Journal of Psychology,* VOL 62, NO 2 (June, 2003), pp. (131-138), ISSN 14210185

Riley, H., & Schutte, N.S. (2003). Low emotional intelligence as a predictor of substance-use problems. *Journal of Drug Education,* VOL 33, NO 4 (2003), pp. (391-398), ISSN 00472379

Roberts, R.D., Zeidner, M., & Matthews, G. (2001). Does emotional intelligence meet traditional standards for intelligence? Some new data and conclusions. *Emotion,* VOL 1, NO 3 (September, 2001), pp. (196-231), ISSN 12934681

Salovey, P., & Mayer, J.D. (1990). Emotional intelligence. *Imagination, Cognition, & Personality,* VOL 9, NO 3 (1990), pp. (185-211), ISSN 15414477

Saucier, G. (2002). Orthogonal markers for orthoganol factors: The case of the Big Five. *Journal of Research in Personality,* VOL 36, NO 1 (February, 2002), pp. (1-31), ISSN 20012335

Schmidt, J.E., & Andrykowski, M.A. (2004). The role of social and dispositional variables associated with emotional processing in adjustment to breast cancer: An internet-based survey. *Health Psychology,* VOL 23, NO 3 (May, 2004), pp. (259-266), ISSN 02786133

Schutte, N. S., Malouff, J. M., Hall, L. E., Haggerty, D. J., Cooper, J. T., Golden, C. J., et al., (1998). Development and validation of a measure of emotional intelligence. *Personality and Individual Differences,* VOL 25, NO 2 (August, 1998), pp. (167-177), ISSN 01918869

Schutte, N. S., Malouff, J. M, Simunek, M., McKenley, J., & Hollander, S. (2002). Characteristic emotional intelligence and emotional well-being. *Cognition and Emotion,* VOL 16, NO 6 (November, 2002), pp. (769-785), ISSN 02699930

Sternberg, R. J., Forsythe, G. B., Hedlund, J., Horvath, J. A., Wagner, R. K., Williams, W. M., Snook, S. A., & Grigorenko, E. L. (2000). *Practical intelligence in everyday life.* Cambridge, ISBN 978-0521659581, New York

Trinidad, D. R., & Johnson, C. A. (2002). The association between emotional intelligence and early adolescent tobacco and alcohol use. *Personality and Individual Differences,* VOL 32, NO 1(January, 2002), pp. (95-105), ISSN 01918869

Van Rooy, D.L., & Viswesvaran, C. (2004). Emotional intelligence: A meta-analytic investigation of predictive validity and nomological net. *Journal of Vocational Behavior,* VOL 65, NO 1 (August, 2004), pp. (71-95), ISSN 00018791

Wilhelm, O. (2005). Measures of emotional intelligence: Practice and standards. In, *Emotional intelligence: An international handbook,* R. Schulze & R.D. Roberts (Eds.), pp. (131-154), Hogrefe & Huber, ISBN 978-0889372832, Cambridge, MA

11

Assessing Emotional Intelligence and Its Impact in Caring Professions: The Value of a Mixed-Methods Approach in Emotional Intelligence Work with Teachers

Roisin P. Corcoran and Roland Tormey
¹Yale University
²École Polytechnique Fédérale de Lausanne
¹USA
²Switzerland

1. Introduction

There has been a growing interest in the concept of emotional intelligence (EI) since it was first identified by Mayer and Salovey (Mayer & Salovey, 1997; Salovey & Mayer, 1990). The concept is one that has attracted many claims including the view that it can be assessed using pen and paper type tests (as with more traditional 'intelligence' models) and that it can predict one or another type of success in life, including academic success. One early account of emotional intelligence – now widely critiqued – even claimed that it "can matter more than IQ" (Goleman, 1995). Even if claims of this magnitude are no longer held to be justifiable, they have in many ways contributed to the popular excitement surrounding the concept. Consequently, academic researchers and theorists are thinking about the concept more critically and using more sophisticated methods of test design, interpretation and application.

Considerations stemming from such debate and concern has led to the development of a number of pen and paper type tests that claim to measure emotional intelligence (though in many cases the concept that is being measured is defined differently and the results of these tests are not really comparable in the way in which different tests of traditional intelligence models would claim to be). At the same time, theorists such as Gardner (1983, 1993) have argued that there is a need for more portfolio forms of assessment for non-traditional intelligences, while others (Sternberg, 1988; Sternberg, Castejón, Prieto, Hautamäki, & Grigorenko, 2001; Thoma, 2002) have argued that there is a need for tests to be framed in more domain specific ways if they are to validly assess cognitive operations. Corcoran (2011) highlights the importance of crossing methodological boundaries when conducting research on emotion and shows how embracing both quantitative and qualitative methods, that is being methodologically ecumenical, can help to make sense of what is actually being measured by such psychometric approaches. Indeed numerous researchers (Denzin, 1984; Sutton & Wheatley, 2003; Zembylas & Schutz, 2009) working on emotion have argued that qualitative or mixed-methods research which offers multi-perspectival answers is now needed in order to understand what is being measured by such tests. A considerable body of research into the impact of having emotional intelligence has also attracted attention to the area. The strength of this research, in many ways, lies in the link between scores on emotional intelligence tests and outcome measures such as performance in work or in other aspects of life (Bar-On, 1997b; Goleman, 1995; Mayer, Salovey, & Caruso, 2002b). Much of the focus in this has been in the use of emotional intelligence measures by management consultants, meaning many studies have been conducted in the context of organisational research and managerial practice with comparatively little attention been given to "caring" professions such as teaching where emotional intelligence is argued to be important (Brackett, Palomera, Mojsa-Kaja, Reyes, & Salovey, 2010; Corcoran & Tormey, 2010; Sutton & Wheatley, 2003). This is all the more important since what data exists on emotional intelligence and teachers suggests that, during their preservice stages of teacher education at least, they typically have a level of emotional intelligence significantly below the average for the wider population (Corcoran & Tormey, 2012). What, then, can be meaningfully said about the ways in which emotionally intelligent people would perform differently than less emotionally intelligent people in a profession like teaching?

This chapter will address these two major issues which are at the cutting edge of emotional intelligence research today. Following an introduction, the next section will evaluate the literature on the use of quantitative approaches to measuring emotional intelligence and will highlight the view that, in order to better understand and contextualise quantitative data on emotional intelligence, qualitative data is also needed. The subsequent section will give a brief overview of the literature on the impact of having emotional intelligence and identify that this too is an area that remains in need of urgent attention from researchers. The final section will present data from the largest ever research study that addresses both these issues. This study, based on the Mayer and Salovey (1997) model of emotional intelligence, will show how the qualitative data highlights the gaps and limitations of relying solely on quantitative data (as measured by the Mayer-Salovey-Caruso Emotional Intelligence Test, MSCEIT; Mayer, Salovey, & Caruso, 2002a), particularly in assessing the extent to which people have developed their emotional capacities. Drawing on interviews from student teachers undertaking a practicum, it will highlight the extent to which students who had undertaken a short emotional intelligence skills program were able to bring a more sophisticated set of emotional intelligence understandings and skills to their practice when compared to those who did not receive such training on emotional intelligence. The chapter will conclude by highlighting the areas in which future researchers should be focusing their attention.

2. Measuring emotional intelligence

In order to measure a concept it is necessary to be clear about what it is we are measuring, and here we come to perhaps the central problem in intelligence research, including emotional intelligence research. As Spearman (1927, p. 4) put it, "The most enthusiastic advocates of intelligence become doubtful of it themselves...the name really has no definite meaning at all; it shows itself to be nothing more than a hypothesised word, applied indiscriminately to all sorts of things." Things have certainly moved on in the last eighty years since these words were written, but not as much as one might have hoped. That said, there is some consensus regarding the qualities comprising intelligence, such as a recognition that it is concerned with learning, with aspects of higher order thinking (for example, reasoning, problem solving and decision making), and that it is concerned with adaptation to the environment (Neisser et al., 1996, p. 77). At the same time there are considerable differences between researchers as to whether intelligence represents just one thing or many different abilities and behaviours (Jensen, 1998; Sternberg, Conway, Ketron, & Bernstein, 1981; Sternberg & Detterman, 1986), and about how intelligence is to be measured (Jensen, 1998; Neisser et al., 1996).

Given the lack of a clear definition in the parent concept of 'intelligence' it is hardly surprising that there is also some lack of agreement in a definition of 'emotional intelligence'. The term, EI, was originally coined and developed over a series of theoretical articles (Mayer & Salovey, 1997; Salovey & Mayer, 1990) to reflect the idea that emotion plays a role in interaction with rationality in adaption and coping in life. Reflecting the idea that 'intelligence' is about learning, using higher order cognitive capacities and about adapting to the environment their definition saw emotional intelligence as being about learning, thinking and adapting using emotional information. Mayer and Salovey gradually refined their definition of EI and argued that it was a real intelligence, that is, it described a cognitive function (Mayer, Caruso, & Salovey, 1999). They came to define EI in working terms as "the ability to perceive and express emotions, to understand and use them, and to manage emotions so as to foster personal growth" (Salovey, Bedwell, Detweiler, & Mayer, 2000, p. 506). This definition encompasses their four-component model of EI with the four components being: (1) *Perception, Appraisal, and Expression of Emotion*, (2) *Using Emotion to Facilitate Thinking*, (3) *Understanding and Analysing Emotional Information* and (4) *Managing the Regulation of Emotion*.

While Mayer and Salovey originated the term EI (Salovey & Mayer, 1990) other approaches to the concept have since developed which has led to inconsistency in the way in which the term is used. Of these, Bar-On's approach – which is credited with coining the term "EQ" (Emotional Quotient; Bar-On, 1988) – is widely referred to in human scientific literature, and Goleman's (1995) is perhaps the most popularly known approach. Bar-On has broadly defined EI as addressing,

> the emotional, personal, social, and survival dimensions of intelligence, which are often more important for daily functioning than the more traditional cognitive aspects of intelligence. Emotional intelligence is concerned with understanding oneself and others, relating to people, and adapting to and coping with the immediate surroundings to be more successful in dealing with environmental demands...In a way, to measure emotional intelligence is to measure one's "common sense" and ability to get along in the world. (Bar-On, 1997b, p. 1)

This definition is what is sometimes called a 'mixed-model' of emotional intelligence, that is, it includes cognitive ('intelligence'-type) functions but also personality-type characteristics (Mayer, Salovey, & Caruso, 2000). This is even more evident when one sees that the Bar-On 'Emotional Quotient Inventory' (EQ-i; Bar-On, 1997a) includes sections which refer to personality-type factors such as optimism. As Mayer et al. (1999, p. 268) have put it:

> Such qualities as problem solving and reality testing seem more closely related to ego strength or social competence than to emotional intelligence. Mixed models must be

analysed carefully so as to distinguish the concepts that are a part of emotional intelligence from the concepts that are mixed in, or confounded, with it.

They, along with other researchers in the field (Roberts, Zeidner, & Matthews, 2001), have asserted that the term EI has become "unmoored" from both emotion and intelligence because so-called mixed models combine mental abilities (the ability to perceive emotion, for example) with self-reported qualities, such as optimism and well-being, that are clearly distinct from mental abilities. Mayer et al. (1999) have argued that EI should be conceptualised as an ability rather than a mix of traits and characteristics. Petrides and Furnham (2001, p. 426) also differentiate between 'trait EI' and 'ability EI', arguing that "ability EI should be studied primarily with respect to psychometric intelligence. Given that intelligence and personality are essentially independent domains... one would expect trait EI to be related to personality, but not to ability factors."

The second question which arises in measuring EI is how this measurement is to be done. Here four different positions emerge. A first position is to argue that emotionality can only really be assessed qualitatively. Denzin (1984), for example, argues that emotionality has best been accessed by phenomenological methods, and that "human emotional interaction must be situated in the natural world. That is, interaction must be confronted and examined in its natural fullness in the world of lived experience" (1984, p. 7). Much of the sociological work on emotions have taken this approach (for example, Hargreaves, 1998; Hochschild, 1983), seeing emotions (and, as a consequence, cognition with emotions) as being culturally-bounded phenomena that can only be described and understood in culturally-specific contexts. With respect to seeking to measure intelligences, Gardner (1995, p. 202) has claimed with respect to his multiple intelligences model that each of his intelligences can be measured, but not through traditional IQ tests (for example, he recommends portfolio models). He outlines that any assessments must be, "'intelligent fair'; that is, in ways that examine the intelligence directly rather than through the lens of linguistic or logical intelligence (as ordinary pencil and paper tests do)." This approach has been subject to considerable criticism, however, with researchers questioning whether some of Gardner's intelligences (for example, bodily-kinaesthetic and interpersonal intelligences which involve motor skills and personality traits respectively) can be considered mental abilities (Neisser et al., 1996). Other simply identify a lack of empirical evidence with respect to the theory (see for example, Sternberg, 1999). As Deary has argued (2001, p. xiv), "statistics is central to research on intelligence...discovering the pattern and significance of the differences between people cannot be done without statistical examination of the data."

A second position is to see emotional intelligence (like the parent concept of 'intelligence') as a general human capacity that can be assessed in ways similar to intelligence tests. One such test is the Mayer-Salovey-Caruso Emotional Intelligence Test (MSCEIT; Mayer et al., 2002a). The MSCEIT was designed, according to Roberts et al. (2001), as a result of several authors (including Mayer and Salovey) having advocated the development of objective, ability-based indicators of EI. The MSCEIT is a 141-item instrument, which provides skills scores for the four core emotional abilities that form the basis of the Mayer and Salovey model of EI. The MSCEIT asks the respondent to solve problems about emotions, or problems that require the use of emotion (Mayer et al., 2002b, p. 70). For example, respondents must view pictures of faces and indicate which emotions are present in the face. Using a five-point rating scale, the MSCEIT interprets respondents' ability to accurately identify the emotions expressed in the face. According to Mayer, Salovey and Caruso (2004, p. 200) true intelligence tests must have answers that can be evaluated as more or less correct, meaning some of the possible answers must be better than others. The 'correctness' of a particular answer on the MSCEIT is determined by either expert or normative sample consensus scoring methods (Mayer, Salovey, Caruso, & Sitarenios, 2003). Item scores reflect the percentage of people in the comparison sample (experts or the normative sample) who provided the same response. For example, if 70% of the expert sample (which included a panel of emotions researchers) indicated that a particular emotion regulation strategy was highly effective and a person chooses that answer, his or her score is incremented by .70. Researchers typically use expert scoring (Mayer et al., 2003).

A third model, also based on a pencil and paper approach to testing EI is the use of self-report questionnaires. The Bar-On EQ-i, for example, is a self-report measure of emotional and social functioning. Responses are based on a five-point Likert scale which range from "very seldom or not true of me" to "very often true of me or true of me"(Bar-On, 2000, p. 365). In this respect it is similar to many of the personality-type inventories that are widely used and, as was noted above, it does seem to contain some personality-type components. There are obvious validity questions which arise in relation to such an approach and Roberts et al. (2001, p. 200) have argued that, "self-report scales rely on a person's self-understanding; if the self-reports are inaccurate, these measures yield information concerning only the person's self-perception (rather than his or her actual level) of EI." This suggests that self-understanding is a key component of self-report measures. However, if self-understanding is inaccurate to begin with, this may affect the overall validity of the measure. With respect to discriminant validity, O'Connor and Little (2003, p. 1901) concluded that while the MSCEIT appeared to be measuring EI as a construct distinct from that of personality, the EQ-i appeared to be measuring personality traits. In assessing both measures Roberts et al. (2001, p. 227) conclude that, "EI is a real quality of the person, distinct from existing personality and ability factors and best measured by performance-based tests."

The fourth model is to look to combine different methods for studying and measuring emotions and emotional intelligence. Mixing qualitative and quantitiative research methods potentially has the capacity to draw on the strengths of both approaches. While qualitative studies of emotion have typically provided rich descriptions and an understanding of the social and cultural contexts within which emotions are experienced they have typically not gone on to identify the differences between better or worse approaches to using emotional information in the process of adapting to one's environment (this will be explored in the next section). At the same time, quantitative approaches have tended to insufficiently deal with cultural and social contexts entirely. Sternberg (1999) and Thoma (2002) have, in different ways, both drawn attention to the need for quantitative measures to be constructed in ways that pay more attention to the context within which decisions or actions are taken. After all, if intelligence is about the ability to adapt to the environment (and not simply about higher cognitive functions) then context needs to be part of the understanding of the operation of such cognitive functions. There is now a growing recognition – particularly among researchers working in emotion in education (Corcoran & Tormey, in press; Sutton & Wheatley, 2003; Zembylas & Schutz, 2009) - that mixed-methods research offers the multi-perspectival answers that are now needed in order to make sense of what is actually being measured by such psychometric approaches.

3. What is the impact of having emotional intelligence in caring professions?

While academic researchers were coining and studying the concept of EI it would certainly not have given rise to such public interest were it not for the work of Daniel Goleman in popularising the term. A key part of public interest in the concept is probably related to Goleman's claims for the predictive validity of his model and that EI can matter more than IQ (Goleman, 1995). Goleman claimed that EI - which included, in his conceptualization, zeal, self-control and persistence – could be taught to children, could enable them to unlock their intellectual potential, and could at the same time counteract a sense of moral deficiency and enhance altruism in wider society (1995, p. xii). Few ideas can ever have been subject to so many claims as EI. Goleman followed the success of *Emotional Intelligence* with a second book, this time on emotional intelligence in the workplace in which more claims were made including the claim that, compared to IQ and expertise, emotional competences mattered twice as much in contributing to excellence in work (1998, p. 31). Independent reviews of Goleman's popular writings have since shown that many of his claims are unsubstantiated or excessive (Epstein, 1998; Hedlund & Sternberg, 2000; Roberts et al., 2001). Nonetheless the question remains valuable because, if EI is not found to be useful in helping people adapt to their world then it is not, by definition, a form of intelligence at all.

There has been considerable focus on the potential of emotional intelligence and its utility for managers (Caruso & Salovey, 2004; Goleman, 1998). However, there has been rather less focus on the role of emotional intelligence in other areas such as in caring professions, like teaching. This is, perhaps, surprising because emotions are inherent to teaching and it is considered one of the most stressful occupations (Hargreaves, 1998; Johnson et al., 2005; Kyriacou, 1987). Yet despite this, until quite recently there was relatively little focus on emotion in educational studies research. Indeed, the mention of the term "emotion" is absent from mainstream literature advocating educational reform (Hargreaves, 1998). As Rosiek has noted:

> Human experience is an emotional affair...It is distressing, therefore, that we find ourselves in a moment when the public discourse about education is so exclusively focused on measurable cognitive outcomes of teaching. (2003, p. 399)

One of the reasons for the paucity of research in this area is the recency of the "emotional revolution" in psychology which began in the early 1980s (Sutton & Wheatley, 2003, p. 328). By the mid to late 1990s this had impacted on teacher education. The special edition of the *Cambridge Journal of Education* (edited by Nias, *1996),* along with several articles by Hargreaves (1998, 2000), attracted some much needed attention to the area. However, according to Sutton and Wheatley (2003), broad sociological studies of beginning and experienced teachers' lives underpin much of the empirical literature on emotions in teaching. For example, recent studies have focused on a variety of pleasant (positive) and unpleasant (negative) emotions teachers confront while teaching (Hargreaves, 1998; Sutton & Wheatley, 2003). Good teachers are described by Hargreaves as being not just, "well-oiled machines" (1998, p. 835). At various times teachers, "worry, hope, enthuse, become bored, doubt, envy, brood, love, feel proud, get anxious, are despondent, become frustrated, and so on" (Hargreaves, 2000, p. 812). The experience of positive emotions can enhance teacher health and well-being (Fredrickson, 2000) as well as self-efficacy (Sutton & Wheatley, 2003). Teachers' experience of positive emotions also may help young students adjust to school

(Birch & Ladd, 1996), cultivate a stronger sense of community in the classroom (Schaps, Battistich, & Solomon, 1996), enhance academic performance and increase socially competent behavior in students (Wentzel, 2002). Unfortunately, according to Emmer (1994) teachers report experiencing negative emotions more frequently than positive ones. For example, teachers experience negative emotions due to the complexities and uncertainties of their work (Helsing, 2007). Teachers experience feelings of anger or frustration particularly when colleagues are uncooperative (Bullough, Knowles, & Crow, 1991), when students interrupt classroom activities or behave aggressively (Blase, 1986; Emmer, 1994), while guilt arises from failure to achieve goals associated with nurturing students and accountability demands (Hargreaves & Tucker, 1991; Oplatka, 2007). Lortie (1975, pp. 143-144) refers to "a kind of emotional flooding" and "a sense of inadequacy, the bitter taste of failure, anger at the students, despair, and other dark emotions" that teachers experienced when asked to assess the outcomes of their own teaching. A number of authors discuss teachers' ability to regulate their own and their students' emotions. Hochschild (1983, p. 7), for example, discusses the "emotional labour" involved in occupations such as teaching which requires an individual to induce or suppress feelings to maintain an appropriate public and professional identity. Others similarly refer to teachers' attempts to "put up a front," or "pretend" they are feeling a particular way even when they are not (Hargreaves, 1998; Sutton, 2004) or that they are expected to, by the culture of teaching, express love, sympathy, concern (Oplatka, 2007) and communicate in a more personal and moral manner with students (Klaassen, 2002). The ability to regulate and manage emotions is often related to the stress that teachers experience which has increasingly been recognised as an international phenomenon, as studies on teacher stress have been conducted in Canada (Klassen, 2010), France (Pedrabissi, Rolland, & Santinello, 1993), Italy (Pisanti, Gagliardi, Razzino, & Bertini, 2003), the Netherlands (de Heus & Diekstra, 1999), China (Hui & Chan, 1996), Australia (Pithers & Soden, 1998), and many other developed countries (Boyle, Borg, Falzon, & Baglioni, 1995; Kyriacou, 1987, 1998; van Dick & Wagner, 2001). In one study, Travers and Cooper (1993) found that more than thirty-percent of British teachers perceived their jobs as stressful with reports of increasing pressure, while Borg (1990) found about as many as a third of the teachers surveyed in various studies around the world reported that they regarded teaching as highly stressful (cited in Chan, 2006, p. 1042). It is therefore not surprising that reports (Alliance of Excellent Education, 2004; Ingersol, 2003) estimate as many as 50% of teachers leave the profession within five years of entering it with stress and poor emotion management continually ranking as the primary reasons why teachers become dissatisfied with the profession and end up leaving their positions (Darling-Hammond, 2001). Research into various aspects of teachers' emotions is becoming increasingly important because of the increasing number of teachers leaving the profession, but also because negative emotions and experiences can reduce motivation (Pekrun, Goetz, Titz, & Perry, 2002), lower the quality of instruction (Helsing, 2007), and the "quality" of education (Schutz & Zembylas, 2009).

If emotions are an important part of teaching, this is likely to be seen nowhere so much as among beginning and preservice teachers. Positive and negative emotion experienced by beginning teachers has been well documented. According to Evelein et al. teachers, "express feelings ranging from resistance, powerlessness, fatigue in teaching to no problems and self-confidence" (2008, p. 1137). Erb likened beginning teachers' emotions to a whirlpool:

From one experience to another, the world of the beginning teacher is never still. Although the direction of a whirlpool may be predictable, the degree of activity is less predictable. Opposing currents may create small or large whirlpools. Objects may stay afloat in gentle currents, or get sucked underneath the waters' surface by the overwhelming intensity of the force. (2002, p. 1)

A number of studies also report anxiety encountered by beginning teachers due to the complexities and uncertainties of learning to teach (Bullough et al., 1991; Erb, 2002; Lortie, 1975; Sutton & Wheatley, 2003; Tickle, 1991). Meyer (2009b) examined student teachers' emotions during the teaching practice experience (or internship) through written reflections from and interviews with student teachers. She outlines that:

Student teachers are introduced to teaching in a highly controlled environment and frequently feel powerless at the same time they are being asked to assume more control. In addition, it is common for student teachers' university supervisors and classroom mentors to sympathize with the myriad of emotions being experienced. At the same time, it is also common for supervisors and mentors to urge student teachers to manage their emotions and conform to professional expectations. (Meyer, 2009b)

It is emotional tensions such as these which make the student teaching practice experience worthy of further exploration. At the same time it would appear that little has changed since Lortie's (1975) work on teachers' lives. He wrote (1975, p. 237), "the way most beginners are inducted into teaching leaves them doubly alone; they confront a 'sink-or-swim' situation in physical isolation and get only occasional cultural support in the process." This raises questions regarding how well preservice teacher education programs deal with emotion. Critics of the current system have suggested that the negative emotions experienced by novice teachers could be as a result of the lack of preparation. Stuart and Thurlow (2000) argue that undergraduate education programs inadequately prepare student teachers for the demands of teaching. Meyer (2009b) highlights the gaps in teacher education programs in addressing some of the current work on teachers' emotions, while Zembylas and Schutz (2009) highlight the need to develop teachers' (including beginning and student teachers') strategies to manage the emotional challenges associated with their work.

As we noted above, the – typically qualitative – studies that exist are certainly useful in highlighting that teaching is an emotional affair, and that the capacity to learn about and use emotional information in solving problems and in adapting to the environment is likely to be enormously valuable. However what these studies do not do is provide a framework which would allow us to clarify what are the specific ability-sets around emotion that teachers would need to have to achieve this. Nor do they allow us to test which emotional skills are of value to teachers in practice by identifying which teachers have more or less of these abilities and how that impacts upon their practice. This is where the qualitative research on teachers can benefit from and be complemented by a more quantitative approach to emotional intelligence. The EI concept is particularly of value here as it would allow us to clarify particular sets of skills, measure them and to see their impact in practice. Drawing on the four component (or branch) model of Mayer and Salovey, it is immediately evident how these skills could be relevant to the classroom teacher.

- *Perception, Appraisal, and Expression of Emotion (PEIQ)*. The skills associated with this area refer to an individual's ability to recognise, appraise and express their own emotional states (congruence) as well as the ability to empathise with and recognise the emotional states of others. This is a core skill for teachers because emotions are a signalling system and contain important data required for decision making and actions (Caruso & Salovey, 2004, p. 37). If teachers are unable to read these signals, then their information about a situation, about where both they and their students are at, is incorrect.

- *Using Emotion to Facilitate Thinking (FEIQ).* Emotional states can often be harnessed by individuals towards a number of ends. The skills associated with this area refer to the individual's ability to use emotional states to aid problem solving and creativity as well as the individual's ability to capitalise on mood swings in the knowledge that moods generate a mental set which in some cases (happy moods) are useful for thinking intuitively or creative thinking and in others (sad moods) are useful when one needs to solve problems slowly with more attention to specific details. This skill area is important both in lesson planning and in responding to mood shifts within the classroom and taking these into account in enabling different types of thinking tasks. Positive moods help generate new ideas, facilitate creative thinking and inductive problem solving, whereas more negative moods may facilitate attention to detail and help in solving deductive reasoning problems (Isen, Daubman, & Nowicki, 1987; Palfai & Salovey, 1993).
- *Understanding and Analysing Emotional Information (UEIQ).* Skills identified under this heading include the individual's ability to label and recognise emotions and also the relationships between various emotions, one's awareness of core relational themes that underlie the various emotions and also the transitions between various emotions. This skill area enables teachers to understand the way in which they and their pupils' emotions change and transition, as well as the underlying causes of these emotions. It is relevant in classroom management, for example, in recognising how emotions can progress from one to another (for example, from annoyance to anger to rage) and in recognising how to prevent issues arising by early and appropriate intervention.
- *Managing the Regulation of Emotion (MEIQ).* Skills associated with this particular section are primarily concerned with the individual's openness to experience various moods and emotions and to generate or mange emotions in oneself and others towards desired ends. According to Intrator (2006, p. 234), "classrooms in particular, are awash in emotional energy." Teachers evaluate and respond to emotionally charged situations using a range of emotional regulation strategies (Sutton, 2004). This skill area enables teachers to effectively manage conflict type situations with pupils and strategize alternative, more desired outcomes.

It is evident that the EI model provides a framework for (a) clarifying what emotional skills are potentially of value to teachers, (b) for assessing the extent to which teachers have such skills (c) and to assessing if, in practice, having these abilities are in fact associated with success in teaching. According to emotional intelligence research, high EI in adults in general has been associated with less aggressive behavior; less drug, alcohol, and tobacco consumption; lower rates of anxiety and depression; higher empathy and well-being; and higher job satisfaction (Brackett, Mayer, & Warner, 2004; Mayer et al., 2002b). The ability to regulate emotions also should influence how teachers express emotions, manage stress, and interact with others (Gil-Olarte Marquez, Palomera, & Brackett, 2006; Gross, 2002; Lopes, Salovey, Côté, & Beers, 2005). At the same time, there are few studies looking at emotional intelligence in teaching. Byron (2001) reported that novice teachers scored no differently on measures of emotional intelligence than the normative sample. Byron used an early version of the test (MSCEIT version 1.1). A contrary view is found in more recent research with secondary school teachers in England (Brackett et al., 2010). Using just one branch of the MSCEIT-Branch 4, this study shows that the mean MEIQ score (which they refer to as emotion-regulation ability) for participants was slightly lower (about 0.5 of a standard deviation) than those reported in the normative sample. They also found that teachers who are more skilled at regulating their emotions tended to report less burnout and job satisfaction; they also experienced greater positive affect while teaching and receive more support from the principals with whom they worked (Brackett et al., 2010). Corcoran and Tormey (2010) found, using a sample of 60 Irish student teachers, that their overall EI score was about 0.3 of a standard deviation below international norms.

While one should be slow to read too much into a small number of studies, carried out with relatively small samples, these findings are notable. They do suggest that some aspects of EI (such as emotional regulation) are associated with potentially valuable teacher outcomes. They also tell us that it is possible that teachers – perhaps especially beginning teachers – may actually have comparatively low levels of EI. Critics of current systems for preservice teacher education have suggested that the negative emotions experienced by novice teachers could be as a result of the lack of preparation. Stuart and Thurlow (2000) argue that undergraduate education programs inadequately prepare student teachers for the demands of teaching. Meyer (2009b) highlights the gaps in teacher education programs in addressing some of the current work on teachers' emotions, while Zembylas and Schutz (2009) highlight the need to develop teachers' (including beginning and student teachers') strategies to manage the emotional challenges associated with their work. It is to a study based on an attempt to equip beginning teachers with just such emotional competences that we now turn.

4. The impact of emotional competence training in preservice teacher education

As identified above, the concept of emotional intelligence holds significant promise for teachers in that it could help to identify what are the particular emotional abilities that are of value to teachers (such as the four component model seeks to achieve). If these abilities can be assessed (as the EI framework implies and as tests such as the MSCEIT seek to accomplish) and if these abilities are found to be particularly useful to teachers, then this knowledge would be of significant value to teachers and to those who work with them. Ideally, in such a scenario, teacher educators may look at how their programs could help develop EI in students – if that is possible. These were the ideas that this research sought to address.

The first aim of this research project was to see if an emotional intelligence or emotional competences program, integrated within a program of preservice teacher education, could increase EI in student teachers as measured by the MSCEIT. A second aim was to see if participation in the emotional competences workshop program had any impact upon students during their teaching practice placement. Recognising the need for mixed-methods approaches, both quantitative and qualitative data was collected from the students.

4.1 The emotional competences workshop program

The students who participated in the workshop series were in the third year of a four-year preservice teacher education program for second-level teachers in physical education, engineering education and science education. The purpose was to see if the workshops could be effectively integrated into a teacher education program which was already perceived to be a busy and intense program. The workshop series was offered as a normal part of the teacher education program (not as an additional workshop offered outside of the normal timetable), and was integrated into the tutorials offered to students on the module. It was offered as an option to students within an existing module, so that some students took the 'traditional' module tutorials (the control group), while others took the 'traditional' module tutorials that integrated the EI or emotional competences skills (the experimental group). All students were assessed in the same way on the module on the material addressed in the 'traditional' tutorials (in other words, EI skills were not part of the module assessment). The EI skills workshops had to be quite limited since the students who participated in the workshop series could not be disadvantaged in assessment when compared to other students.

The intervention involved a short emotional competences workshop program consisting of a two-hour class every second week for 12 weeks (six classes in all). It aimed to develop students' emotional intelligence capacity through a range of activities. Some of these activities were developed as part of the EI skill-building workshop (Caruso, Kornacki, & Brackett, 2005) – an application-based training course for MSCEIT certified individuals – most of which were modified to include a teaching and teacher education lens. In the intervening weeks, students had to engage with content relating to the compulsory preservice teacher education module to ensure coherency with other tutorial groups. During this time students were encouraged to develop and apply their emotional intelligence skills. Some of the activities included in the workshops are listed below.

- *Perception, appraisal, and expression of emotion:* The mood meter (Caruso et al., 2005) plots emotions along two dimensions: feelings (negative to positive) and energy (high to low). This activity helps students to monitor and track change in their own and other students' moods.
- *Emotional Facilitation of thinking:* In groups, one member (the storyteller) had to pick a card with an emotion word and tell a story from their previous teaching practice/ practicum experience regarding that emotion, without using the word. The storyteller had to generate emotions in themselves and in the listener. The listener had to engage in active listening, ask question that reflected the storyteller's emotion and make empathic comments throughout. The third member of the group used a people watching chart, similar to that outlined by Caruso et al. (2004) to observer and evaluate the listener.
- *Understanding and analysing emotional information:* Students had to review a list of causes of emotions and reflect on times from teaching practice/practicum when they experienced that emotion. They had to indicate specific events that gave rise to a particular emotion. They also had to discuss the behaviour the emotion gave rise to, whether the emotion intensified or changed and so on.
- *Regulation of emotion:* Students watched video clips of teachers using preventative and responsive emotional management strategies and had to evaluate the emotionally

charged situations between the teacher and pupils. The aim of the activity was to identify how the teacher managed a conflict type situation with a pupil and strategise alternative more desired outcomes. Students also engaged in various relaxation techniques throughout the workshops and were also given a C.D. of relaxation exercises.

Overall, the Mayer and Salovey model of EI has a number of distinct strengths that make it suitable for work in this area; the EI model provides a framework for conceptualising emotional skills or competences, and the MSCEIT as a way of testing those skills.

4.2 The study design

Third-year undergraduate student teachers were invited to participate in a series of workshops aimed at developing their emotional intelligence capacity through a range of activities. Of the students who applied, 30 were selected at random (through the process of random allocation to tutorial groups by the university administration). These 30 were further divided into an experimental and a control group, again using a random selection methodology. The MSCEIT was administered (test 1) to these two groups of students. One group then undertook the emotional competences workshops, while the other did not and continued with their studies as normal. At the end of the process, the MSCEIT was re-administered (test 2) to both the experimental group and control group to identify what changes (if any) had occurred. Most of these students also participated in qualitative interviews exploring their own perceptions of emotion, of emotional skills and of their learning through their course. At this time the MSCEIT was also administered to another group of 70 undergraduate students (control group 2) selected using a stratified random

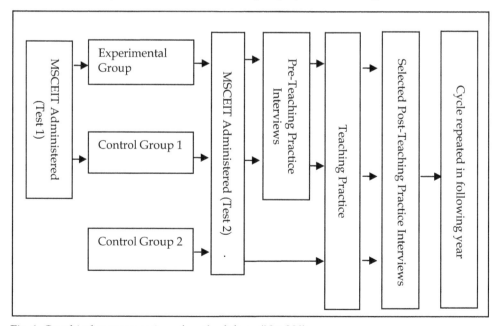

Fig. 1. Graphical representation of methodology ($N = 200$)

sampling methodology. This provided MSCEIT (emotional intelligence) scores for 100 students in total. In the later phase of the work, students were interviewed again after undertaking teaching practice to identify if their increased awareness of the skills of emotional intelligence had impacted upon their teaching. This entire process was then repeated the following year after careful review and planning. The second cohort (in cycle two) were students on the same education courses at the same point in their studies and drawn from the same applicant pool as the previous participants.

The college courses represented were as follows: Physical Education, Engineering and Construction Education and Science Education. Given the gender imbalance in the courses of study, the male student teachers were largely drawn from the Engineering and Construction programs and female students were largely drawn from Physical Education and Science programs.

4.3 Findings

As was reported elsewhere (Corcoran & Tormey, 2010; Corcoran & Tormey, 2011) the student teachers who participated in the emotional intelligence skills workshop did not show any significant increase in their measured MSCEIT during the course of their participation in the workshop program. Total EIQ for the experimental group remained static between test 1 and test 2, while for the control group it actually declined slightly (but not significantly). However, this apparent stability in fact hid some notable shifts at the level of what is referred to as branch scores (or ability areas). So, while the participants' scores for perceiving emotions in self and others (PEIQ) actually reduced over the course of the workshop series (perhaps as a result of over thinking their perceptions by the time they took test 2 or the absence of a parallel alternate test form), their scores for emotional regulation (MEIQ) increased by one third of a standard deviation. Although notable, however, this increase was marginally non-significant ($t=1.928$; $df = 29$; $p=0.064$). No comparable pattern of increase was seen in the control group.

This finding was disappointing, but at the same time it was hardly surprising. EI is described as being an 'intelligence' and so, some would argue, should not really be teachable, especially given the limited nature and duration of the workshop series. At the same time, the notable (if non-statistically significant) increase in the MEIQ score for the experimental group was encouraging and the fact that it was not seen among those in the control group hinted that more was going on than simply the typical maturation process of the students.

When students were interviewed about their experiences, a clearer sense of the impact of the workshop series began to emerge. The first set of interviews took place after the MSCEIT had been administered to the group for the second time (see Fig. 1) and before their teaching practice experience. The interviews addressed issues relating to the four components identified by Mayer and Salovey, and students who had participated in the workshops showed a greater sense of awareness of these skills than those who had not. With respect to recognising emotions in self and others (PEIQ), for example, nine of the twenty-seven students who had participated in the workshops interviewed reported an awareness of body language, with seven of these students indicating that they had developed their awareness as a result of activities in the workshops. For example, one student demonstrated an awareness of his own body language and appraised how it might be interpreted by others.

> I suppose recognising people's emotions, even the way I'm sitting here with you, I could be like this [student folds arms and crosses leg] whereas I'm probably more open this way just chatting away to you. So yes I'd recognise that even afterwards when I came into class if I was talking to you I'd be like "she's sussing me out now."

Six students identified empathy as an important skill which they felt they had developed. For example, one student described how he managed an interaction with his niece differently after taking part in the workshops. He described how his ability to empathise not only helped him to see and understand things from her perspective, but also to reach a shared understanding.

> Put myself in her position the next time it happened and then just talked it through as to why it couldn't happen. Like, see where she was coming from, accept that her thing was valid and then put your own point across and reach a compromise. That was a much better outcome, we both got what we wanted and it worked out fairly well.

Another student similarly reported how the workshops helped him to consider other people's emotions. He articulated the value of allowing people to express themselves and indicated that the ability to empathise with others was highly beneficial.

> I certainly take more time to consider the emotions of the people I'm dealing with. This is something I feel will be very useful… In the past I may have found I might be a little too invasive, but if you consider that someone is coming to you say to speak about something that concerns them or whatever, they perhaps want you to investigate a little further. That they don't want to come out with directly how they're feeling or what's affecting them. They want you to perhaps draw them out a little bit, it makes it easier for them to speak of it. Certainly empathy is something of huge benefit if you can develop that. If this module is showing that that's developing within me that can't be bad.

Students who had participated in the workshops also showed an awareness of emotional management. Fifteen students highlighted strategies that involved modifying the situation as important regulation strategies. For example, they highlighted modifying lesson plans, modifying teaching methods, and refocusing lessons based on their own and their pupils' emotions. One student said, "Just look at the different things and how it could affect your class; you might have to change your whole plan depending on the day. I didn't really look into that in [previous teaching practicum experience] at all". In total, twenty-four of the twenty-seven students who were interviewed reported cognitive change strategies as important emotional regulation strategies. For example, they highlighted using relaxation techniques, shifting perspectives, self-talk, looking at things more positively and putting things into perspective.

Twenty-three of the thirty students in the control group were also interviewed. Obviously, given that they had not participated in the workshops they were unlikely to refer to emotional skills development through their tutorials; however, they were given opportunities to describe how they had developed emotional skills over the course of their program more generally. They had also taken the MSCEIT and received feedback on it and were able to reflect upon its meaning for them. These students tended to highlight what they perceived to be gaps in their knowledge and skills rather than highlighting what they felt they had learned about emotional skills during their teacher education program. A typical response came, for example, from one student who said she never, "thought about how to construct an atmosphere that is positive or if you need loads of energy how to do that." She discussed her surprise when pupils were not as excited about participating in an experiment she had organised on a previous teaching practice placement and said, "You would need to know the atmosphere there and try to increase their perception of the task and get them into the mood for doing it."

Students were again interviewed after their next teaching practicum experience in order to identify if they had used the skills developed in the workshop series or if indeed they had 'washed out' when they were faced with the complex reality of classroom life once more. Those who had participated in the workshop series typically identified that they used some of the skills developed through the workshop series while on teaching practice. As one put it:

> For me it definitely was effective for teaching practice. I know myself I did learn from it. At the start I was sceptical, I was thinking how will this work, how is it going to change and I said well if I learn one thing from it I will be happy, and I learned a lot from it, and it really did affect, compared to second year, teaching practice. I'm definitely more aware of it and it did help me teaching because I could tell where the [pupils] were like, he is going to drift now because I'm saying something that he is not interested in. You would ask them a question and you would see them looking away and you would spot them, just little things like that. Definitely reading emotions was a big thing for me. That was what the most part of the course that I used on teaching practice. It was the most effective.

Students that had participated in the workshops highlighted an increased awareness of their own and other people's body language on teaching practice. Students highlighted activities in the workshops such as storytelling from teaching practice and group work activities as important in terms of developing these emotional skills. Students in the experimental group highlighted an increased awareness of their own tone of voice and of the tone of voice of others on teaching practice. While many students demonstrated a vague awareness of how emotions can enhance thinking, nobody directly highlighted which emotions were associated with success in different types of thinking tasks. Students were more likely to indicate that pupils' moods changed at particular times of the day. Some indicated that activities in the workshops, such as the match the mood to the task activity, had made them more aware of this emotional issue. While a number of students indicated that they tried to see things from another perspective on teaching practice, students tended to be vague in articulating how they shifted perspectives. Students indicated that they were more aware of the relationships and transitions between various emotions in relation to themselves and others. They highlighted activities in the workshops as important in terms of making them more aware of emotional progressions on teaching practice. Students were more likely to focus on basic emotions such as anger, happiness and sadness with some demonstrating a limited emotional vocabulary, which may have inhibited their reasoning about emotion. Students also demonstrated some understanding of the causes of emotions, and an ability to engage in emotional what-if analysis.

Students in the control group tended to be very limited in the understanding of emotional processes that they displayed in the interviews post-teaching practice. Few students in the control group discussed an awareness of various skills relating to themselves and to others on teaching practice. Six students in the control group reported difficulties in regulating their emotions on teaching practice. Students highlighted the difficulty in taking pupils' behaviour and comments less personally and in regulating their pupils' emotions, with one student questioning whether the teacher education program adequately prepares students in terms of emotional regulation. While students in the control group were able to describe the strategies they used to regulate emotions while on teaching practice, some strategies were obviously less appropriate than others, with some students expressing regret when reflecting on their response to certain situations.

Overall, while the quantitative data showed little or no change in the group who had taken the EI skills workshop, and measured them as broadly comparable to the control group, the qualitative data showed some quite interesting differences. The group who had taken the EI-skills workshops showed a greater sensitivity to and awareness of emotions and emotional information in relation to teaching. This was true both before their teaching practice (that is, a short period after the workshop series) and after their teaching practice (a period of some months after the workshop series). The group who had not taken the workshop tended to speak about emotion issues with respect to what they felt they still needed to learn to be an effective teacher, rather than with respect to what they had learned over the course of their program. While the knowledge and awareness of those who had taken the workshops was sometimes presented in general and vague terms, it was far more specific and framed much more clearly than the views of those who had been in the control group.

5. Limitations and future directions

In this study the MSCEIT was used as a means of assessing EI in student teachers, as it appears to offer higher levels of discriminant validity and construct validity than alternative measures of EI. It was investigated whether or not a short EI-skills workshop, integrated into a teacher education program, would lead to an increase in measured EI. It did not, though it did hint at a possible increase in the emotional regulation score for those who participated in the workshops. This was combined with a qualitative approach to data collection, based on interviews with students who had participated in the EI skills workshop and those who had not. The findings indicate that despite the similarity of their average EI scores, the two groups showed notable differences with those who had taken the workshops showing a greater awareness of emotional issues and of emotional skills when compared to those who had not taken the workshops.

Despite considerable methodological strengths, these findings need to be interpreted in the context of some important conceptual and methodological limitations. First, it is possible that the MSCEIT is not sensitive enough to detect what were some important changes in students between their first and second testing. In addition to this, these data have been collected in an Irish context. As with all quantitative tests it is still open to question as to whether or not the norms are genuinely transferable across different ethnic groups or national origins (Sue, 1999). However, the test was reviewed for cultural applicability before its use and no issues with language were reported by participants during the testing. A

Assessing Emotional Intelligence and Its Impact in Caring Professions: The Value of a Mixed-Methods
Approach in Emotional Intelligence Work with Teachers

211

Confirmatory Factor Analysis (CFA) involving a larger sample was performed also to see if the factor structure remains valid in an Irish context. Second, another possible explanation is that the MSCEIT measures something that is more or less fixed ('emotional intelligence') and that the qualitative interviews were in fact picking up changes in something more malleable ('emotional competences' or 'emotional awareness'). Given that the changes noted in the students (whether they are deemed to be 'emotional intelligence' or 'emotional competences') were seen by the students to be quite meaningful in shaping and helping their practice in schools, it is clear that they were worth knowing about. Third, the MSCEIT asks participants to solve problems about emotions, or problems that require the use of emotion, and is based on scenarios typical of everyday life (Mayer et al., 2002b). However, presenting participants with broad social scenarios that lack any educational and teaching content (that is, they are not context-specific) may result in the participants abandoning their teaching role when taking the test and thereby compromise the results. For example, participants' responses may depend on their ability to empathize with the character in the scenario or understand the problem fully, owing to similar personal experience or familiarity with particular scenarios. This in turn raises methodological considerations and potential for future research; ideally scenarios should closely mimic reality (Roberts, MacCann, Matthews, & Zeidner, 2010; Sternberg, 1999; Thoma, 2002). This may mean a need to develop context-specific versions of tests, such as test specifically designed for teachers, for example. Fourth, it is possible that students' responses in the interviews may have been positively biased. Possible reasons for such bias include the relationship between the students and interviewer (who also facilitated the emotional intelligence skills education program). While techniques were used to overcome such bias, it is important to acknowledge that factors such as these may have influenced their responses. For these reasons, it seems clear that supplementing the quantitative data collection with qualitative data was quite valuable. Finally, this study investigates the impact of having emotional intelligence in a profession like teaching. However, future research needs to determine whether there is a relationship between students' levels of emotional intelligence (as measured on the MSCEIT), and both their performance as a teacher in schools (as measured by grades on teaching practicum) and their academic scores (Corcoran & Tormey, 2012). Given that teaching practice is considered a core component within teacher education programs across Europe (Drudy, 2004) and in the U.S. (Darling-Hammond & Baratz-Snowden, 2005), such research would explicitly uncover the EI skills that are associated with both teaching performance and academic scores.

6. Conclusion

The emotional intelligence concept is one that is of potentially enormous value to those in caring professions, like teaching. It provides a framework for making clear what emotional skills might be thought to be of particular value to teachers and why. It also provides a framework for assessing which teachers have more or less of these skills or abilities and for identifying if, in practice, these skills are actually associated with a superior teaching performance. Given the emotional workload involved in learning to be a teacher, the role of emotional intelligence at this stage in a teacher's career is of particular interest. However, the concept of emotional intelligence is still in its early stages, and there is a particular need, at this stage, for using mixed-methods approaches to looking at the role of emotional skills or capacities in teaching.

It is also worth noting that the data suggests that a very short input (six two-hour classes over twelve weeks, on top of an already full and intense program) was found by student teachers to be of real value to them in learning to teach. Critics of the current system recognise the need to better prepare student teachers to meet the challenges associated with the profession and have highlighted the gaps in teacher education programs in addressing some of the current research on teachers' emotions (Brookhart & Freeman, 1992; Fullan & Stiegelbauer, 1991; Goodlad, 1990; Kagan, 1992; Meyer, 2009a; Stuart & Thurlow, 2000). Some of the work that has been done on emotion in teacher education has proposed models that would require considerable change to and investment from programs, such as coaching/counselling models (Hoekstra & Korthagen, 2011) or teacher retreat models (Whitcomb, Borko, & Liston, 2008). This research shows that emotional competences and skills can be readily developed in preservice teacher education by providing students with a framework with which to make sense of and process the emotional experiences of being a student teacher.

7. Acknowledgment

This research was based on Roisin Corcoran's doctoral dissertation and written with the support of a Postgraduate Award (IRCHSS; Irish Research Council for Humanities and Social Sciences) to Roisin Corcoran. The authors also wish to acknowledge the support of Tom Geary and Jim Glesson in the University of Limerick for facilitating this research, and the Ubuntu Network which also funded this project as part of a study of the role of emotional intelligence in enabling student teachers to engage with overseas development issues and moral education. Correspondence concerning this article should be addressed to Roisin Corcoran, Ph.D., Health, Emotion and Behavior Laboratory, Department of Psychology, Yale University, CT 06511. Email: roisin.corcoran@yale.edu

8. References

Bar-On, R. (1988). The development of a concept of psychological well-being. Unpublished Doctoral Dissertation, Rhodes University, South Africa.

Bar-On, R. (1997a). Bar-On Emotional Quotient Inventory (EQ-i): A test of emotional intelligence. Toronto, Canada: Multi-Health Systems.

Bar-On, R. (1997b). Bar-On Emotional Quotient Inventory (EQ-i): Technical manual. Toronto, Canada: Multi-Health Systems.

Bar-On, R. (2000). Emotional and social intelligence: Insights from the the emotional quotient inventory. In R. Bar-On & J. D. A. Parker (Eds.), The handbook of emotional intelligence: Theory, development, assessment, and application at home, school, and in the workplace (pp. 363-388). San Francisco: Jossey-Bass.

Birch, S. H., & Ladd, G. W. (1996). Interpersonal relationships in the school environment and children's early school adjustment: The role of teachers and peers. In J. Juvonen & K. R. Wentzel (Eds.), Social motivation: Understanding children's school adjustment (pp. 199-225). Cambridge, England: Cambridge University Press

Blase, J. J. (1986). A qualitative analysis of sources of teacher stress: Consequences for performance. American Educational Research Journal, 23(1), 13-40.

Assessing Emotional Intelligence and Its Impact in Caring Professions: The Value of a Mixed-Methods
Approach in Emotional Intelligence Work with Teachers
213

Borg, M. G. (1990). Occupational stress in British educational settings: A review. Educational Psychology: An International Journal of Experimental Educational Psychology, 10(2), 103-126.

Boyle, G. J., Borg, M. G., Falzon, J. M., & Baglioni, A. J. (1995). A structural model of the dimensions of teacher stress. British Journal of Educational Psychology, 65(1), 49-67.

Brackett, M. A., Mayer, J. D., & Warner, R. M. (2004). Emotional intelligence and its relation to everyday behaviour. Personality and Individual Differences, 36(6), 1387-1402.

Brackett, M. A., Palomera, R., Mojsa-Kaja, J., Reyes, M. R., & Salovey, P. (2010). Emotion-regulation ability, burnout, and job satisfaction among British secondary-school teachers. Psychology in the Schools, 47(4), 406-417.

Brookhart, S. M., & Freeman, D. J. (1992). Characteristics of entering teacher candidates. Review of Educational Research, 62(1), 37-60.

Bullough, R. V., Knowles, J. G., & Crow, N. A. (1991). Emerging as a teacher. London; New York: Routledge.

Byron, C. M. (2001). The effects of emotional knowledge education in the training of novice teachers. Unpublished Doctoral thesis, Teachers College, Columbia University, New York.

Caruso, D. R., Kornacki, S., & Brackett, M. A. (2005). Understanding and developing your emotional intelligence skills. MSCEIT certification workshop, London school of business: unpublished.

Caruso, D. R., & Salovey, P. (2004). The emotionally intelligent manager: How to develop and use the four key emotional skills of leadership. San Francisco: Jossey-Bass.

Chan, D. W. (2006). Emotional intelligence and components of burnout among Chinese secondary school teachers in Hong Kong. Teaching and Teacher Education, 22(8), 1042-1054.

Corcoran, R. P. (2011). Investigating the role of emotional competencies in initial teacher education. Unpublished Doctoral Dissertation, University of Limerick, Ireland.

Corcoran, R. P., & Tormey, R. (2010). Teacher education, emotional competencies and development education. Procedia - Social and Behavioral Sciences, 2(2), 2448-2457.

Corcoran, R. P., & Tormey, R. (2011). Developing emotional intelligence in initial teacher education: An action research approach, Paper presented at the American Educational Research Association annual conference. New Orleans, Louisiana.

Corcoran, R. P., & Tormey, R. (2012). Teaching practice, academic grades and emotional intelligence among preservice teachers, American Educational Research Association annual conference. British Columbia, Vancouver, Canada.

Corcoran, R. P., & Tormey, R. (in press). Developing emotionally intelligent teachers: Emotional intelligence and initial teacher education. U.K.: Peter Lang Publishing.

Darling-Hammond, L. (2001). The challenge of staffing our schools. Educational Leadership, 58(8), 12-17.

Darling-Hammond, L., & Baratz-Snowden, J. C. (Eds.). (2005). A good teacher in every classroom: Preparing the highly qualified teachers our children deserve. San Francisco, CA: Jossey-Bass.

de Heus, P., & Diekstra, R. F. W. (1999). Do teachers burn out more easily? A comparison of teachers with other social professions on work stress and burnout symptoms. In R.

Vandenberghe & A. M. Huberman (Eds.), Understanding and preventing teacher burnout: A sourcebook of international research and practice (pp. 269-284): New York, US: Cambridge University Press.

Deary, I. J. (2001). Intelligence: A very short introduction. Oxford: Oxford University Press.

Denzin, N. K. (1984). On Understanding Emotion. London: McGraw-Hill.

Drudy, S. (2004). Second-level teacher education in the Republic of Ireland: Consecutive programmes. Armagh: Centre for Cross-Border Studies.

Emmer, E. T. (1994). Towards an understanding of the primacy of classroom management and discipline. Teaching Education, 6(1), 65-69.

Epstein, S. (1998). Constructive thinking: The key to emotional intelligence. Westport, Connecticut: Praeger Publishers.

Erb, C. S. (2002). The emotional whirlpool of beginning teachers' work, Paper presented at the annual meeting of the Canadian Society of Studies in Education. Toronto, Canada.

Evelein, F., Korthagen, F., & Brekelmans, M. (2008). Fulfilment of the basic psychological needs of student teachers during their first teaching experiences. Teaching and Teacher Education, 24(5), 1137-1148.

Fredrickson, B. L. (2000). Cultivating positive emotions to optimize health and well-being. Prevention & Treatment, 3(1), Article 0001a.

Fullan, M., & Stiegelbauer, S. (1991). The new meaning of educational change (second ed.). London: Cassell.

Gardner, H. (1983). Frames of mind: The theory of multiple intelligences. New York: Basic Books.

Gardner, H. (1993). Multiple intelligences: The theory in practice. New York: Basic Books.

Gardner, H. (1995). Reflections on multiple intelligences: Myths and messages. Phi Delta Kappan, 77(3), 200-209.

Gil-Olarte Marquez, P., Palomera, M. R., & Brackett, M. A. (2006). Relating emotional intelligence to social competence and academic achievement in high school students. Psicothema, 18 Suppl, 118-123.

Goleman, D. (1995). Emotional intelligence: Why it can matter more than IQ. New York: Bantam Books.

Goleman, D. (1998). Working with emotional intelligence. London: Bloomsbury.

Goodlad, J. I. (1990). Teachers for our nation's schools. San Franscisco: Jossey-Bass.

Gross, J. J. (2002). Emotion regulation: Affective, cognitive, and social consequences. Psychophysiology, 39(3), 281.

Hargreaves, A. (1998). The emotional practicum of teaching. Teaching and Teacher Education, 14(8), 835-854.

Hargreaves, A. (2000). Mixed emotions: Teachers' perceptions of their interactions with students. Teaching and Teacher Education, 16(8), 811-826.

Hargreaves, A., & Tucker, E. (1991). Teaching and guilt: Exploring the feelings of teaching. Teaching and Teacher Education, 7(5-6), 491-505.

Hedlund, J., & Sternberg, R. J. (2000). Too many intelligences? Integrating social, emotional, and practical intelligence. In R. Bar-On & J. D. A. Parker (Eds.), The handbook of emotional intelligence: Theory, development, assessment, and application at home, school, and in the workplace (pp. 136-168). San Francisco: Jossey-Bass.

Assessing Emotional Intelligence and Its Impact in Caring Professions: The Value of a Mixed-Methods
Approach in Emotional Intelligence Work with Teachers

215

Helsing, D. (2007). Regarding uncertainty in teachers and teaching. Teaching and Teacher Education, 23(8), 1317-1333.

Hochschild, A. R. (1983). The managed heart: Commercialization of human feeling. Berkeley: University of California Press.

Hoekstra, A., & Korthagen, F. (2011). Teacher learning in a context of educational change: Informal learning versus systematically supported learning. Journal of Teacher Education, 62(1), 76-92.

Hui, E. K. P., & Chan, D. W. (1996). Teacher stress and guidance work in Hong Kong secondary school teachers. British Journal of Guidance and Counselling, 24(2), 199-211.

Intrator, S. M. (2006). Beginning teachers and the emotional drama of the classroom. Journal of Teacher Education, 57(3), 232-239.

Isen, A. M., Daubman, K. A., & Nowicki, G. P. (1987). Positive affect facilitates creative problem solving. Journal of Personality and Social Psychology, 52(6), 1122-1131.

Jensen, A. R. (1998). The g factor: The science of mental ability. Westport, CT: Praeger.

Johnson, S., Cooper, C., Cartwright, S., Donald, I., Taylor, P., & Millet, C. (2005). The experience of work-related stress across occupations. Journal of managerial psychology, 20(2), 178.

Kagan, D. M. (1992). Professional growth among preservice and beginning teachers. Review of Educational Research, 62(2), 129-169.

Klaassen, C. A. (2002). Teacher pedagogical competence and sensibility. Teaching and Teacher Education, 18(2), 151-158.

Klassen, R. M. (2010). Teacher stress: The mediating role of collective efficacy beliefs. The Journal of educational research, 103(5), 342.

Kyriacou, C. (1987). Teacher stress and burnout: An international review. Educational Research, 29(2), 146-152.

Kyriacou, C. (1998). Teacher stress: Past and present. In J. Dunham & V. Varma (Eds.), Stress in teachers: Past, present and future (pp. 1-13). London: Whurr.

Lopes, P. N., Salovey, P., Côté, S., & Beers, M. (2005). Emotion Regulation Abilities and the Quality of Social Interaction. Emotion, 5(1), 113.

Lortie, D. C. (1975). School teacher: A sociological study. Chicago: University of Chicago Press.

Mayer, J. D., Caruso, D. R., & Salovey, P. (1999). Emotional intelligence meets traditional standards for an intelligence. Intelligence, 27(4), 267-298.

Mayer, J. D., & Salovey, P. (1997). What is emotional intelligence? In P. Salovey & D. Sluyter (Eds.), Emotional development and emotional intelligence: Educational implications (pp. 3-31). New York: Basic Books.

Mayer, J. D., Salovey, P., & Caruso, D. R. (2000). Models of emotional intelligence. In R. J. Sternberg (Ed.), Handbook of intelligence (pp. 396-420). Cambridge: Cambridge University Press.

Mayer, J. D., Salovey, P., & Caruso, D. R. (2002a). The Mayer-Salovey-Caruso Emotional Intelligence Test (MSCEIT): Item booklet. Toronto, Canada: Multi-Health Systems.

Mayer, J. D., Salovey, P., & Caruso, D. R. (2002b). The Mayer-Salovey-Caruso Emotional Intelligence Test (MSCEIT): User's manual. Toronto, Canada: Multi-Health Systems.

Mayer, J. D., Salovey, P., & Caruso, D. R. (2004). Emotional intelligence: Theory, findings, and implications. Psychological Inquiry, 15(3), 197-215.

Mayer, J. D., Salovey, P., Caruso, D. R., & Sitarenios, G. (2003). Measuring emotional intelligence with the MSCEIT V2.0. Emotion, 3(1), 97-105.

Meyer, D. K. (2009a). Entering the emotional practices of teaching. In P. A. Schutz & M. Zembylas (Eds.), Advances in teacher emotion research (pp. 73-91)). New York: Springer.

Meyer, D. K. (2009b). Entering the emotional practices of teaching. In P. A. Schutz & M. Zembylas (Eds.), Advances in teacher emotion research (pp. 73-91). New York: Springer.

Neisser, U., Boodoo, G., Bouchard, T. J., Boykin, A. W., Brody, N., Ceci, S. J., et al. (1996). Intelligence: Knowns and unknowns. American Psychologist, 51(2), 77-101.

Nias, J. (1996). Thinking about feeling: The emotions in teaching. Cambridge Journal of Education, 26(3), 293-306.

O'Connor, R. M., & Little, I. S. (2003). Revisiting the predictive validity of emotional intelligence: Self-report versus ability-based measures. Personality and Individual Differences, 35(8), 1893-1902.

Oplatka, I. (2007). Managing emotions in teaching: Toward an understanding of emotion displays and caring as nonprescribed role elements. The Teachers College Record, 109(6), 1374-1400.

Palfai, T. P., & Salovey, P. (1993). The influence of depressed and elated mood on deductive and inductive reasoning. Imagination, Cognition and Personality, 13(1), 57-71.

Pedrabissi, L., Rolland, J. P., & Santinello, M. (1993). Stress and burnout among teachers in Italy and France. Journal of Psychology, 127(5), 529-535.

Pekrun, R., Goetz, T., Titz, W., & Perry, R. P. (2002). Academic emotions in students' self-regulated learning and achievement: A program of qualitative and quantitative research. Educational Psychologist, 37(2), 91-105.

Petrides, K. V., & Furnham, A. (2001). Trait emotional intelligence: Psychometric investigation with reference to established trait taxonomies. European Journal of Personality, 15(6), 425-448.

Pisanti, R., Gagliardi, M. P., Razzino, S., & Bertini, M. (2003). Occupational stress and wellness among Italian secondary school teachers. Psychology & health, 18(4), 523-536.

Pithers, R. T., & Soden, R. (1998). Scottish and Australian teacher stress and strain: A comparative study. British Journal of Educational Psychology, 68(2), 269-279.

Roberts, R. D., MacCann, C., Matthews, G., & Zeidner, M. (2010). Emotional intelligence: Toward a consensus of models and measures. Social and Personality Psychology Compass, 4(10), 821-840.

Roberts, R. D., Zeidner, M., & Matthews, G. (2001). Does emotional intelligence meet traditional standards for an intelligence? Some new data and conclusions. Emotion, 1(3), 196-231.

Rosiek, J. (2003). Emotional scaffolding: An exploration of the teacher knowledge at the intersection of student emotion and the subject matter. Journal of Teacher Education, 54(5), 399-412.

Salovey, P., Bedwell, T. B., Detweiler, J. B., & Mayer, J. D. (2000). Current directions in emotional intelligence research. In M. J. Lewis & J. M. Haviland-Jones (Eds.), Handbook of emotions (second ed., pp. 504-520). New York: Guilford Press.

Salovey, P., & Mayer, J. D. (1990). Emotional intelligence. Imagination, Cognition and Personality, 9(3), 185-211.

Schaps, E., Battistich, V., & Solomon, D. (1996). School as a caring community: A key to character education. In A. Molnar (Ed.), Ninety-sixth yearbook of the National Society for the Study of Education (pp. 127-139). Chicago: University of Chicago Press.

Schutz, P. A., & Zembylas, M. (2009). Introduction to advances in teacher emotion research: The impact on teachers' lives. In P. A. Schutz & M. Zembylas (Eds.), Advances in teacher emotion research (pp. 3-11). New York: Springer.

Spearman, C. (1927). The abilities of man. New York: Macmillan.

Sternberg, R. J. (1988). The triarchic mind: A new theory of human intelligence. New York: Cambridge University Press.

Sternberg, R. J. (1999). Successful intelligence: Finding a balance. Trends in Cognitive Sciences, 3(11), 436-442.

Sternberg, R. J., Castejón, J. L., Prieto, M. D., Hautamäki, J., & Grigorenko, E. L. (2001). Confirmatory factor analysis of the Sternberg Triarchic Abilities Test in three international samples: An empirical test of the Triarchic Theory of Intelligence. European Journal of Psychological Assessment, 17(1), 1-16.

Sternberg, R. J., Conway, B. E., Ketron, J. L., & Bernstein, M. (1981). People's conceptions of intelligence. Journal of Personality and Social Psychology, 41(1), 37-55.

Sternberg, R. J., & Detterman, D. K. (1986). What is intelligence? Norwood, N.J.: Ablex.

Stuart, C., & Thurlow, D. (2000). Making it their own: Preservice teachers' experiences, beliefs, and classroom practices. Journal of Teacher Education, 51(2), 113-121.

Sue, S. (1999). Science, ethnicity, and bias: Where have we gone wrong? American Psychologist, 54(12), 1070-1077.

Sutton, R. (2004). Emotional regulation goals and strategies of teachers. Social Psychology of Education, 7(4), 379-398.

Sutton, R., & Wheatley, K. (2003). Teachers' emotions and teaching: A review of the literature and directions for future research. Educational Psychology Review, 15(4), 327-358.

Thoma, S. J. (2002). An overview of the Minnesota approach to research in moral development. Journal of Moral education, 31(3), 225-245.

Tickle, L. (1991). New teachers and the emotions of learning teaching. Cambridge Journal of Education, 21(3), 319-329.

Travers, C., & Cooper, C. (1993). Mental health, job satisfaction and occupational stress among UK teachers. Work and Stress, 7(3), 203-219.

van Dick, R., & Wagner, U. (2001). Stress and strain in teaching: A structural equation approach. British Journal of Educational Psychology, 71(2), 243-259.

Wentzel, K. R. (2002). Are effective teachers like good parents? Teaching styles and student adjustment in early adolescence. Child Development, 73(1), 287-301.

Whitcomb, J., Borko, H., & Liston, D. (2008). Why Teach? Part II. Journal of Teacher Education, 59(4), 267-272.

Zembylas, M., & Schutz, P. A. (2009). Research on teachers' emotions in education: Findings, practical implications and future agenda. In P. A. Schutz & M. Zembylas (Eds.), Advances in teacher emotion research (pp. 367-377). New York: Springer.

12

Development of a Chinese Emotional Intelligence Inventory and Its Association with Physical Activity

Gladys Shuk-fong Li, Wei Ting Li and Hsiu Hua Wang
Department of Athletic Sports, National Chung Cheng University
Taiwan

1. Introduction

This chapter aims to report the development of a Chinese Emotional Intelligence Inventory (CEII) that suits specifically to Taiwan society and culture; CEII items were created synthesizing the western and Chinese theoretical structure of emotional intelligence; next, we provided a detailed description of its psychometric properties, and finally, we examine the association of EI and physical activity for Taiwan university students.

1.1 Emotional intelligence and university students

Emotions, an integral and significant aspect of human nature and the motivation for behavior, has been recognized by psychology scholars as being an advanced topic of great significance; Emotional Intelligence is also a topic that has gained significant recognition from psychologists, scholars in education, management, and health studies over the past decade. emotional intelligence is concerned with understanding oneself and others, relating to people, and adapting to and coping more successfully in dealing with environmental demands (BarOn, 2002), and therefore, is an important indicator of future success in many aspects of life, including academic performance, career achievement (Saarni 1999; Goleman 1995; BarOn, 2002), and contributes to individual life satisfaction (Law, Wong, & Song, 2004).

Numerous studies have indicated that the ability to help predict academic performance and future achievements and success has given rise to why EI is critical for university students (Brackett, Mayer, and Warner, 2004; Bar-On, 1997; Parker, Summerfeldt, Hogan, & Majes, 2004). In their research, Parker, Summerfeldt, Hogan, and Majes (2004) conducted a study on 372 university students. They found that profound changes were experienced during the period between senior high school or college and university because of the influence of emotional intelligence and social abilities; a correlation was evident between these emotional and social factors and university students' future achievements and performances.

Nowadays, Taiwanese university students are often referred to as the "strawberry generation." This term implies that university students tend to display characteristics such as low stress tolerance difficult to adjust to changing situation, and poor emotional management skills; and they tend to evade reality. The reason for such behaviors is that university students are experiencing the transitional phase between adolescence and adulthood; the self-inflicted or external stimulants that they experience cause changes in their intrinsic or extrinsic emotion and behavior. Since emotion is a part of human life, emotion is undoubtedly one of the most critical factors that significantly influence university students' daily lives and their social interactions. Therefore, it would be interesting in examining the emotional intelligence of university student in Taiwan.

1.2 What have been done in the past literature of emotional intelligence?

Currently, the definition and theoretical construct of emotional intelligence has not reached consensus to date. In the academia of international psychology, some scholars (Emmerling and Goleman, 2003; Shi & Wang, 2007) categorized the construct of EI into three main schools of theory, including ability, mixed model, or trait.; while the other scholars (Mayer, Salovey, & Caruso, 2000; Petrides & Furnham, 2000) reported that there are two dominant approaches to conceptualizing and measuring EI (Keele & Bell, 2007; Petrides & Furnham, 2000; Tett & Fox, 2006), including ability-based EI (Mayer, Salovey, & Caruso, 2000); and an alternative to ability EI, namely, trait EI (BarOn, 2002; Schutte et al., 1998), which are used interchangeably with the other EI models, such as socio-emotional, mixed, personal factors or as trait EI.

The first distinct concept of emotional intelligence from the literature is the 'ability' theory represented by Mayer-Salovey; as measured by Mayer, Salovey, Caruso Emotional Intelligence Test, MSCEIT; Mayer, Salovey, & Caruso, 2000). Mayer, Salovey, and Caruso (2000) defined emotional intelligence as the mental ability (ability EI) to perceive emotions; to recognize, use and regulate emotional, personal and social information in an adaptive way, and to use this information to guide one's thinking and actions (Mayer, Caruso, and Salovey, 1999). The second distinct conceptual framework of EI construct evolved is the multifactorial approach of 'traits' or 'personality' theory, represented by BarOn (BarOn, 2002), and Goleman (2001). Bar-On defined emotional intelligence as the emotional, personal, social, and survival dimensions of intelligence (BarOn, 2002); it concerned with understanding oneself and others, relating to people, and adapting to and coping with the immediate surroundings to be more successful in dealing with environmental demands; and he included the personality dimensions of impulse control, optimism, and stress tolerance…in the Bar-On emotional intelligence inventory (BarOn EQ-i).

The third perspective of emotional intelligence is proposed as the mixed models, which combine mental ability with personality characteristics such as optimism and well-being; this mixed models of EI conceptualized EI as a combination of cognitive, motivational, and affective constructs (Goleman, 2001).

Proposed a four-domain framework of emotional intelligence reflecting how an individual master the skills and competencies of Self-awareness, Self-Management, Social Awareness, and Relationship Management, Goleman (2001) stressed the critical distinction of this model that these skills and competencies could be learned, and allow individuals achieve greater effectiveness in the workplace. In sum, BarOn attempts to develop a general measure of social and emotional intelligence predictive of emotional well-being and adaptation, and

Mayer and Salovey seek to establish the validity and utility of a new form of intelligence, and Goleman put forward a theory that is specific to the domain of work performance based on social and emotional competencies (Emmerling & Goleman, 2003). In sum, the definition, theory, and the measurement of 'Emotional Intelligence (EI)' developed or adopted have been distinct and controversial among researchers, however, all theories within the EI research paradigm seek to understand how individuals perceive, understand, utilize and manage emotions in an effort to predict and foster personal effectiveness (Emmerling & Goleman, 2003).

The current literature available on the topic of emotional intelligence focuses on one or some of the following four research directions and objectives: (1) the effectiveness of different variables for predicting EI; (2) the determination of emotional intelligence scales and the verification of their reliability and validity; (3) the impact that EI has on academic or work performance, on health (including physical and mental health), and recently, on sport; and/or (4) the relationship between EI and other intelligence tests or other related studies. However, empirical studies and literature on EI rarely discuss its application. In fact, only when EI-induced abilities are cultivated and promoted can the significance and value of the topic of EI be truly demonstrated. If EI is the result of a series of interrelated capabilities developing and as advocated by human development theory that life experiences influence and enhance emotional intelligence (Wong, Foo, Wang, & Wong, 2007), then it is beneficial for us to investigate into the factors that affect the development of emotional intelligence.

As we currently know, life experiences already determined as predictors of EI include age (BarOn, 1997), gender, full-time parents, and parents' EI (Wong, Foo, Wang, & Wong, 2007) . Although two indicators of EI, age, and having a full-time parent implicate the nurture effects of experience, however, these variables, with its specific nature, couldn't be modified or acquired easily. If emotional intelligence could be nurtured or trained through certain life experiences, and use these experiences to design effective EI training program, thus, lead to the development of EI, the value of emotional intelligence could then be magnified, Wong, Foo, Wang, & Wong (2007) suggested that other potential nurture effects should be examined in the future studies.

The studies of the association of EI and physical activity received attention recently (Adhia, Nagendra, & Mahadevan, 2010; Dietrich & Audiffren, 2011; Li, Lu, & Wang (2009). Dietrich & Audiffren, 2011 reported the underlying mechanisms of the relationship between EI and exercise, while Li, Lu, & Wang (2009) found that physical activity was one of the predictor variables of emotional intelligence. Nevertheless, the topic of how the experience of physical activity influences emotional intelligence and whether emotional intelligence could be mediator of physical activity behavior change, or directly leads to changes in exercise behavior has yet to be discussed.

1.3 Does emotional intelligence lead to changes in exercise behavior?

Engaging in regular physical activity (PA) which plays an essential role in enhancing physical fitness and health-related behavior, has become the prime health indicator (ACSM, 2009; Nieman, 1998; World Health Organization, 2004). However, the prevalence of inactivity among Taiwan college students has increased for the last decade; there are only 10.7% who exercise regularly enough to the recommended level that can reap the health benefits (Lin et al. 2006), thus, those inactive may lead to adverse health consequences early in life (Racette et al. 2007). While Taymoori and Lubans (2008) suggested that the lack of knowledge regarding the mechanisms responsible for behavior change may explain the low levels of effectiveness in PA interventions among individuals, Dishman (2004) indicated that emotional changes related to exercise are an important part of exercise adherence. Thus, hypothesizing EI as a key component for the development of regular exercise behavior seems rationale.

The impact of emotional intelligence towards optimal health has been well documented. Through a comprehensive meta-analysis of the correlational studies of emotional intelligence and health, higher EI is linked with better health, thus, the value of EI as a plausible health predictor had been recognized (Martins, Ramalho, & Morin, 2010; Schutte, et. al. 2007). If EI might lead to changes in healthy behavior, hypothesizing a connection between EI and exercise behavior seems rational. However, emotional intelligence (EI) has received scant attention from researchers in the sport or exercise domain to date (Laborde, Brull, Weber, & Anders, 2011; Lu, Li, Hsu, & Williams, 2010), yet some researchers agreed that emotions are key to exercise and sport performance (Biddle, 2000; Laborde, Brull, Weber, & Anders, 2011; Vallerand & Blanchard, 2000). Vallerand & Blanchard (2000) suggested that emotional processes typically play an adaptive role in sport and exercise settings, high levels of emotional experience may facilitate participation in sport and exercise activities from both an intra- and an interpersonal perspective.

Recently, the studies of EI in the sport context began to receive some attention. Sizzi, Deaner,, & Hirschhorn (2003) indicated that an athlete must recognize one's emotions, as well as teammates' and opponents' emotions, in order to perform well in team sports. Moreover, Laborde, Brull, Weber, & Anders (2011) confirmed the link between EI and stress coping in athletes, Laborde, Brull, Weber, & Anders (2011) found that high trait EI athletes (handball players) experienced a lower increase of stress compared to their low trait EI counterparts, indicating trait EI may help athletes cope better with stress. In comparing the emotional intelligence, body image and disordered eating attitudes in combat sport athletes and non-athletes, Costarelli, & Stamou (2009) found the athletes having high emotional intelligence had higher emotional intelligence than non-athletes. While the impacts of EI in sport began to emerge, the empirical study of the association between physical activity and EI is scarce (Li, Lu, & Wang, 2009); to the best of our knowledge, the effects of EI on physical activity, and the importance of how physical activity plays an important role in enhancing emotional health of individuals has been overlooked in the past.

1.4 The effects of physical activity towards emotion

Some researchers strived to seek the linkage of exercise and emotional well-being, and reported the following emotional benefits that attribute to regular PA from the past studies (Reed, & Ones, 2006; Leith 2002; Kerr & Kuk 2001; Fox 1990; Biddle 2000; ASCM 2009). The effects of physical activity towards emotion include enhanced positive activated affect (Reed, & Ones, 2006) ; pleasant emotions (Kerr & Kuk 2001), positive mood, moderate anxiety-reduction effects (Biddle 2000), elevating their sense of happiness (Szabo 2003), and have higher score in optimistic levels (Kavussanu & Mcauley 1995), and increased in emotional intelligence (Adhia, Nagendra, & Mahadevan, 2010). Yet, very few empirical studies have investigated the influence of physical activity or exercise participation on emotional intelligence (Li, Lu, & Wang, 2008). Not until recently has there been one empirical study investigate the impact of exercise participation on emotional intelligence. Adhia, Nagendra, & Mahadevan (2010) examined the impact of yoga on EI and managerial performance in managers from a business enterprise, and reported that yoga practice enhanced both of the EI and managerial performance in managers

1.5 Measurement of emotional intelligence

While currently no consensus exists on the definition and theoretical construct of EI, the suitability of various EI-measuring methods suffer from controversial debate (Keele and Bell, 2007). The main EI-measuring methods proposed by scholars include measurement by trait (EIS, Schutte), by a mixed approach: personality and ability (BarOn EQi, BarOn), by ability (intelligence and ability, Goleman), or by trait and personality (WLEIS, Wong and Law) (Shi and Wong, 2007). Moreover, indigenization is currently missing in EI construct adopted in Taiwan; The majority of existing research studies on EI in Taiwan tends to adopt Western EI concepts, theories, methodologies, and testing instruments in a haphazard and even irrational manner, and ignores the significance and heterogeneity of Chinese culture. (Yang, 2004), Yang further stated that to establish and adopt the concept of indigenization, and apply indigenized methodologies and instruments in empirical research studies designed for Chinese people is needed for revealing a true emotional culture for Taiwan Chinese.

1.5.1 Theoretical framework for developing Chinese Emotional Intelligence Inventory (CEII)

Psychology scholars in Taiwan indicated that Chinese society adopts the thinking of Confucianism, Taoism, and Buddhism. Our society is particularly influenced by Confucianism; hence, the social orientation of Chinese culture is based on the Confucian concept of "interdependent self-construal," which emphasizes the connection between social relationships and our dependence on other people. By contrast, Western countries are strongly influenced by humanism and people in Western countries tend to display self-orientation largely based on individualism with an emphasis on self-independence (Yang, 2004). Modern Chinese people now adopt a mixture of self-orientation and social-orientation in their concept of self. For example, Yang (2004) asserted that people in Taiwan and Hong Kong currently adopt a way of life that is both self- and society-orientated. Over time they have developed "composite self" behavior. This type of psychological behavior now exists in the Chinese cognitive system and people's composite selves coexist and interact.

This research uses the four-factor theory of the Chinese self proposed by Yang (2007) as a reference to discuss whether we can use the concept of self-esteem as a medium to integrate and build a systematic model of emotion for an emotion theory more applicable to Taiwanese people. The four-factor theory of the Chinese self proposed by Yang (2007) suggests that the majority of people in Chinese societies (including Taiwanese people) demonstrate both "traditional self" (socially-oriented self that focuses on the collective and relationships) and "modern self" (individually-oriented self) traits and behaviors. The combined self-concept type is referred to as the "traditional-modern bicultural self." Thus, Yang suggested that the four-factor theory of the Chinese self be used as the basis for designing scales related to the concept of self. Such scales include the basic individually-oriented self emotion scale and socially-oriented self emotion scale.

Having summarized the concepts and definitions of EI proposed by various scholars, we realize that EI can occur on a "personal" and "interpersonal" level. In this study, the emotional intelligence inventory designed for Taiwanese university students incorporated the preceding EI theories suggested by Emmerling and Goleman (2003); and adopted the concept of "individually-oriented self" and "socially-oriented self" in the "four-factor theory of the Chinese self" proposed by Yang (2004). This research categorizes university students' ability to integrate emotion during intrapersonal and social interaction into four main concepts; we developed a scale for measuring university students' EI. The proposed scale comprises four main dimensions: "Cognition and understanding of self-emotion," "Application and management of self-emotion," "Cognition and understanding of social interaction," and "Application and management of social interaction". Regarding social interaction, this research not only discusses the relationship between interpersonal EI, but it also incorporates life, external environment, and academic factors into the design of the scale questions. Using the construct of social interaction, this study presents a more extensive discussion of EI and university students' cognition, understanding, application, and management abilities under the influence of the social environment. Each of the four concepts is described below:

Cognition and understanding of self-emotion

This refers to university students' ability to recognize and understand their emotions, and whether they can realize changes in their emotions. For example, their ability to identify the delight, anger, sorrow, and happiness they experience, to determine whether they feel happy or sad, and to understand whether their emotions have changed.

Application and management of self-emotion

This refers to university students' ability to appropriately manage their emotions and avoid the adverse influence of negative emotions. For example, their ability to adopt solutions when negative emotions arise, controls their emotions, and remains upbeat despite experiencing adverse situations.

Cognition and understanding of social interaction

This refers to university students' ability to recognize other people's emotions, understand changes in their own emotions in certain environments, and identify the external factors that influence their emotions.

Application and management of social interaction

This refers to university students' interpersonal communication skills and ability to interact with others and emotionally cope with external changes in their environment (situational changes, such as to their education, personal relationships, friendships, and family). For example, whether they can remain composed under stress, have healthy interactions with others, and appropriately show empathy to other's emotions.

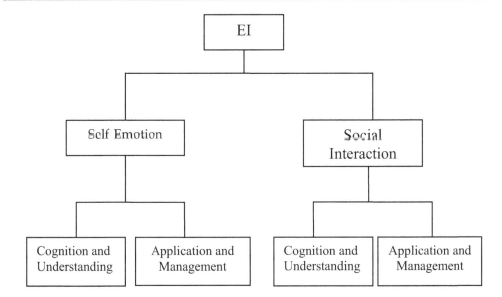

Fig. 1. Theoretical framework for the Chinese Emotional Intelligence Scale (CEII)

1.6 Significance of this research

In summary, this study does not directly adopt the theories and methodologies used in previous studies by Western scholars; instead, this study demonstrates sufficient indigenous compatibility and is conducted from the perspective of indigenous psychology and exercise science. Since the topic of emotional intelligence and physical activity has not yet been empirically examined, as an exploratory effort, this study attempts to examine a possible nurture factor, physical activity, in the development of EI. Therefore, the objective of this research is to develop an instrument that is easy to use, suitable, valid, and reliable for measuring emotional intelligence of Taiwan Chinese university students, and furthermore, to explore the associations of emotional intelligence and physical activity by utilizing this emotional intelligence Inventory.

1.7 Research objectives

This research has two main objectives:

- To develop a Chinese Emotional Intelligence Inventory (CEII) with good reliability and validity that is appropriate for university students,
- To explore the relationship of physical activity and emotional intelligence.

2. Method

2.1 Participants

In the pilot test, the student respondents included 613 university students, and 50 university students were selected to be tested again 1-week later to obtain the test-retest reliability. For the official test, we selected eight national and private universities in Northern, Central, and Southern and eastern part of Taiwan using a cluster and convenience sampling approach. This study distributed 100 questionnaires to each of the selected universities, for a total of 800 questionnaires. Then, 743 completed questionnaires (92.88 %) were collected; of these, 727 questionnaires were valid (for a validity rate of 97.85 %). Student participants were asked to fill in self-response questionnaires including Chinese Emotional Intelligence Inventory and self-report containing sections on demographic characteristics, and physical activity questionnaire. The description of the student participating is shown in Table 1.

Variable	Group	N	%
Gender	male	269	37.0
	female	458	63.0
Grade	freshman	216	29.7
	sophomore	185	25.4
	Junior	212	29.2
	Senior	101	13.9
	Fifth Year	13	1.8
Total		**727**	**100**

Table 1. Gender and Grade of the student participants

2.2 Measurement

2.2.1 Chinese Emotional Intelligence Inventory

Based on the theoretical framework for the Chinese Emotional Intelligence Inventory mentioned above, this research designed a Chinese Emotional Intelligence Inventory for Taiwan university students. 108 items for the initial questionnaire was derived in reference to the four main dimensions: "cognition and understanding of self-emotion," "application and management of self-emotion," "cognition and understanding of social interaction," and 'application and management of social interaction." Content validity of EQ items were obtained through consultation and verification of a focus group including emotional experts and relevant scholars, we then modified and deleting those ambiguous or non self-explanatory items by obtaining feedback from 50 university students who answered the questions, 96 items were finally obtained for the empirical research. We employed a six-point Likert scale for the responses to each item; 1, denotes "strongly disagree", 2 denotes "disagree", 3 denotes "somewhat disagree", 4 denotes "slightly agree", 5 denotes "agree", to 6 denotes "strongly agree" for positively or negatively-keyed items.

2.2.2 Physical activity

We adopted the physical activity formula used by Fox (1999) to measure the level of exercise participation, subjects were asked to recollect the exercise they performed within the past seven days, and the information was recorded under "exercise participation" in the section of demographic background. Exercise participation is measured by the multiplication of weekly exercise frequency, the duration of how long they exercise, and the intensity of the exercise (according to the Ratings of Perceived Exertion, RPE). The calculation formula is:

Exercise Participation = Frequency × (Average Intensity + Duration). The higher the score for exercise participation, the more the subject involved and engaged in exercise. The scoring method is described as follow:

Exercise intensity

This is measured using the rating instrument devised by Borg (1983), namely the Ratings of Perceived Exertion (RPE). RPE measures the level of perceived lethargy On 15 levels (from 6-20) here, numerals are used to represent the intensity of the exercise as perceived by subjective cognition. The result obtained by comparing the perceived intensity and actual intensity indicated by the heart rate can be used as the basis for calculating exercise intensity if the two results are consistent (Hoeger and Hoeger, 2002).

Exercise frequency

This is the number of times a student exercises per week. 1 denotes one or no exercise sessions per week, whereas 5 denotes five or more exercise sessions per week. The larger the number, the more frequently the student exercises.

Exercise duration

This is the average continuous duration of time spent exercising excluding breaks. 1 denotes a duration of 0 to 15 min for each session, whereas 5 denotes a duration of 61 min or over for each session. The larger the number, the longer the student exercises each session.

For example, if the average intensity indicated by the RPE scale is 10, the subject perceives the exercise to be fairly moderate; a frequency of 3 means the subject exercises 3 times or more per week; and duration of 3 means the subject exercises for an average of 31 to 45 min per session. Given the formula, the exercise participation of the particular subject is: 3× (10+3) = 39.

2.3 Procedure

For the pilot test, we tested the reliability and validity of the initial Chinese Emotional Intelligence Inventory on a sample of 613 university students using exploratory factor analysis. 50 students selected from sample participants completed the Chinese Emotional Intelligence Inventory one week after the first test in order to obtain the test-retest reliability of the proposed inventory. We also analyzed the criterion-related validity of the proposed inventory using WLEIS developed by Wong and Law (2002). 100 students were selected from the participants to fill in the Wong and Law's Emotional Intelligence Scale (WLEIS) (Wong & Law, 2002), this allowed us to determine the concurrent validity of the Chinese emotional intelligence inventory. We used the analytical results from the pilot test to adjust and finalize the official scale items which comprised 16 positively phrased items and 6 negatively phrased items. A higher test score indicates better emotional intelligence.

On the verification stage, by using a cluster and convenience sampling approach, we distributed the resulting 22-items official Chinese Emotional Intelligence Inventory and self-report containing sections on demographic characteristics, and physical activity categories to students at eight national and private universities in Northern, Central, Southern, and Eastern Taiwan, and collected 727 valid questionnaires.

2.4 Data analyses

Being aware of the imperativeness of having a reliable, valid, and sound measuring instrument, the statistical analysis was performed utilizing SPSS for Windows 15.0 and AMOS 7.0. We conducted an exploratory factor analysis (EFA) to obtain the construct validity of the scale; and Confirmatory factor analysis (CFA) to assess the goodness of fit of the hypothetical measurement model of Chinese Emotional Intelligence Inventory, and to verify whether the scale conforms to the theoretical framework. This approach was used to develop an established and consistent emotional intelligence scale for university students, so that this measure can be used as a suitable measuring instrument in future studies. The majority of the scholars suggest using the absolute fit measure (including χ^2, GFI, RMR, SRMR, and RMSEA), incremental fit measure (including AGFI, CFI, NFI, RFI, and IFI), and parsimony goodness of fit (including PNFI, AIC, and χ^2/df) for goodness-of-fit measures (Jöreskog & Sörbom, 1993). Of the proposed measures, χ^2 may be affected by the sample size and, therefore, precaution should be taken when using it. Considering this potential situation, we prioritized other indices and approaches less susceptible to sample size and model complexity. These indices include GFI, RMR, RMSEA, AGFI, CFI, NFI, and χ^2/df. Lastly, Pearson product moment correlation coefficient was used to examine the relationship between university students' emotional intelligence and their levels of physical activity.

3. Results

3.1 Exploratory factor analyses

We used exploratory factor analysis to obtain the construct validity of the scale. Item analysis was conducted to determine the level of difficulty and to discriminate item that cannot reflect the response level of different test subjects. We extracted the factors using principle axis factoring, and then performed Promax oblique rotations to better explain factor loading. Based on this process, we retained items with item loading value higher than 0.4. After seven rotations, we obtained 22 items comprising two scales, four factors. In total, the four factors accounted for 48.74 % of the explained variance of emotional intelligence. The factors were labeled as "cognition and understanding of self-emotion" (6 items), "application and management of self-emotion (6 items)", "cognition and understanding of social interaction" (5 items), and "application and management of social interaction (5 items)". Please refer to Table 2 for the results for the factor analysis of the Chinese Emotional Intelligence Inventory.

3.1.1 Internal consistency

We used Cronbach's α to determine for internal consistency, to examine whether the questions in the same subscales actually test the same category of emotional intelligence; the *a* value of the subscale factors and the entire scale were between .78 and .86, and the Cronbach's α for the whole inventory was .89. As shown in Table 4, internal consistency reliability is adequate for the whole scale and 4 subscales (range = .74 - .87). See table 3. Test-retest reliability was employed to obtain the coefficient of stability which assesses the consistency of the testing results on the same group of test subjects using the same measuring instrument obtained over time, the test-retest reliability in this study was $r = .73$ ($p < .05$).

No.	Question	Factor			
		1	2	3	4
6	I deal with the majority of issues with an optimistic attitude.	.810			
13	I am an optimistic person.	.781			
9	I can face challenges and difficulties with an optimistic mindset.	.740			
3	I am able to maintain a positive mood most of the time.	.721			
4	I am able to maintain a good mood regardless of whether I am in a positive or negative situation.	.645			
2	I can rid myself of unpleasant feelings.	.518			
10	I actively console others when they are sad.		.839		
7	I actively show my concern for others when they encounter difficulties or adverse situations.		.795		
8	I try to calm others when they are experiencing anger.		.708		
21	I like to help other people relieve stress or manage their emotional issues.		.575		
18	I can appreciate the feeling when my friends feel sad.		.522		
11*	I do not manage unexpected situations well.			.656	
1*	I have no patience for complicated issues.			.621	
12*	I do not wish to try when I encounter unfamiliar things.			.603	
5*	When under stress, I feel choosing to avoid the issue is easier than choosing to face it.			.587	
20*	I am dissatisfied with myself, yet I do not know how to change the situation.			.571	
14*	I do not know how to identify my true emotions.			.570	
16	I constantly encourage myself to overcome difficulties.				.857
15	When I encounter difficulties, I focus all my energy and effort to resolve them.				.635
22	When I encounter difficulties, I try to figure out the solutions.				.633
19	I strive to achieve my objectives.				.617
17	When other people show little faith in what I do, I actually become more motivated.				.609
	Eigenvalues	7.16	2.30	1.92	1.33
	Explained variance accounted for (%)	30.36	8.05	6.34	3.99
	Total explained variance	48.74			

Note: * questions are negatively phrased items

Table 2. Factor loadings pertaining to the Chinese Emotional Intelligence Inventory

Subscale (item no.)	Item number	a
Cognition and understand of self-emotion (6)	1, 5, 11, 12, 14, 20	.74
Application and management of self-emotion (6)	2, 3, 4, 6, 9, 13	.87
Cognition and understand of social interaction (5)	15, 16, 17, 19, 22	.84
Application and management of social interaction (5)	7, 8, 10, 18, 21	.83
Self-emotion (12)	1, 2, 3, 4, 5, 6, 9, 11, 12, 13, 14, 20	.84
Social Interaction (10)	7, 8, 9, 10, 15, 16, 17, 18, 19, 21, 22	.86
Total scale (22-items)		.89

Table 3. Internal consistency of the whole scale and subscales of the CEII (n = 727)

3.1.2 Concurrent validity

For the criterion-related validity, we employed the Wong and Law Emotional Intelligence Scale (WLEIS) designed by Wong and Law (2002) to obtain the concurrent validity of the proposed Chinese emotional intelligence inventory. The correlation between CEII and WLEIS was $r = .51$ ($p < .05$), and the correlation coefficients of the four subscale to WLEIS ranged $r = .22 - .43$ ($p < .05$) indicating a satisfied concurrent validity. See table 4.

	EI total	Self Cogn Understanding	Self Apply & Man	Social Cogn & Understanding	Social Apply & Man
WLEIS total	.506*	.223*	.423*	.350*	.427*

$P < .05$

Table 4. Correlations of the CEII and WLEIS

In summary, the results of the exploratory factor analysis successfully to support the 4-factor structure of the Chinese emotional intelligence inventory. As a result, the official scale comprised 16 positively phrased items and 6 negatively phrased items.

3.2 Structure validity

We conducted confirmatory factor analysis (CFA) on the 22 item to examine the structure validity of Chinese emotional intelligence inventory. The four-factor model fit well. These results meet the criteria for goodness of fit indices (>.90) and root mean square residual (RMR < .05), which means that the Chinese emotional intelligence Inventory contain a four-factor structure in Taiwan Chinese university students sample. See table 4 and Fig. 2, and. As shown in Fig. 1, the scale developed in this research contains two main latent variables, namely "self-emotion" and "social interaction." These two variable categories each comprise two first-order latent factors, including "cognition and understanding", and "application and management" that made up four factors.

For the scores of the Chinese emotional intelligence inventory to display a normal distribution, the skewness should be smaller than ±3.0 and the kurtosis should be smaller than ±8.0 (Pedhazur & Schmelkin,1991). Our analysis confirmed that all the factor and scale values in the inventory fell between the required critical values, meaning they demonstrated a normal distribution and were fit for use in confirmatory factor analysis. As Table 5 demonstrate, the goodness of fit shown by the index values of the hypothetical measurement model, RMR=.038, GFI=.937, AGFI=.922, NFI=.917, CFI=.946, RMSEA=.047, and χ^2/df=2.637, are all within the acceptable range (Jöreskog & Sörbom, 1993). Therefore, the hypothetical measurement model adopted by this research requires no adjustment. The university student emotional intelligence scale devised by this study is proven to conform to the theoretical model and possess good construct validity. Therefore, we can conclude that this scale is appropriate for future studies when measuring emotional intelligence of university students.

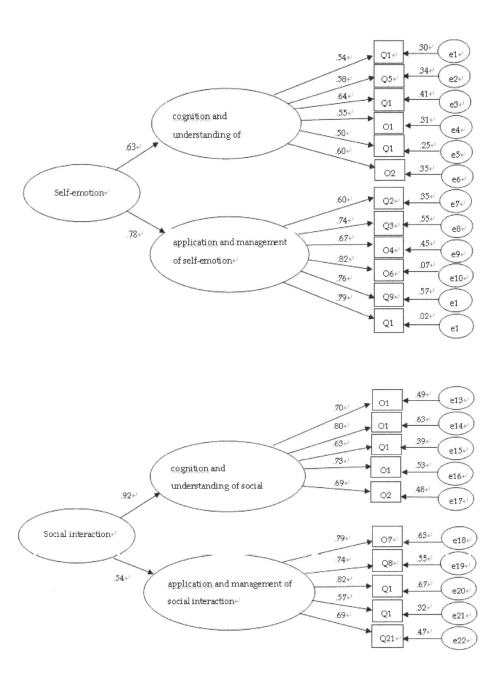

Fig. 2. Second order four-factor model of Chinese Emotional Intelligence Inventory (CEII)

Test Statistic	Index	Result	Criteria	Result
Absolute Fit Measure	GFI	.937	>.90	Accept
	RMR	.038	<.05, better if <.025	Accept
	RMSEA	.047	Excellent if <.05, good if between .05 and .08	Accept
Incremental Fit Measure	AGFI	.922	>.90	Accept
	CFI	.946	>.90	Accept
	NFI	.917	>.90	Accept
Parsimony Goodness of Fit	χ^2/df	2.637	1.0 - 3.0	Accept

Table 5. Summary of the Confirmatory Factor Analysis Result of the four-factor model of CEII

3.3 The association of emotional intelligence and physical activity

Pearson product moment correlation coefficient was performed to examine the relationship of emotional intelligence and physical activity. The results indicated that significant ($p < .05$) associations were found between physical activity and total emotional intelligence score ($r = .145$, $p < .05$), subscale score of self-emotion ($r = .112$, $p < .05$), subscale score of social interaction ($r = .156$, $p < .05$), and 3 factors, including "Application and management of self-emotion" ($r = .162$, $p < .05$) "Cognition and understanding of social interaction," ($r = .101$, $p < .05$), and "Application and management of social interaction ($r = .164$, $p < .05$)"; indicating a low to moderate positive association between physical activity and emotional intelligence.

	EI Total	Self Emotion	Social Interaction	Self-cognition	Self-management	Social-cognition	Social-management
Physical Activity	.145*	.112*	.156*	.023	.162*	.101*	.164*

$p < .05$

Table 6. Correlations of emotional intelligence and physical activity

4. Discussion

In this chapter, we attempted to describe the development of a Chinese Emotional Intelligence Inventory (CEII) that suited specifically to Taiwan society and culture. The result of the current study provided support for the reliability and validity of Chinese emotional intelligence inventory; the psychometric features of the Chinese emotional intelligence Inventory supported its feasibility as a research instrument to measure emotional intelligence appropriately for Taiwan Chinese university students. The results of confirmatory factor analysis of the CEIII verify the four-factor structure of the theoretical framework we previously proposed, that incorporated the preceding western EI theories and the concept of "individually-oriented self" and "socially-oriented self" in the "four-factor theory of the Chinese self" proposed by Yang (2004). The correlation between total emotional intelligence scores and the scores of four subscales of CEII and WLEIS were positive. The results showed that higher scores on general emotional intelligence, as measured by CEII, were substantially associated with higher scores on the WLEIS, demonstrating good concurrent validity for CEII in a Taiwan Chinese university student population. In summary, the CEII was shown to possess good psychometric properties. In order to enhance the explanatory power of CEII, further research is required to establish the norm and validate the instrument.

The second purpose in this study was to examine the association of CEII and physical activity for university students in Taiwan. There has been very few study on the association between physical activity and emotional intelligence in the past, only recently has there been two empirical studies linking emotional intelligence to exercise participation (Adhia, Nagendra, & Mahadevan, 2010; Li, Lu & Wang, 2009). In our study, a positive relationship was found between physical activity and emotional intelligence, indicating that the more physical activity participation the university students have, the higher their emotional intelligence. The finding of our study are in line with the finding from the other studies (Adhia, Nagendra, & Mahadevan, 2010; Li, Lu, & Wang, 2009) that yoga exercise enhanced both of the emotional scores in managers, Adhia, Nagendra, & Mahadevan (2010) further explained that yoga provides a means to de-stress individuals and improve personal satisfaction, also help them to disengage from the negative role and unhappy involvement one has created for oneself, moreover, becoming more self-aware, self-regulated, and with a proper perspective of life and various relationships through yoga practice might lead to the enhancement of EI.

In an attempt to explore the associations of physical activity and emotional intelligence in Taiwan college students, Li, Lu, & Wang (2009) found that College students who reported a recommended level of physical activity scored significantly higher than insufficient and inactive counterparts in emotional intelligence; and physical activity was found to be one of the predictor variables towards emotional intelligence. Li, Lu, & Wang (2009) concluded that exercise participation or physical activity might be an effective way for the enhancement of emotional health in college students.

Several plausible mechanisms for PA effects on emotional consequences have been identified (Dietrich & Audiffren, 2011; Carron et al. 2003; Biddle & Mutrie, 2001); including having higher level of self-perception and body image through improvements in physical fitness or weight loss that resulted from exercise (Fox 2000); attaining positive emotions by changing in self-esteem due to mastering new exercise skills, or from an increased sense of intra-personal control (Biddle, 2000). In explaining the underlying neurobehavioral mechanism of how exercise could be beneficial towards emotions, Dietrich & Audiffren (2011) presented an evolutionary model of reticular-activating hypofrontality model of acute exercise; Dietrich & Audiffren (2011) noted that exercise first engages arousal mechanisms in the reticular-activating system by releasing a number of neurotransmitters (mainly norephinephine, dopamine, and serotonin) which shed positive effect on emotion; then secondly, since exercise motion demands enormously on motor, sensory, and autonomic structures of exercised individuals, thus, deactivate the higher-order functions of the prefrontal cortex by decreasing neural activity, thus, might help exercisers to mitigate the negative and unhelpful emotions. The study from Dietrich & Audiffren (2011) gave rationale support to the connection of exercise and EI from a neuroscience perspective.

There are, however, two limitations in our research. First, this study is cross-sectional in design; therefore, inferring causal relationships of physical activity towards emotional intelligence enhancement should not be feasible. Furthermore, all the data in this research were collected in Taiwan universities; we still don't know whether our finding could expand generalization into university population from other culture, and we also don't know if Chinese emotional intelligence inventory can be used in other cultures, or even for the entire Chinese population, for substantial discrepancy still exists between Oriental and Western prototypes of ideal cultures (Yang, 2004) .Therefore the cross-cultural validity of this Chinese emotional intelligence inventory needs further verification.

Recommendations for future study are suggested as follow:

- Conducting a comparative study and/or cross-cultural validity study using Chinese emotional intelligence inventory among different Chinese communities (such as Hong Kong, China, Macao, and Taiwan)
- We recommend that future studies explore the relationship between EI and physical activity using path analysis. If correlation exists between their paths then use structural equation modeling to verify the direct and indirect effects of exercise participation on EI. Through this approach (using SEM to verify the direct and indirect effects of exercise on EI, or the impact of EI on physical activity), the research findings will be even more valuable. These are all imperative exploratory research topics that require further investigation.
- If predictions regarding the effect of exercise participation on emotional intelligence can be inferred, then research studies concerning emotional intelligence and physical activity will be highly applicable and practical. To enhance the explanatory power of Chinese emotional intelligence inventory, the construction of norm models for university students are necessary.
- We suggest that the scale proposed by this research be applied in a more holistic manner in future studies. Not only can the scale be used to assess and understand the emotional intelligence of university students, it can also be used to discuss a range of different background variances, such as explaining the heterogeneity between different genders, years of study, schools and colleges, and family structures.

5. Conclusions

In this study, the psychometric features of the Chinese emotional intelligence Inventory supported its feasibility as a research instrument to measure EI appropriately in Taiwan Chinese university students. All statistical indexes, coefficients, and values indicated that the 4-factor, 22 items Chinese Emotional Intelligence Inventory was a reliable and valid measure for physical activity study in Chinese settings. In sum, whether EI ability can be learned through physical activity participation? Or Whether EI can influence physical activity participation are still the research topics that need constant effort, our study provided a useful reference for future studies.

6. References

ACSM (2009). *ACSM's resource manual for guidelines for exercise testing and prescription*, (6th ed.). Baltimore, MD: Williams & Wilkins.

Adhia, H., Nagendra, H. R., Mahadevan, B. (2010). Impact of adoption of yoga way of life on the emotional intelligence of manager, IIMB Management Review, 22, 32-41.

BarOn, R. (2002). *BarOn Emotional Quotient Inventory: Technical Manual*. North Tonawanda, NY: Multi-Health Systems.

Bar-On, R., Maree, J. G., & Elias, M. J. (2007). *Educating People to Be Emotionally Intelligence*. Westport Connecticut, London: Praeger. ISBN-13: 978-0-275-99363-4

Biddle, S. J. H. (2000). Exercise, emotions, and mental health. In Y. L. Hann (ed). *Emotions in sport*. Human Kinetics, Champaign, IL, pp 267-292. ISBN 0-88011-879-2

Biddle, S. J. H., & Mutrie, N. (2001). *Psychology of Physical Activity: Determinants, well-being and interventions*. New York, NY: Routledge.

Birkeland, M. S., Torbjorn, T., & Wold, B. (2009). A longitudinal study of the relationship betweenleisure-time physical activity and depressed mood among adolescents, Psychology of Sport and Exercise, 10, 25-34.

Borg, G. (1983). Perceived exertion: A note on history and method. *Medicine and Science in Sport and Exercise, 5*, 90-93.

Brackett, M., Mayer, J. D., & Warner, R. M. (2004). Emotional intelligence and its relation to everyday behaviour, *Personality and Individual Differences, 36*(6), 1387-1402.

Carron, A.V., Hausenblas, H. A., Estabrooks, P.A. (2003). *The psychology of physical activity*. New York, NY: McGraw-Hill Higher Education,.

Costarelli, V., & Stamou, D. (2009). Emotioanl intelligence, body image and disordered eating attitudes in combat sport athletes, Journal of Exercise Science and Fitness, 7(2), 104-111.

Dishman, R. K. (1997). The norepinephrine hypothesis. In W. P. Morgan (ed.). *Physical activity and mental health*, pp 199-212.Washington, DC : Taylor & Francis.

Dishman, R. k., Washburn, R. A., & Health, G. W. (2004). *Physical activity epidemiology*. Champaign, IL: Human Kinetics.

Dietrich, A., & Audiffren, M. (2011). The reticular-activating hypofrontality (RAH) model of acute exercise. Neuroscience and Biobehavioral Reviews, 35(6), 1305-1325.

Emmerling, R. J., & Goleman, D. (2003). *Emotional intelligence: Issues and common misunderstandings*. Retrieved Jun 16, 2011 from The Consortium for Research on Emotional intelligence in Organizations web site:
https://www.talentsmart.com/media/uploads/pdfs/EI_Issues_And_Common_Misunderstandings.pdf

Fox, K. R. (1999). The influence of physical activity on mental well-being. Public Health and Nutrition, 2(3), 411-418.

Fox, K. R. (2000). The effects of exercise on self-perceptions and self-esteem. In S. J. Biddle, K. R. Fox, S. H. Boutcher (eds.). pp 88-117. *Physical activity and psychological well-being*. New York, NY: Routledge..

Goleman, D. (1995). Emotional intelligence: Why it can matter more than IQ. Bantam, NY: Books.

Goleman, D. (2001). Emotional intelligence: Issues in paradigm building. In C. Cherniss & D. Goleman (Eds.), The emotionally intelligent workplace, pp. 13-26. San Francisco, LA: Jossey-Bass.

Hoeger, W. W. K., & Hoeger, S. A. (2002). *Principles and Labs for Fitness and Wellness (6th ed.)*. Belmont, CA: Wadsworth.

Jöreskog, K., & Sörbom, D. (1993). *LISREL 8: Structural equation modeling with the SIMPLIS common language.* Hillsdale, NJ: Lawrence Erlbaum Association Publishers.

Kafetsios, K. (2004). Attachment and emotional intelligence abilities across the life course, *Personality and Individual Differences, 37*(1), 129-145.

Kavussanu , M., & McAuley, E. (1995). Exercise and optimism: Are highly active individuals more optimistic. *Journal of Sport and Exercise Psychology, 17*, 246-58.

Keele, S. M., & Bell, R. C. (2007). The factorial validity of emotional intelligence: An unresolved issue. *Personality and Individual Differences, 44*(2), 487-500.

Kerr, J. H., & Kuk, G. (2001). The effects of low and high intensity exercise on emotions, stress and effort. *Psychology of Sport and Exercise, 2*, 173-186.

Kerr, J. H., Wilson, G. V., Svebak, S., & Kirkcaldy, B. D. (2006) Matches and mismatches between telic dominance and type of sport: Changes in emotions and stress pre- to post-performance. *Personality and Individual Differences, 40*, 1557-1567.

Leith, L. M. (2002). *Foundations of exercise and mental health.* Morgantown, WV: Fitness Information Technology,.

Laborde, S., Brull, A., Weber, J., & Anders, L. S. (2011). Trait emotional intelligence in sports: A protective role against stress through heart rate variability? *Personality and Individual Differences, 51*, 23-27.

Law, K. S., Wong, C. S., & Song, L. J. (2004). The construct and criterion validity of emotional intelligence and its potential utility for management studies, Journal of applied Psychology, 89(3), 483-496.

Li, G. S. F., Lu, F. J. H., & Wang, H. H. (2009). Exploring the relationships of Physical Activity, Emotional Intelligence, and health in Taiwan college students, Journal of Exercise Science and Fitness, 7(1), 55-63.

Lin, M. S., Lee, C. H., & Miu, P. R. (2006). Exercise habit and health-related physical fitness in college students participating in physical education class. *National Changhua University of Education Bulletin of Physical Education, 6*, 302-310.

Lu, F. J. H., Li. G. S. F., Hsu, E. Y. W., & Williams, L. (2010). Relationship between athletes' emotional intelligence and precompetitive anxiety, *Perceptual and Motor Skills, 110*(2), 1-16.

Martins, A., Ramalho, N., & Morin, E. (2010). A comprehensive meta-analysis of the relationship between emotional intelligence and health. Personality and Individual Differences, 49(6), 554-564.

Mayer, J. D. & Salovy, P. (1990). *Emotional intelligence and the self-regulation of affect.* Englewood Cliffs, NJ: Prentice-Hall.

Mayer, J. D. & Salovy, P. (1993). The intelligence of emotional intelligence. *Intelligence, 17*, 433-442.

Mayer, J. D., & Salovey, P. (1997). What is emotional intelligence. Emotional development and emotional intelligence: Educational implications. New York, NY: Basic Books.

Mayer, J. D., Salovy, P., & Caruso, D. R. (2002). *Mayer-Salovey-Caruso Emotional Intelligence Test (MSCEIT) Users Manual.* Toronto, Canada: MHS Publishers.

Mayer, J. D., Caruso, D. R., & Salovy, P. (1999). Emotional intelligence meets traditional standards for an intelligence. Intelligence, 27, 267-298.

Nieman, D. C. (1998). *Exercise-health connection.* Champaign, IL: Human Kinetics.

Palmer, B. R., Manocha, R., Gignac, G., & Stough, C. (2003). Examining the factor structure of the Bar-On Emotional Quotient Inventory with an Australian general population sample. *Personality and Individual Differences, 35,* 1191-1210.

Parker, J. D. A., Summerfeldt, L. J., Hogan, M. J., & Majeski, S. A. (2004). Emotional intelligence and academic success: examining the transition from high school to university. Personality and Individual Differences, 36, 163-172.

Pedhazur, E. J., & Schmelkin, L. P. (1991). Measurement, design, and analysis: An integrated approach. Hillsdale, NJ: Lawrence Erlbaum.

Petrides, K. V., & Furnham, A. (2000). On the dimensional structure of emotional intelligence. Personality and Individual Differences, 29, 313-320.

Racette, S. B., Deusinger, S. S., Strube, M. J., Highstein, G. R., & Deusinger, R. H. (2007). Changes in weight and health behaviors from freshman through senior year of college. *Journal of Nutrition Education and Behavior, 40,* 39-42.

Reed, J., & Ones, D. S. (2006). The effect of acute aerobic exercise on positive activasted affect: A meta-analysis, *Psychology of Sport and Exercise, 7,* 477-514.

Saarni, C. (1999). The development of emotional competence. New York, NY: Guilford

Schutte, N. S., Malouff., J. M., Thorsteinsson, E. B., Bhullar, N., & Rooke, S. E. (2007). A meta-analytic investigation of the relationship between emotional intelligence and health. *Personality and Individual Differences, 42*(6), 921-933.

Shi, J., & Wang, L. (2007). Validation of emotional intelligence scale in Chinese university students. *Personality and Individual Differences, 43,* 377-387.

Szabo, A (2003). The acute effects of humor and exercise on mood and anxiety. *Journal of Leisure Research, 35,* 152-162.

Taylor, C. B., Coffey, T., Berra, K., Iaffaldano, R., Casey, K., & Haskell, W. L. (1984). Seven day activity and self-report compared to a direct measure of physical activity. *American Journal of Epidemiology, 120,* 818-824.

Taymoori, P., & Lubans, D. R. (2008). Mediators of behavior change in two tailored physical activity interventions for adolescent girls. Psychology of Sports and Exercise, 9, 605-619.

Tett, R. P., & Fox, K. E. (2006). Confirmatory factor structure of trait emotional intelligence in student and worker samples, Personality and Individual Differences, 41, 1155-1168.

Vallerand, R. J., & Blanchard, C. M. (2000). The study of emotion in sport and exercise: Historical, definitional, and conceptual perspectives. In Y. L. Hann (ed). *Emotions in sport.* Human Kinetics, Champaign, IL, pp 3-38. ISBN 0-88011-879-2

Wong, C. S., & Law, K. S. (2002). The effects of leader and follower emotional intelligence on performance and attitude: An exploratory study. *Leadership Quarterly, 13,* 243-274.

Wong, C. S., Foo, M. D., Wang, C. W., & Wong, P. M. (2007). The feasibility of training and development of EI: An exploratory study in Singapore, Hong Kong and Taiwan. *Intelligence, 35,* 141-150.

World Health Organization (2004). *Global strategy on diet, physical activity and health.* Available from http://www.who.int/dietphysicalactivity/publications/facts/pa/en/index.html (Date accessed: Aug 15, 2011)

Yang, K. S. (2004). Chinese Self theory analysis and empirical research: From socially-oriented and self-oriented viewpoints. *Indigenous psychology Research, 22,* 11-80.

Zizzi, S. J., Deaner, H. R., & Hirschhorn, D. K. (2003). The relationship between emotional intelligence and performance among college baseball players. Journal of Applied Sport Psychology, 15, 262-269.

13

Developing Emotional Intelligence for Healthcare Leaders

Claudia S. P. Fernandez[1], Herbert B. Peterson[1],
Shelly W. Holmström[2] and AnnaMarie Connolly[1]
[1]The University of North Carolina at Chapel Hill
[2]The University of South Florida
USA

1. Introduction

Skills in emotional intelligence (EI) help healthcare leaders understand, engage and motivate their team. They are essential for dealing well with conflict and creating workable solutions to complex problems. EI skills are grounded in *personal competence*, upon which build the skills for *social competence,* including social awareness and relationship management. The leader's EI skills strongly impact the culture of the organization. This article lists example strategies for building seventeen key emotional intelligence skills that are the foundations for personal and work success and provides examples of their appropriate use as well as their destructive under-use and over-use. Many examples are those incorporated into our healthcare-related leadership development institutes offered at the University of North Carolina's Gillings School of Global Public Health.

2. EI and EQ in healthcare leaders

"More than prescriptions, medicine involves communication, tolerance, flexibility, listening, hard work and a passion for the practice."

--Floyd Loop, MD (Loop 2009)

In the world of healthcare, as with many other sectors, equating intelligence with leadership can be a significant error. While intelligence is a critical building block of success for healthcare leaders, and for physicians in particular, to rely upon sheer intelligence to manage the complexities inherent in modern healthcare is tantamount to inviting career derailment. Healthcare as a field is cast against a background of patient and family anxiety, often challenging diagnosis and treatment, and financial as well as regulatory complexity. Intellect is helpful, but is only one of many keys to success for healthcare leaders.

In considering challenging work situations encountered by physicians, nurses and other healthcare leaders with colleagues or staff, many center on: 1) misunderstandings of either word or intent; 2) the inability of an individual to grasp the impact of their actions on others; or 3) the "grit-in-the-gears" hurdles created by organizational culture issues. While healthcare leaders face clinical and financial challenges, interpersonal issues frequently prove the most time- and resource-consuming (Pfifferling 2008, Freshman & Rubino 2002, Gifford, et al 2002, Cummings 2009).

Tools required for healthcare leaders to succeed generally fall into two categories: *hard* and *soft* (Klaus 2008). For physicians in particular, but also for many other healthcare leaders, "hard skills" are the technical skills traditionally emphasized in training. Medical schools and residency programs, as well as advanced nursing and allied health training programs, and public health focus on clinical fund-of-knowledge and clinical skill acquisition. For healthcare administrators these hard skills typically fall under financial, systems, and facilities management. Development of these skills requires an intellectual capacity to absorb, process, and integrate knowledge which, at times, is referred to as the intelligence quotient or "IQ".

The "soft skills" are more nuanced and include interpersonal and communication skills and professionalism (Porath & Pearson 2009, O'Toole & Bennis 2009, Awad 2004) which, until recently, have received far less attention in formal training for either medicine (Awad 2004, Horwitz 2008, Mrkonjic & Grondin 2011, Wagner 2002), nursing (Cummings 2009), or healthcare administration (____ 2011). These skills are strategic in nature, and as such, cross disciplines rather than being the province of any single profession. Differentiated from IQ, these skills rely much more on "emotional intelligence", sometimes referred to as EI, or emotional quotient (EQ). Emotional Intelligence as a differentiated construct is made up of the personal-emotional-social components of general intelligence (Bar-On 1997, Bar-On 2002, Pearman 2003). Thus, EI generally refers to a broad range of competencies, often addressed from a theory standpoint. By contrast, EQ generally refers to a quantification of skills in practice, and in particular to measures of emotional intelligence captured by commonly used psychological assessment instruments (Ackley 2006, Bar-On 1997, Bar-On 2002, Mayer et al 2002, Pearman 2003, Stein 2011).

In practice, and axiomatically, leaders can only get things done by working with and through others. While the most senior clinical leaders in healthcare may be marginally involved in the actual clinical setting, most healthcare leaders coordinate or oversee the direct-care efforts of their teams or organizations. At all levels, leaders set the EI culture in their enterprise and this culture directly impacts patient relationships (Levinson 2002, Mrkonjic & Grondin 2011, Wagner 2002), staff morale (Freshman & Rubino 2002), turnover (Gifford, et al 2002, Hill 2002), and relationships with colleagues (Freshman & Rubino 2002, Porath & Pearson, O'Toole & Bennis 2009, Cummings 2009, Awad 2004, Mrkonjic & Grondin 2011). When development of the EI of the culture is ignored in favor of a view that "intellect rules", organizations make themselves susceptible to disruptive behavior—from incivility to outright hostility (Porath & Pearson 2009, Loop 2009, Lewis 2010). This disruptive behavior often provides examples of poor application of emotional intelligence skills, which can cause direct organizational harm. For example, when leaders fail to deal directly with disruptive physician behavior, it negatively impacts medical quality, safety, team work, creativity, and commitment (Porath & Pearson 2009, Pfifferling 2008). Consequently organizations expend an inordinate amount of effort and resources in stopping, neutralizing, or correcting disruptive behavior, (Pfifferling 2008, Loop 2009). An overt disruptive behavior and those cultures failing to embrace and implement emotional intelligence directly cause significant detrimental effects to the bottom line of an enterprise (Porath & Pearson 2009, Pfifferling 2008). Creating leadership environments that are non-relational (task focused) has been related to poorer emotional health and emotional exhaustion in nurses, while creating those that are founded upon EI-associated relational leadership has been found by many studies to enhance nurse satisfaction, recruitment, and retention (Cummings 2009). Poor application of EI in healthcare settings specifically will harm the organization's reputation, its patient care, and increase staff turnover, all of which can impact financial health (Porath & Pearson 2009, Pfifferling 2008).

Recent work from the Center for Creative Leadership (CCL; Greensboro, NC) reports that the healthcare sector's top priority for leadership development is improving the ability to lead employees and work in teams (CCL 2010). However, this skill, along with self-awareness, was rated *lowest* of skills actually *demonstrated* by healthcare leaders (CCL 2010). Other recent CCL research indicates that the interpersonal soft-skills are rising in importance among leaders, with participative management, building and mending relationships, and change management replacing former top-rated skills such as resourcefulness, decisiveness, and "doing whatever it takes" (Martin 2005). Clearly EI is a foundational skill that is a pre-requisite for good leadership in healthcare situations (Horowitz 2008, Schwartz 2000, Levinson 2002, Lattore 2005).

At the University of North Carolina at Chapel Hill, the Gillings School of Global Public Health is heavily invested in teaching leadership skills to health system professionals. As an essential component of leadership, our development programs for physicians, nurses, allied health, public health, public academic institutions, and health administrators all center on the concept of emotional intelligence. Reuven Bar-On, a pioneer researcher in the field of EI, offers a compelling definition of emotional intelligence as, *"an array of non-cognitive* (emotional and social) *capabilities, competencies, and skills that influence one's ability to succeed in coping with environmental demands and pressures"* (Stein & Book 2006, Bar-On 1997, Bar-On 2006, Pearman 2003). Certainly healthcare and public health as well are fields fraught with environmental demands and pressures with which leaders must endlessly cope. EI skills are essential tools for healthcare leaders since they enable groups to advance interests that serve the team. These skills are crucial because healthcare is rarely delivered in isolation of the rest of a team. Indeed, even the currently heralded medical home model is patient-centered and community-connected (Rosenthal 2008, O'Malley et al 2008, Fisher 2008): a strong blend of the values of both the health care and public health fields.

Emotional Intelligence is a strong tool for building bridges and alliances and, importantly, for repairing those relationships when they are damaged (Fernandez 2007a). Leaders in healthcare and public health must realize the challenging nature of distributing scarce resources in difficult times: relationships can become frayed due to internal competition for those resources, recognition, or opportunity. However, the same groups that compete in one arena often need to partner in another or at another time to survive. The ability to mend relationships is particularly crucial to leaders in today's rapidly changing healthcare world (Lombardo and Eichinger 1989).

Goleman, another leading researcher in EI, suggests that 67% of the competencies needed by successful leaders fall into the emotional intelligence realm (Goleman 1996). In The EQ Edge, (Stein & Book 2006) Stein and Book report on one of the first studies to use a valid measure of emotional and social intelligence to examine the relationship between intelligence and self-perceived success at work. They found that IQ predicted an average of

6% and EQ an average of 27%-45% of success in a given position. Stein and Book conclude, "regardless of how brainy we may be, if we turn others off with abrasive behavior, are unaware of how we are presenting ourselves or cave in under minimal stress, no one will stick around long enough to notice our high IQs" (Stein & Book 2006).

While EI skills might not be innate, they can be developed, learned and taught (Porath & Pearson 2009, CCL 2010, Stein & Book 2006, Bar-On 1997, Bar-On 2006, Goleman 1996, Fernandez 2007a, Lombardo & Eichinger 1989, Mayer et al 2002, Lynn 2002, Pearman 2002, Goleman 2000, Goleman 2001, Goleman 2008, Thumm 2008). When engaging in leadership development of healthcare leaders, regardless of the discipline, basing skill development on both a theoretical *and* practical basis of EI skills is crucial (Pagnini 2009). Two components should be taken into consideration: the development program itself, with the elements of skill development incorporated, and the desire of the participant to learn and grow. In particular, EI development requires a desire for self-improvement, a willingness to face personal blind spots or shortcomings, and a sense of humility. When mastering cognitive or hard skills, an error can be corrected by simply learning facts or honing a behavioral skill, like suturing, wound dressing, budget reconciliation, or statistical analysis. In contrast, when correcting an EI problem the feedback can feel far more personal, identity-based, or even painful to the individual. It can be perceived as being about the individual and not simply about the behavior or the executed skills of the individual. Thus, creating a learning environment that is safe, non-judgmental, and conducive to self-insight without fostering a sense of shame is crucial.

For EI self-improvement in our work, the focii are *personal competence* and *social competence*. Personal competence is characterized by a broad range of abilities, including how one perceives and expresses oneself, makes decisions and manages stress. In our construction of development programs and coaching these basic skills serve as the foundation for *social competence*, which itself is comprised of *social awareness* and *relationship management* (CCL 2010, Stein & Book 2006, Bar-On 1997, Bar-On 2006, Goleman 1996). Based on our review of the literature (Goleman 1996, Goleman 2000, Goleman et al 2001, Stein & Book 2006, Bar-On 1997, Bar-On 2006, Collins 2001, Pearman 2003, Heifetz 1994) and assessment tools, our work with hundreds of physician leaders through six years of providing leadership development institutes, and our work with hundreds of public health, allied health, health system, and public sector leaders, we have created an EI development model (Figure 1). This model is the foundation for our leadership skills development work with healthcare and other leaders. These programs are offered as intensive training leadership institutes offered at or in conjunction with the Department of Maternal and Child Health, the Gillings School of Global Public Health, at the University of North Carolina at Chapel Hill.

It is easier to "talk the EI talk" than to "walk the EI walk" and putting EI into practice requires an understanding of how to execute the related skills, particularly in difficult or uncomfortable situations. This chapter will focus on the major components of EI, how weak and strong skills might manifest in the workplace, and how EI skills can be enhanced. For this exploration we will use the model of EI that serves as the basis for the construction of our programs (Figure 1). This model has been inspired by and adapted from the research of Goleman, Bar-On, Stein, and others. Examples of EI skills development from the leadership training institutes will be offered as EI development strategies. One important point is that

EI skills can be *over*-used as well as *under*-used — especially when not used in balance. When under-used the effects are often dramatic and easy to observe. Although over-use can manifest more subtly, the results can be equally problematic to the individual and the organization, though perhaps harder to identify or "diagnose". Several examples of both effective use of EI skills and potential EI "mis-steps" are presented below.

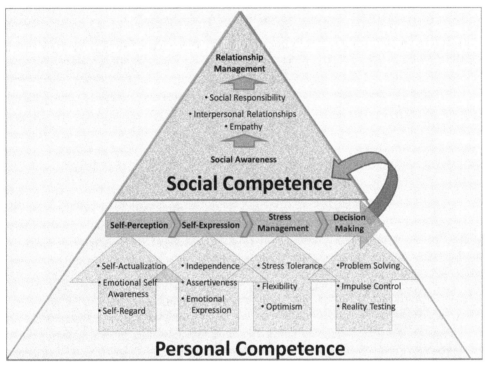

Fig. 1. The Model of EI for physician leaders that serves as the basis for UNC's Leadership Development Institutes

3. Personal competence

Personal competence is the foundation of EI and is characterized by knowing, understanding and expressing oneself. In terms of operationalizing these concepts we embrace the EQ-i theory as originally proposed by Bar-On (Stein & Book 2006, Bar-On 1997, Bar-On 2006) and recently updated as EQ-i 2.0 (Stein 2011). Personal competence can be sub-divided into categories of 1. *Self-Perception*, 2. *Self Expression*, 3. Stress Management skills, and 4. Decision Making (Stein 2011) In many ways these skills successively build on one another, with skills in self perception being necessary for those in self expression, and those serving as a basis for stress management. Stress management, itself helps lay the groundwork for skills in decision making. In this way, our model is a "stacked" one, in which some skills create leverage points for the development of others. In our leadership programs we focus on the development of those leverage skills prior to addressing the more sophisticated and advanced ones at the higher levels of the pyramid.

1. *Self-Perception* is an essential component required for effective EI skill development and consists of *self-regard, emotional self-awareness,* and *self-actualization.*
    a. *Self-regard,* is "the ability to respect and accept (one)self as basically good" (Stein & Book 2006), and that one has strengths and weaknesses (Stein 2011). Consider, as an example, knowing that one remains a good person, a caring and competent nurse or physician, even after facing disappointment in a job search, being laid off during a health system's downsizing, or experiencing a divorce. The ability to maintain respect for oneself and to identify with ethically grounded principles and values while facing the common difficulties of life, or even failing at some of them, is key to maintaining integrity of self, personal identity, and a feeling of self-confidence. The capacity to see oneself as good is essential for relating well to others. If over-used or over-developed, self regard may be interpreted by others as arrogance or cockiness, egotism, and ignoring feedback (Bar-On 1997, Bar-On 2003, Mayer et al 2002, Pearman 2003)–when behaviors are seen in this light leadership derailment is a risk (Lombardo & Eichinger 1989).

The leadership training programs offered through our Department of Maternal and Child Health work to support and develop each of these components of emotional intelligence. In terms of *self-regard,* there are many strategies used to role model this foundational component of EI. The programs are held at executive education centers or resort-type hotels, which cater to individual dietary or disability needs. Conducting the programs at these type of facilities is based on the concept that people learn better when the environment is conducive to the program purpose (learning) and individual comfort. Less-than-comfortable and adequate surroundings strongly distract from the ability of participants to fully focus and learn. Participants are treated respectfully and with exceptional care by the Institute staff: those behaviors are taught and reinforced in training exercises, becoming a behavioral norm. All program content areas are delivered from a non-judgmental perspective, with sessions placing a strong value on cultural competence, tolerance, mutual understanding, and creating a culture of thought diversity (Fernandez 2007b). Participants receive extensive feedback on a variety of psychological and leadership assessments and individual coaching from both the Institute staff and external professional executive coaches—all of which comes from a non-judgmental, supportive, confidential, and positive perspective.

    b. *Emotional self-awareness* is the ability to understand how one is feeling and why (Stein & Book 2006). It further allows one to grasp the nuance of emotions and the potential "impacts they have on the thoughts and actions of oneself and others" (Stein 2011). Decades ago, Eskin noted the concept of self awareness (understanding the self in terms of beliefs, attitudes, norms, and values) as an essential and fundamental quality for a physician to act as a change agent and related lack of these qualities as detrimental to the physician's ability to serve in that capcity (Eskin 1980). Understanding how one personally feels may help one to effectively support oneself and then be able to support others through difficult times. Emotional self awareness allows one's contributions to conversations to revolve around the root issues, rather than to be distracted by the behaviors that can result from the issues. However, when over-used, emotional self-awareness can lead one to being seen as weak or self-absorbed, focused on negativity, melodrama or threats (Bar-On 1997, Bar-On 2002, Mayer et al 2002, Pearman 2003). Leadership development institutes for healthcare-related professions should not only help participants understand how they are feeling, they should also teach how those feelings are similar to and dissimilar from the feelings of others. Our experience indicates that physician leaders tend to be aware of their own emotions—yet they can be surprised that while their feelings and perceptions are logical to them they are not necessarily the same as others whom they admire and respect. We use a variety of psychological assessment instruments to great effect in teaching diversity of perspective, and these contribute greatly to participants' emotional self awareness. For example, our Leadership Institute programs teach differences in how people gather information, make decisions, and deal with change (Jung 1971, Myers and McCaulley 1985, Musselwhite & Ingram 2003, Musselwhite and Jones 2004)—and examine the emotions that arise over these differences. The programs support the value of decision making both from a logical/critical thinking standpoint as well as a values/feeling oriented one (Jung 1971, Myers and McCaulley 1985).

c. *Self-actualization,* is "the ability to lead a rich and meaningful life", and an enjoyable life, through the willingness to persistently strive to improve oneself towards the maximum development of one's abilities and talents (Stein & Book 2006, Bar-On 1997, Bar-On 2006, Stein 2011). Poor EI skills in this area leave one feeling as though life is a treadmill, with no inherent meaning or purpose. One can develop this ability through learning new skills (related or unrelated to clinical practice or administration) or through engaging in selfless activities that benefit others. Many find such personal fulfillment and meaning through volunteer, charity, or medical mission work. When over-used, leaders can appear resistant to the ideas of others, overly self-assured, or intolerant. Healthcare leaders are in danger of personal burnout when very engaged yet going it alone (Bar-On 1997, Bar-On 2002, Mayer et al 2002, Pearman 2003). In our leadership training programs, the nature of support, connection with others, and creation of meaning in life is approached through outdoor experiences and low-ropes course training as well as other team building exercises and sessions that are specifically designed to teach through the experience of fun. Some of our leadership programs include artistic expression and reward as well.

2. *Self-Expression* is the second core area of Personal Competence and contains three elements: *emotional expression, assertiveness, and independence.*

a. *Emotional expression* is a constructive expression of emotions based in an ability to openly convey one's feelings both verbally and non-verbally (Stein 2011). The basic ability to *perceive* these emotions (described above) undergirds the ability to give expression to them. Poor skills in emotional expression leave one with either unexpressed or inappropriately expressed feelings, which can lead to isolation, disengagement, anger or unfounded anxiety. The professional is at risk of being regarded as moody, emotional, too tough or too weak to function appropriately in the organization. At its worst, underdeveloped skills in emotional expression can result in abusive outbursts that are rooted in personal frustration—and clearly lead to derailment (Porath & Pearson 2009, Loop 2009, Pfifferling 2008, Lombardo & Eichinger 1989). Overused skills in this area can lead to team members feeling overwhelmed by the depth of self-revelation (Bar-On 1997, Bar-On 2002, Mayer et al 2002, Pearman 2003). In many organizational cultures having too low a threshold of privacy or confusing honesty with candor can lead to derailment or limited opportunities for advancement as well. The task for the leader is to titrate their degree of emotional self awareness and their response to it, taking into consideration the situation, others involved, the culture of the individuals and their personality as well as the culture of the organization. Circumstances in the healthcare or academic workplace can create a bevy of negative feelings, particularly when organizations or policy issues are undergoing significant change or budgets are strained. In our leadership development programs, we operationalize this construct of emotional expression by teaching participants to "speak the language" of those who see the world differently, building upon the basic investigation of interpersonal differences, as described above (Jung 1971, Myers and McCaulley 1985, Musselwhite & Ingram 2003, Musselwhite and Jones 2004, Fernandez 2007b). We build skills in managing difficult conversations (Fernandez 2010b) and in helping others to gain insight and understanding through negotiation and conflict resolution skills. The programs support the value of decision making both from a logical/critical thinking standpoint as well as a values/feeling oriented one. Creating strong organizational cultures that maximize thought diversity (Fernandez 2007b) is a central tenet of all the leadership programs we offer. Tolerance, respect and civility are behaviors that are often commonly associated with emotional intelligence (Lewis 2010, Fernandez 2010a) and have a strong root in well managed emotional expression.

b. *Assertiveness* is the ability to openly communicate feelings, beliefs, and thoughts and defend personal rights and values in a socially acceptable, non-destructive, non-offensive manner (Stein 2011), and to maintain the ability to do so even if the stance taken is not necessarily admired or accepted by others as the norm (Stein & Book 2006, Lombardo & Eichinger 1989). Certainly, honesty and candor are needed in order to support transparency and information sharing during decision making (O'Toole & Bennis 2009). EI helps one share information and self-advocate with eloquence and grace. When done appropriately, assertiveness allows individuals to respectfully disagree with others and helps in the defense of deeply held beliefs without resorting to subterfuge (Stein & Book 2006). However, when assertiveness is misused individuals may be seen as blunt, abrasive, intimidating, and alienating (Bar-On 1997, Bar-On 2002, Mayer et al 2002, Pearman 2003). Those who are overly zealous can be interpreted or labeled as not being a team player or as a poor listener (Bar-On 1997, Bar-On 2002, Mayer et al 2002, Pearman 2003). The UNC-based leadership training programs teach concepts such as "Managing Difficult Conversations", "Negotiation Skills", "Advocacy", and "High Stress Communications". Each of these sophisticated sessions gives skills-based practice and feedback in appropriate EI-based implementation of assertiveness.

c. *Independence* is being self-controlled and self-directed in one's actions. Freedom from emotional dependency is central to independence (Stein & Book 2006, Bar-On 1997, Bar-On 2006), as is the ability to autonomously engage in decision making, planning and daily tasks (Stein 2011). When independence is under-used or even under-developed, one is more likely to "go along to get along", to succumb to peer pressure, or to refrain from speaking up. When overused, independence is similarly dysfunctional and can lead to isolation, an inability to function well on teams, alienating others, failing to ask for help when needed, or a fear of loss of control (Bar-On 1997, Bar-On 2002, Mayer et al 2002, Pearman 2003). This latter quality may manifest as micromanaging or failure to delegate appropriately. Resisting the bureaucracy inherent in many healthcare organizations—to the detriment of communication and data management—can also be a manifestation of overly relied-upon independence. Our healthcare leadership development programs foster confidence-building and self-efficacy through skills-based training sessions, such as Peer Coaching, which help participants understand the degree of influence they allow from others and how they might work more collaboratively. Sessions that focus on building thought diverse cultures also help those participants who might over-rely on independence to become more collaborative.

3.   *Stress Management* is characterized by the ability to weather difficult situations without becoming overwhelmed (Stein & Book 2006), and is the third core area of Personal Competence. As with the other dimensions of EI it also contains three sub-components: *optimism, stress tolerance,* and *flexibility.*

   a.   *Optimism* is an indicator of one's positive attitude and outlook on life. It is related to remaining resilient and hopeful despite occasional setbacks (Stein 2011), and characterized by the ability to weather difficult situations without becoming overwhelmed (Stein & Book 2006). Adversity and challenge do not defeat or demoralize those who see the proverbial "light at the end of the tunnel". Optimism in the face of stress greatly facilitates learning from mistakes and is positively associated with success, both for the individual and for the group (Stein & Book 2006, Seligman 1998). Optimistic people are sure of themselves in most circumstances, believe they can stay on top of difficult situations through their ability to handle even upsetting problems. When over-used, this skill manifests as a "Pollyana-ish" or unrealistic perspective in which the individual is at risk of failing since they do not take issues seriously enough (Bar-On 1997, Bar-On 2002, Mayer et al 2002, Pearman 2003). When under-used, individuals can become cynical or jaded (Heifetz et al 2009, Pearman 2003). In our physicians leadership training program in particular, optimism is addressed through motivational sessions with prominent athletic coaches, who use a great deal of inspiration in their work with team members. Participants also meet privately with a professional executive coach who can help them explore their own feelings and perceptions as well as their feedback from others.

   b.   *Stress tolerance* is the ability to withstand adverse events and stressful situations without falling apart by actively and positively coping with stress (Stein & Book 2006, Stein 2011). Another term for stress tolerance is "resilience". The risks of having inadequate stress tolerance skills are obvious, yet many are surprised when they learn that these could be over-used as well as under-used. When coping skills are over-used, one does not react with the appropriate sense of urgency or is unaware of being overloaded (Bar-On 1997, Bar-On 2002, Mayer et al 2002, Pearman 2003). This method of coping can lead to burnout and failure to deliver on objectives, a major cause of derailment (Lombardo & Eichinger 1989). Indecisiveness can also result from poor EI skill development in this area (Bar-On 1997, Bar-On 2002, Mayer et al 2002, Pearman 2003). Our leadership training programs offer the opportunity for participants to discuss stress management in their individual coaching sessions as well as to receive feedback on stress management-related behaviors via 360-assessment tools. Some of our programs offer segments in stress management theory and skills.

c. *Flexibility* is the ability to adjust one's thoughts, emotions, and behavior to dynamic circumstances that are unpredictable or unfamiliar (Stein 2011, Stein & Book 2006). Being able to see a situation objectively, as described below in *reality testing*, is related to the ability to capitalize on this EI skill of *flexibility*. Martin (Martin 2007) holds that the ability to hold two opposing ideas in mind and generate a new idea "that contains elements of the others but is superior to both" is a hallmark of exceptional leadership. This ability requires a keen flexibility of the mind. When executed well, flexibility leads to openness and tolerance (Stein & Book 2006, Bar-On 1997, Bar-On 2006, Lewis 2010). Additionally, flexibility allows the iterative process of seeing and embarking on a defined course, re-assessing its effectiveness, and re-directing beliefs and feelings in the light of data accordingly and as necessary. When executed poorly, there is over dependence on routine, a lack of desire to learn new skills, or a refusal to make changes despite the clear need to do so. Over-use of flexibility can result in being taken advantage of, being scattered, or being too easily swayed from one's own good ideas (Bar-On 1997, Bar-On 2002, Mayer et al 2002, Pearman 2003). Participating in a leadership retreat is itself an exercise in flexibility. Program Fellows must constantly adapt to new learning situations, simulations, participative events, and styles. Understanding thought diversity (Fernandez 2007b) and valuing the contributions brought by others who have different skills or perspectives is a foundation of the programs and fosters flexibility. Further, receiving assessment feedback data and understanding how others experience the world or view interpersonal interactions differently from oneself helps many participants become more flexible and less rooted in their own perspective or experience.

4. *Decision Making* is the fourth core area of Personal Competence, containing three sub-elements: *reality testing*, *impulse control*, and *problem solving*.

a. *Reality testing* is the capacity to remain objective by seeing things as they really are (Stein 2011). The ability to recognize when emotions or personal bias can cause one to be less objective is key to this EI construct as well (Stein 2011). This skill includes one's ability to accurately and objectively "size up" a situation (Stein & Book 2006). For example, the ability to depersonalize a situation and gain "a balcony perspective" is a sentinel leadership skill (Heifetz 2009, Linsky & Heifetz 2002, Heifetz et al1994). Increased reality testing proficiency requires taking a step back from situations and refraining from making judgments about them, yet still confronting the truth and facts that are evident (Collins 2001). Effective reality testing can include observing others by their actions and words, and considering the perspectives, needs, biases and beliefs that motivate them. When used poorly, this EI skill appears as overly linear thinking or too "all or none" (Bar-On 1997, Bar-On 2002, Mayer et al 2002, Pearman 2003). Poor reality testing can cause cynicism, pessimism, and over analysis, which can deflate team morale and effectively destroy innovation (Bar-On 1997). UNC leadership development retreats support reality testing through inclusion of several valid and reliable leadership assessment tools, including 360-degree assessments, and tools that measure emotional intelligence. These assessments help participants understand how others view a situation, thus promoting gaining that "balcony perspective". Institutes also include data and fact-based discipline-related sessions, teaching participants how to make decisions and recommendations based on complex data. The ability to use data and fact to depersonalize a situation can help improve reality testing skills.

b. *Impulse control* is the ability to resist or delay an impulse, drive or temptation to act (Stein 2011). It involves managing a temptation, halting an angry or aggressive outburst, or avoiding a hostile or irresponsible behavior (Stein & Book 2006). Examples of poor impulse control include angry outbursts, emotional tempers, insensitive statements, vindictiveness, passive aggressiveness, incivility (Porath & Pearson 2009, Lewis 2010), or uncontrolled passions: these examples are hallmarks of poor emotional intelligence. Low impulse control can have serious implications for organizational culture and productivity. In Leadership and Medicine, (Loop 2009) Loop makes the connection between problematic behavior and career derailment, noting that deficits in impulse control were the biggest executive management problem experienced in the Cleveland Clinic health system (Loop 2009). There is a highly destructive link between incivility and team work, creativity, innovation and commitment (Porath & Pearson 2009, CCL 2010, Lewis 2010). Poor EI skills are evident when one acts in haste, is overly spontaneous, or quick to jump to conclusions. It may seem surprising that impulse control can be over-utilized as well as under-utilized. However over-used impulse control risks failing to react quickly enough, being too aloof, being seen as too unengaged, not being committed to the team, or being unable to be in the present moment (Bar-On 1997, Bar-On 2002, Mayer et al 2002, Pearman 2003). Too much control of self can manifest as inhibition and dissuade one from using assertiveness skills (Bar-On 1997, Bar-On 2002, Mayer et al 2002, Pearman 2003), which, for example, can impair a leader from successfully implementing an organizational culture allowing for zero tolerance of incivility or hostility (Porath & Pearson 2009, Lewis 2010). Similar to stress management skills, the leadership training programs we provide give feedback on many impulse control-related behaviors via 360-assessment tools. Experiential learning sessions and simulations also illicit behaviors around this skill area, allowing the participant to both see the effects of their behaviors and to receive constructive feedback on them.

c. *Problem solving* is "the ability to find solutions to problems in situations where emotions are involved" (Stein 2011). It involves generating and implementing potentially effective solutions (Stein & Book 2006) that take into account how emotions impact decision making (Stein 2011). Problem solving has seven steps, including identifying that a problem exists and gathering the necessary information about that problem (both subjectively and objectively). Subsequently, a list of solutions (assessment/analysis) are generated, and then the alternatives are evaluated. The next steps involve choosing an optimal solution and then implementing it (planning), followed by assessing the outcome. Clinicians, in particular, may relate clinical problem solving with the "SOAP" process, which looks at the Subjective (what the patient says), the Objective (what the clinician measures), the Assessment (what the clinician deduces), and the Plan (diagnostic work up plan, treatment, etc). While this approach is an imminently useful framework for clinical settings, it has more limited uses in general interpersonal situations. Emotional Intelligence skills relate to non-clinical situations as well as clinical ones, and this seven step process an iterative one. Implemented plans need subjective and objective review. At the same time, understanding that some implemented plans are adaptive and require human behaviors for success, achieving changes may need persistence and heavy reliance in EI skills (Heifetz et al 2009, Linsky & Heifetz 2002, Heifetz 1994).

However logical and constructive this skill may seem, common symptoms of overuse are focusing on minutiae, over-analysis, and apparent indecisiveness. At the other extreme, over-reliance on intuition, without sufficient investigation and data gathering, may lead to derailment (Bar-On 1997, Bar-On 2002, Mayer et al 2002, Pearman 2003).

As an example of one strategy for supporting EI problem solving skills, the UNC-based leadership training institutes teach participants to make decisions from a 4-point perspective and to utilize viewpoints that might not be innately natural to them. They are taught how to assess the decision making process in groups, to ascertain when the quality of thought is too homogeneous, and how to introduce questions that will broaden the considerations when solving problems and making decisions (Fernandez 2007b). Additionally a series of outdoor, physical activities force physician leaders to solve complex problems facing the group. These specific situations are designed to lead to team success only when the physicians function as participating and contributing team members — individual, competing leadership styles in these team situations will lead to team failure. Physician leaders engage their problem solving skills and many other EI assets during these exercises.

4. Social competence

As depicted in Figure 1, in the EI development model we follow *Personal Competence* provides the psychological foundation upon which the skills of *Social Competence* are built, following the theories of Goleman (Goleman 1996, Goleman 2000). Social competence is a complex of *social awareness* and *relationship management* that allows a healthcare leader to understand the emotional tenor of her or his group, to communicate effectively and compassionately with members of the group, and to solicit input from them. The ability of healthcare leaders to manage relationships is crucial to their capacity to create impact in their organizations and communities — and for providers, with their patients. In the end, much of success is rooted in successfully managing relationships.

1. *Social awareness* is the ability to understand the social networks and unspoken norms of a group, often through attending to both verbal and non-verbal cues. It is appreciating a group's values and culture (Goleman 2008) and considering the motivations, allegiances and stakeholders which affect others (Heifetz et al 2009, Heifetz 1994). Well-developed EI in this arena allows one to speak with tact and empathy, implementing skills in cultural competence and cultural elasticity. Skills in social awareness allow one to ask for the perspectives of others while listening attentively and non-judgmentally. While critically important for leaders, particularly those in diverse communities or who serve as boundary spanning ambassadors for their organizations, over-use of this skill can lead to unnecessary deference to the group norms and an inability to push group

members with competing or incompatible views toward solutions (Bar-On 1997, Bar-On 2002, Mayer et al 2002, Pearman 2003). Over use of this skill, particularly in combination with poorly used assertiveness and relationship management skills, can lead to organizations that are less culturally competent, flexible, and elastic, and can contribute to "groupthink". (Janis 1972, Janis 1982, Fernandez 2007b, Bosjoly 1987, NASA). In addition to our sessions teaching the concepts of thought diversity, the group-based leadership risk-taking activities and the outdoor experience of low ropes gives participants concrete practice in concepts, behaviors, perspectives and skills around social awareness.

a. *Empathy*. A subcomponent of *Social Awareness* that bridges to *Relationship Management* is *empathy*, which is the ability to recognize, understand, and appreciate the way others feel (Stein 2011). This is considered by many to be a crucial leadership skill (Stein 2011, Stein & Book 2006, Goleman & Boyatzis 2008, Ackley 2006, Goleman 2000, Cummings et al 2010, Levinson et al 2002, Wagner et al 2002). When underused, one risks being perceived as cold, uncaring, self-centered or overly task-focused (Bar-On 1997, Bar-On 2002, Mayer et al 2002, Pearman 2003). Lack of empathy can cause a lack of trust from others or lack of confidence in the ability to confide in the leader. Poorly developed skills in empathy can lead one to be surprised in other people's reactions as well (Bar-On 1997, Bar-On 2002, Mayer et al 2002, Pearman 2003). However, empathy can be overused, causing challenges in separating feelings from business, inability to make tough decisions, an inability to say no, and denying one's own feelings (Bar-On 1997, Bar-On 2002, Mayer et al 2002, Pearman 2003). In our leadership development programs, physician leaders gain skills in empathy through dialogue and psychological assessment feedback instruments as well as coaching. A variety of interactive exercises, as well as intensive emotional exploration around communication and the feelings of others during the outdoor activities promote development of this EI skill.

b. *Interpersonal Relationships* is also an EI skill that bridges the gap between *Social Awareness* and *Relationship Management*, and exists within the larger domain of *Social Competence*. This component is based on developing and maintaining mutually satisfying relationships that are characterized by trust and compassion (Stein & Book 2006, Stein 2010). When this skill is underdeveloped or under-used individuals can be seen as self-absorbed, being more concerned with their own interests or welfare than with that of the team (Bar-On 1997, Bar-On 2002, Mayer et al 2002, Pearman 2003). They can also been seen as cautious when it comes to human interactions and potentially secretive. Conversely, when overused as an EI skill, one can struggle with individual performance and seem incapable of working without a team. Failure to progress with tasks becomes a risk. When so poorly developed that derailment becomes an issue, the behaviors seen can manifest as providing too much personal information, using work relationships inappropriately, violating the personal space of others, or sexual harassment (Bar-On 1997, Bar-On 2002, Mayer et al 2002, Pearman 2003). Our physician leadership programs foster interpersonal relationship skills through 360-feedback, individual coaching, team building exercises and simulations around negotiation skills, and leadership success and derailment, among others.

2. *Relationship management* is the pinnacle of our EI pyramid: as the most sophisticated of the EI skills it relies heavily on the hierarchy of skills upon which it is built (Figure 1). In *relationship management*, one attends to and nurtures interactions with others to create an environment where group behavior can be directed towards a positive course and/or effectively meet difficult challenges. The ability to manage relationships fosters information sharing (O'Toole & Bennis 2009) and creativity (Amabile & Khaire 2008). When relationship management is poorly developed or executed, group competition abounds and problem solving comes from a narrower perspective. When poor relationship management is combined with poor impulse control skills, passive aggression or explosive behavior is likely to manifest. To develop and hone relationship management, a healthcare leader can practice articulating a compelling and unifying vision for the group and specifically one that is grounded in shared values and shared success. Effective mentoring, including providing tactful, sympathetic, contextualized and useful feedback will further support relationship management in professional settings. Cultivating a positive emotional tone among the team, creating a safe environment where ideas can be shared non-judgmentally, and supporting members while fostering their cooperation will likewise further one's relationship management skills and so improve team performance. (Pfifferling 2008, Fernandez 2007a,Goleman 2000, Goleman 2008, Goleman 2001,Thumm 2008). Our UNC-based leadership programs foster relationship management skills through team building exercises and simulations around negotiation skills, among others. Programs also include a mentoring session, which address how to be both a successful mentor as well as mentee.

    a. *Social Responsibility.* The final construct that we capitalize upon in our leadership development programs is social responsibility, which reflects behaviors of willingly contributing to society, to one's social groups, and generally to the welfare of others. It includes acting responsibly, having a social consciousness and showing concern for the greater community (Stein 2011). We find that this is a common strength in our physician leaders, who are all engaged in leadership on an unpaid, volunteer basis, to advocate for the welfare of the patients they serve. In general when this skill is underused or under-developed individuals can be seen as overly self-reliant, willing to bend the rules to favor their own desired outcome, or having a lack of involvement with the greater organizational community or team (Bar-On 1997, Bar-On 2002, Mayer et al 2002, Pearman 2003). When this is an overly-relied upon skill, it can manifest as burnout through taking on too many tasks, adopting other's problems as one's own, making an incorrect — yet popular — choice, or having no tolerance for rule flexibility even when warranted (Bar-On 1997, Bar-On 2002, Mayer et al 2002, Pearman 2003). Leadership development can address issues around social responsibility through interactive values-based exercises. We use a Peer Coaching interaction to approach organizational problems and social responsibility issues, as well as 360-feedback and sessions on leadership success and derailment.

5. The role of well-being and happiness in emotional intelligence

Research in EI formerly characterized *Happiness* as a component of general mood, and a background skill that set the stage for EI development (Bar-On 1997, Stein & Book 2006).

However recent research characterizes *happiness* as an outcome of adequate EI development and an indicator of well-being (Stein 2011). As such it is now seen as separate from the central concept of EI skills (Stein 2011). Happiness is defined as "the ability to feel satisfied with (one's) life, to enjoy (one)self and others and to have fun" (Stein & Book 2006). While these abilities help leaders focus on and play to a team's strengths, there are also interesting supporting relationships between happiness and *self-regard, optimism, interpersonal relationships, and self-actualization* (Stein 2011). The ability to have fun positively impacts a work culture and improves work performance (Stein & Book 2006, Goleman 2008, Goleman 2001). The happiness of the team and its leaders can be a critical element of a healthcare team's success (Porath & Pearson 2009, Pfifferling 2008) and should not be overlooked as a leadership asset. Interestingly, happiness has been found to have a positive, if limited, relationship with physicians' scores on emotional intelligence instruments and patient satisfaction (Wagner et al 2002). In our programs we focus on life satisfaction and interpersonal relationships through a variety of teaching strategies, including one-on-one individual coaching, creating learning sessions that are fun in addition to challenging and thoughtful, and role modeling this perspective for participants. In particular, our physician's leadership development institute provides 35 hours of continuing medical education over a 3-½ day immersion. Despite this extremely intensive structure, the program is designed with a premise of fun, social interaction, group based learning, and networking. For six consecutive years physician participants have rated the experience an overall 5 out of 5 on all program evaluations. Participants leave motivated and "with their vessels refilled", as many comment. Our other leadership programs for allied health and public health follow a similar model.

Through the UNC department of Maternal and Child Health we work with about 200 mid- to senior-level leaders a year as of this printing. We strongly believe that leadership training programs can promote the broad array of EI-based skills and foster practical leadership skills in physicians, nurses, public health and other health-related and public sector professionals.

6. Conclusion

Early research in EI has shown that five areas measured by standardized EQ tests (Stein & Book 2006, Bar On 1997, Bar On 2006) relate to workplace success: self-actualization, stress tolerance, happiness, optimism, and assertiveness. While we hold that each of the areas discussed above are crucial for effective EI development, the data that these five areas relate to career success are most interesting. More research is needed to further validate these findings. Table 1 relates these specific five areas to strategies for improvement in both clinical and external-to-work settings. It would be helpful for research to focus on measuring improvement of practical EI skills development in these five areas, however it should be noted that the innate complexity of EI presents significant challenges to its measurement. Rigid tests that determine EI are not available in the same sense that clinical tests can determine the presence of a specific type of virus or a level of a health-risk indicator from a blood sample. Assessments of EI capture a more generalized picture of these *personal competence* and *social competence* skills, and thus research into methodology for developing strongly measureable EI skills, quantified in terms of EQ, remains in the relatively early stages. It may be that definitively measuring emotional intelligence will prove elusive—far more elusive than capturing the interpersonal and organizational impacts on situations in which those skills are underdeveloped in leaders. This dichotomy — the ease of observing the absence of EI skills coupled with the extreme difficulty in measuring the EQ skills—presents interesting challenges to those interested in EI research.

Yet, strategies that facilitate strong EI skill development could prove exceptionally helpful to healthcare leaders, and particularly physician leaders and those in public or academic settings. Promoting one's own emotional intelligence can impact the observed emotional intelligence skills and behaviors of co-workers and team members (Porath & Pearson 2009, Goleman 2001). While the use of logic and reason in decision making and interaction are important, so is the recognition that humans are primarily emotional animals. Being able to give constructive voice to personal opinions while remaining optimistic, tolerating the stresses and challenges of the workplace, and being sensitive to the views and feelings of co-workers are essential skills that facilitate workplace success. We have found that using the model of EI presented herein as a theoretical basis for the creation of a variety of leadership institutes for those in medicine, allied health, academic organizations, and public health, has resulted in very highly rated experiences that are both meaningful to the participants as well as build practical skills for the healthcare and public sector workplace. Thus, in particular, this EI model serves as a helpful guide to creating interactive leadership development programs that build skills in key leadership personnel.

We are starting to evaluate the impacts of leadership training based on this EI model in our most mature programs, which include the physician leadership and academic leaders programs (each entering a seventh cohort in 2011-2012). In our academic leaders programs one of the largest measureable impacts has been professional career development and career progression. Fellows start in this 2-year program primarily at the Chair/Head or Assistant Dean level. As of 2011, 40% of graduates from the first five cohorts have moved into new positions of greater authority, including three serving as University Presidents, two as Provosts, seven as Vice President/Vice Provost, and nine as Deans of their schools. We also have a wealth of qualitative data supporting the effectiveness of these kinds of interventions on developing and honing interpersonal and leadership skills. This qualitative data is still in the collection stages and has yet to be published.

In our physician leadership development programs, one of the primary program goals has served as a measure of success: subsequent commitment to and participation in district and national-level activities in the partnering professional association. Since this participation requires volunteer time of these physicians, which impedes their opportunity for personal financial advancement, allocating time to the professional association requires considerable personal sacrifice. Willingness to make this personal sacrifice after attending the leadership institute has been seen as a strong measure of program success. Qualitative data gathered consistently links the program's personal impact with both the intent to participate and the subsequent participation in leadership activities in the organization. Currently, 21 of the 25 members of the leadership council have completed a district and/or the national leadership institute. Sixteen of these same individuals have completed the training at the national level. Implementation at the District level has been seen as an unexpected measure of success. While the program was initially offered only at the National level, graduates returned to their districts and advocated for this training to be more widely available and offered to the district level membership. As of 2011, half of the professional association's districts have now offered a 1-day version of the larger program, with nearly all of the 11 districts planning to include it over the next few years. Another unexpected measure of success of this type of training occurred in 2009, when budgetary concerns called into question the continuation of the National program. Graduates led a campaign to endow the program themselves by making personal financial contributions. Their advocacy efforts ensured that the National leadership program was allocated for in the permanent budget of the association. While this does not demonstrate a measureable increase in EI skills, it clearly demonstrates the perception of impact and significance of the program by those who have completed the EI-promoting experience. We are currently looking at ways to qualitatively measure behaviorally-demonstrated skills in EI-related areas in participants.

Our public health-sector program is in its second cohort of Fellows and success will be measured by the community and organizational-based impacts of their individual leadership projects. Most of these projects involve coalition building and the creation of partnerships, both of which rely heavily on the successful use of EI-related skills. The impacts of these projects will become increasingly clear over the next few years and will be studied. In this program we are also undertaking an analysis of a "ripple effect" of training—that is how leadership training of one individual impacts the skill development of others in organizational settings. We hope to track the impact of improving EI-related interpersonal skills across organizations through associated learning in addition to tracking improvements in outcomes such as community partnerships and community health indicators.

While participants in our programs provide a wealth of qualitative data, as yet unpublished, of how they have implemented the leadership skills gained through programs based on this EI-model, for practical reasons we have yet to undertake a systematic review or conduct an analysis with a control group. In fact, we are unaware of any published studies that assess the impact of leadership training based on emotional intelligence which include a well-defined control group. However, there is research that evaluates other public-sector impacts of this kind of training that relate to successful implementation of the type of *personal* and *social competence* skills discussed in this chapter. A report by the Lewin Group provides stunning findings on the Management Academy for Public Health (MAPH), also offered at the University of North Carolina at Chapel Hill through the Gillings School of Global Public Health. This program offers leadership training through a practical business skills focus, not an exclusively EI focus, although many of the projects put forth by these public health teams require partnerships and coalitions. In 2003 the Lewin Group analysis reported that nearly 40% of MAPH alumni teams implemented business plans as a result of the Management Academy training. The Lewin Group found that these alumni teams generated $6 million in revenue with those plans, which represents a 300% return on investment of the approximately $2 million spent on the training (Lewin Group 2003). While results of EI-based leadership training would not likely be measured in such stark terms as revenue generated, this study supports the strong impacts that leadership training in general can have in non-profit, health-focused organizations, and how those impacts might be measured and captured.

The importance of the development of EI skills to successful leaders is clear and has been demonstrated in a variety of fields. Yet more research on *measureable strategies* to successfully develop EI-based leadership skills is crucial and would make a significant contribution to the field, as would further research on refined measures of EI itself. Such research could further promote effective leader development and support inclusion of those strategies in succession planning and talent development programs across health care and other non-profit, public sectors.

EQ Skill: **Self Actualization** The ability to lead a rich and meaningful life by persistently striving to improve oneself towards the maximum development of one's abilities and talents (Stein and Book 2006, Stein 2011). *Examples:* • *Deciding to learn how to speak medical Spanish in response to a desire to pursue life long learning and because of an increasing number of Spanish speaking only patients coming from the community to the office for care* • *Learning new skills outside of medicine (dance class, scuba diving, art or music skills)* • *Engaging in selfless activities that benefit others*
EQ Skill: **Stress Tolerance** The ability to withstand adverse events without falling apart or becoming overwhelmed (Stein and Book 2006, Stein 2011). *Examples:* • *Coping with an operative complication and leading staff through the necessary steps to address the complication without panicking or yelling and doing so calmly.* • *Having an outlet for stress reduction (exercise, meditation, yoga, tai chi)* • *Managing difficult patients or patients' families without becoming negatively impacted* • *Practice the ability to "let go" of situations you can't control or that are in the past*
EQ Skill: **Optimism** The ability to maintain a positive attitude despite challenges and setbacks. *Examples:* • *Positively rallying staff and self to temporarily work longer hours than usual in response to receiving unexpected news that a fellow staff person will be out of the office schedule for 3 weeks due to a family emergency* • *Seeking the positive aspects of changes* • *Seeing conflict as an opportunity for change* • *Adapting to changing work environment (mastering a new skill)* • *Confront the truth and facts that are around you and remain firm in your belief that you will prevail in the end (Collins 2001)*
EQ Skill: **Happiness** The ability to feel satisfied with one's life, to enjoy oneself and others, and to have fun (Stein & Book 2006, Stein 2011). *Examples:* • *Taking time to enjoy lunch with staff after a busy office Monday morning and actively participating in the conversation on what everyone did for the weekend.* • *Engaging in an environment of teamwork* • *Creating camaraderie with staff & other colleagues*

EQ Skill: **Assertiveness**

The ability to openly communicate feelings, beliefs, and thoughts and defend personal rights and values in a socially acceptable, non-destructive, non offensive manner, and to maintain the ability to do so even if the stance taken is not admired or accepted by others as the norm, the ability to constructively self-advocate (Stein & Book 2006, Stein 2011)
Examples:
- *Professionally confronting a colleague who is always 15 minutes late to the clinic when s/he comes on call.*
- *Pursuing promotion & tenure*
- *Seeking a raise/bonus*
- *Asking for recognition of one's achievements*
- *Learning to delegate & work as a team*
- *Maintaining principles/ethics even when asked by patient to bend the rules*

Table 1. Strategies for developing the specific EI skills related to work-based success, as measured using EQ instrumentation (Bar-On 1997, Bar-On 2002, Stein 2011).

7. Acknowledgment

The authors would like to thank Dr. Shane Burgess, Dean of the College of Agriculture and Life Sciences at the University of Arizona, for his generous editorial advice on this chapter.

8. References

_____. (2011). Culture is the Key to Execution. H&HN: Hospitals & Health Networks, August, Supplement, p24-25.

Ackley, D. (2006) EQ Leader program manual. Toronto, Canada: Multi-Health Systems

Amabile TM, Khaire M. (2008). Creativity and the role of the leader. *Harvard Business Review*, October 2008, pp 101-109.

Awad SS, Hayley B, Fagan SP, Berger DH, Brunicardi C. (2004). The impact of a novel resident leadership training curriculum. The American Journal of Surgery vol 188, pp 481-481.

Bar-On R. (1997). EQ-I technical manual. Toronto, Canada: Multi Health Systems.

Bar-On R. (2002). EQ-I technical manual. Toronto, Canada: Multi Health Systems.

Bar-On R. (2006).The Bar-On model of emotional-social intelligence (ESI). *Psicothema*. Vol 18 Suppl, pp 13-25.

Boisjoly, Roger M. 1987.Ethical Decisions -- Morton Thiokol and the Space Shuttle Challenger Disaster. American Society of Mechanical Engineers Annual Meetings. Webpages created by Jagruti S. Patel and Phil Sarin, "Engineers and Scientists Behaving Well" Online Ethics Center for Engineering 6/9/2010 National Academy of Engineering URL:*http://www.onlineethics.org/Topics/ProfPractice/Exemplars/BehavingWell/RB-intro.aspx, accessed July 15, 2011.*

Calabrese, RL; Roberts, B. (2001). The promise forsaken: neglecting the ethical implications of leadership. The International Journal of Educational Management, vol 15, issue 6, pp 267-275. This article is available at www.emerald-library.com/ft

Center for Creative Leadership (2010). Addressing the leadership gap in healthcare. What's needed when it comes to leader talent? A white paper. Greensboro, NC: CCL; July.

Center for Studying Health System Change (2008). "Making Medical Homes Work: Moving From Concept to Practice." *Policy Perspective* December, pp 1-20.

Chaudry J, Jain A, Mckenzie S, Schwartz RW. (2008). Physician Leadership: The Competencies of Change. J surg Education, Vol 63, issue 3, pp 213-220.

Collins, J. (2001). Good to Great: why some companies make the leap...and others don't. Harper Business, NY.

Cummings GC; MacGregor T; Davey M; Lee H, Wong CA, Lo E, Muise M, Stafford E. (2010). Leadership styles and outcome patterns for the nursing workforce and work enviornment: A systematic review. International Journal of Nursing Studies. Vol 47, pp 363-385.

Eskin F. (1980). The community physician as change agent. Public Health. Vol 94, pp 44-51.

Fernandez CSP. (2007). Emotional intelligence in the workplace. *J Public Health Pract Manage*; vol 13, issue 1, pp 80-82.

Fernandez, C. (2007). Creating thought diversity: the antidote to group think. *J Public Health Management Practice*, vol 13, issue 6, pp 679–680.

Fernandez, CSP (2010). Emotional Intelligence in the Workplace. In Baker, E.L., Menkens A.J., Porter J.E. (eds), Managing the Public Health Enterprise. Jones and Bartlett Publishers, Boston (MA). Pp 45-50.

Fernandez, CSP (2010). Managing the Difficult Conversation. In Baker, E.L., Menkens A.J., Porter J.E. (eds), Managing the Public Health Enterprise. Jones and Bartlett Publishers, Boston (MA). Pp 145-150.

Fisher, E. (2008). "Building a Medical Neighborhood for the Medical Home." *New England Journal of Medicine vol* 359, issue 12, pp 1202-1205.

Freshman B, Rubino L.(2002). Emotional intelligence: a core competency for health care administrators. Health Care Manag (Frederick). vol 20. pp 1-9.

Goleman D. (1996) Emotional intelligence: why it can matter more than IQ. New York: Bantam Dell.

Goleman D. (2000). Leadership that gets results. *Harvard Bus Rev*. March-April. pp 78-90.

Goleman D, Boyatzis R, McKee A. (2001). Primal leadership: the hidden driver of great performance. *Harvard Bus Rev*. December. pp 42-51.

Goleman D, Boyatzis R. (2008). Social intelligence and the biology of leadership. *Harvard Bus Rev*. September pp 74-81.

Gifford BD, Zammuto RF, Goodman EA. (2002). The relationship between the hospital unit culture and nurses' quality of work life. *J Healthc Manag* vol 47. pp 13-25.

Heifetz R. Leadership without easy answers. (1994). Cambridge (MA): Harvard University Press.

Heifetz R, Linsky M, Grashow A. (2009). The practice of adaptive leadership: tools and tactics for changing your organization and the world. Boston (MA): Harvard Business Press.

Hill KS. (2002). Practitioner Application (organizational culture of nursing units). *J Healthc Manag*. vol 47. pp 25-26.

Horwitz IB, Horwitz SK, Daram P, Brandt ML, Brunicardi FC, Awad SS. (2008). Transformational, transactional, and passive-avoidant leadership characteristics of a surgical resident cohort: analysis using the multifactor leadership questionnaire and implications for improving surgical education curriculums. J Surg Res. Vol 148. pp 49-59

Janis, IL (1972). Victims Of Groupthink. Houghton Mifflin Company Boston, 1972

Janis, IL. (1982). Victims Of Groupthink. Houghton Mifflin Company Boston, 1982

Jung, C. (1971). Psychological Type. Princeton, NJ: Princeton University Press.

Klaus P. (2008). The hard truth about soft skills: workplace lessons smart people wish they'd learned sooner. New York (NY): HarperCollins.

Lattore P, Lumb PD.(2005). Professionalism and interpersonal communications: ACGME competencies and core leadership development qualities. Why are they so important and how should they be taught to anesthesiology residents and fellows? Seminars in Anesthesia, Perioperative Medicine, and Pain. Vol 24. pp 134-137.

The Lewin Group, Inc (Fairfax, VA). Management Academy for Public Health Final Program Evaluation. Submitted to the CDC Foundation; 2003:21. Unpublished report.

Lewis, D. (2010). Promoting a Civil Workplace. In Baker, E.L., Menkens A.J., Porter J.E. (eds), Managing the Public Health Enterprise. Jones and Bartlett Publishers, Boston (MA). Pp 51-56.

Levinson W, D'Aunno T, Gorawara-Bhat R, Stein T, Reifsteck S, Egener B, Dueck R. (2002). Patient-physician communication as organizational innovation in the managed care setting. Am J. Managed Care vol 8 . pp 622-630.

Linsky M, Heifetz R. (2002). Leadership on the line: staying alive through the danger of leading. Boston (MA): Harvard Business Press.

Lombardo MM, Eichinger RW.(1989). Preventing derailment: what to do before it's too late. Greensboro (NC): Center for Creative Leadership.

Loop FD.(2009). Leadership and medicine. Fire Starter Publishing. Gulf Breeze (FL).

Lynn AB. (2002). The emotional intelligence activity book: 50 activities for promoting EQ at work. New York (NY): HRD Press.

Mayer JD, Salovey P, Caruso DR. (2002). Mayer-Salovey Emotional Intelligence Tests (MSCEIT) User's Manual. Toronto. Canada: Multi-Health Systems Inc;.

Martin A. (2005). The changing nature of leadership: A CCL Research Report. The Center for Creative Leadership, Greensboro (NC), pp 1-16.

Martin, R. (2007). How Successful Leaders Think. Harvard Business Review, June, pp 60-67.

Mrkonjic L, Grondin SC. (2011). Introduction to concepts in leadership for the surgeon. Thoracic Surgery Clinics. August, vol 21, pp 323-331.

Musselwhite WC, Ingram R.P. (2003). Change Style Indicator: Facilitator Guide (technical manual). Discovery Learning Press, Greensboro (NC).

Musselwhite, C. Jones R. (2004). Dangerous Opportunity: Making Change Work. Xlibris Corporation. Bloomington (IN).

Myers, I.B. & McCaulley, M.H. (1985). Manual: A guide to the development and use of the Myers-Briggs Type Indicator. Palo Alto, (CA): Consulting Psychology Press.

O'Mallley, A., Peikes, D., & Ginsburg, P. (2008). "Making Medical Homes Work: Moving from Concept to Practice & Qualifying a Physician Practice as a Medical Home." Policy Perspective. vol 1. pp 1-19.

O'Toole J, Bennis W. (2009). What's needed next: a culture of candor. Harvard Business Review. June. pp 54-61.

Pagnini F, Manzoni GM. (2009). Emotional intelligence training and evaluation in physicians. Letter to the editor. JAMA, February 11, 2009; vol 301. Issue 6.

Pearman R. (2003). Emotional Intelligence For Self-Management and Enhanced Performance v 5.2 (Bar-On Emotional Quotient Training Manual). Qualifying.Org. Winston-Salem (NC).

Pearman R. (2002) Introduction to type and emotional intelligence: pathways to performance. Palo Alto (CA): Consulting Psychologists Press.

Pfifferling, JH. (2008). Physicians' "disruptive" behavior: consequences for medical quality and safety. *American Journal of Medical Quality*. Vol 23. pp 165 (URL: *http://ajm.sagepub.com*)

Porath CL, Pearson CM. (2009). The Cost of Bad Behavior. *Organizational Dynamics*. Vol 39. Issue 1.pp 64-71.

Report of the Presidential Commission on the Space Shuttle Challenger Accident, Chapter VII: The Silent Safety Program, URL: *http://history.nasa.gov/rogersrep/genindex.htm* URL:*http://history.nasa.gov/rogersrep/51lcover.htm*, accessed July 15th 2011. Part [70] Findings. 10.c.

Rosenthal, T. (2008). "The Medical Home: Growing Evidence to Support a New Approach to Primary Care." *Journal of the American Board of Family Medicine*. vol 21. Issue 5. pp 427-440.

Schwartz RW, Pogge C. (2000). Physician Leadership: essential skills in a changing environment. Am J Surg. Vol 180. pp 187-192.

Seligman MEP. (1998). Learned optimism. New York (NY): Pocket Books.

Stein SJ, Book HE. (2006). The EQ edge: emotional intelligence and your success, (2nd edition). Toronto, Canada: Multi-Health Systems.

Stein, SJ. (2011). The Complete EQ-I 2.0 Model (technical manual). Toronto, Canada: Multi-Health Systems. Accessed at http://ei.mhs.com/eq20_manual/part1/Intro.html September 21, 2011.

Thumm JE. (2008). Soft skills for tough issues: fostering interpersonal communication in the workplace. Bloomington (IN): Xlibiris.

Wagner PJ, Moseley GC, Grant MM, Gore JR, Owens C. (2002). Physician's emotional intelligence and patient satisfaction. Fam Med vol 34. Issue 10. pp 759-4.

14

Thinking Skill of Emotional Intelligence Education Programme

Müge Yılmaz
Ondokuzmayıs University
Turkey

1. Introduction

Human being is the one that can express his feelings and thoughts which result in behaviour verbally. Emotions have effect that can influence all of one's behaviour at each stage of his life. For long time, it is seen that within the studies concerning intelligence, emotions have not been taken into consideration. However, recently the impact of emotions upon intelligence and behaviour is begun to be discussed with the emerge of the term emotional intelligence. Because the expression "many of the skills that we use in our lives arise from our emotions and thoughts." has become a widely accepted one. As well as the intellectual intelligence, emotional intelligence is also important in order for an individual to reach the desired results and lead a fruitful life (Yavuz,2002).

For researchers, the non-cognitive side of the intelligence is also important and before 1940s intelligence was divided into two as cognitive and non-cognitive elements. Non-cognitive elements indicate the affection(tenderness), personality and social factors (Cherniss, 2000; Ülgen,1995; Gürün, 1991; Brockert & Braun, 2000). Additionally, the personality of the individual and the skills have significant effect upon his behaviour. In relation to this, it is known that emotions effect the personality and the skills (Ackerman & Haggestad, 1997; Salovey&Sluyter, 1997).

The term emotional intelligence primarily focuses on the intelligence potential that reflects from the emotional results in daily life. For most healthy individual, emotions give information about human relations. For instance, responses that arise from emotions like fear and happiness and the view of the relations of the individual with the others help to form emotional laws and emotional generalizations. These general rules help to understand and identify reason of the emotions. Apart from identifying simple emotions, in order to understand emotional intelligence, it is needed to understand the cultural surrounding of the individual (Salovey&Sluyter, 1997).

Understanding the cultural surrounding of the individual will help us to understand how their emotional intelligence work. Firstly, the emotional schemes that cultural cultural environment has created will activate their intellectual functions with the emotions that the individual has.

Emotions take place at the second half of the intellectual functions. The term that is tried to be identified with emotions include the whole of the emotions, emotion situations, evaluations and other emotion expressions. As a result, the identifications of emotional intelligence need to be the ones that associate intelligence and emotion (Mayer et al.,2000). One of the reasons of the intelligence and emotion association is that they both take place in intellectual functions. The schemes that take place in mind and are still being formed function with emotions and construct a basis for our behaviour.

When emotions activate the schemes, they form a special potential. Emotions and thoughts are the parts and parcels of the same operation. A thought activates an emotion and thus emotions direct thoughts (Brocket&Braun, 2000; Damasio, 1999; Ortony et al., 1998).

Emotions effect the individual in many ways. Not only emotions effect the individual, but they also effect the community that the individual lives. As well as the same emotions effect the individuals in different ways, different emotions may cause different emotions upon the same individual. These effects both influence the physical and phenomenological periods. Especially, it effects the memory, thinking, and imagining skills. Perception periods that are effected by emotions are in proportion with cognitive periods. For instance, an angry person just has angry thoughts. Our behaviour is shaped in relation to the organized thoughts and basic perception. At the basis of the emotional reactions there underlie an object or a situation (Izard, 1989).

Emotions improve our adaptation skills to the basic living skills. Basic living skills can be explained as achieving, losing, disappointment. Some general rules (elements) of living skills are made up of emotions. Though, emotions show individual and cultural differences, they are observable phenomenon based upon social learning (Ekman&Davidson, 1994).

In emotional intelligence development, in limited sensation, the usage and the direction of emotions concepts take place. External behaviour like posture, mimic, voice, muscle movements, and etc. can be observed by other people. Behaviour forms that come out as a result of emotions also show the emotional intelligence level of the individual.

Thorndike's "Social Intelligence" and Gardner's "Multiple Intelligence" studies can be placed within the researches that make up the concept of Emotional Intelligence. Salovey and Mayer used the term "Emotional Intelligence" for the first time. Salovey and Mayer (1990) explained emotional intelligence as evaluating the individual's own emotions and others and the ability to use this information effectively. Bar-on (1996) explained it as the individual's ehole emotional, personal, and social abilities. Later, Mayer, Salovey and Caruso (2000) explained emotional intelligence as realizing the emotions, realizing the relations that underlie the emotions, perceiving, ordering, managing the emotions in interpersonal relations, reasoning and problem solving. As it is seen, the other term is based on the usage of the emotions to develop the cognitive activities.

Goleman (1996) explained emotional intelligence as "understanding his own and others' feelings, distinguishing feelings, thinking about these emotions and using them as information for acting". Emotional intelligence can be identified as "auto-control, enthusiasm and constancy and the ability to motivate himself." In this explanation it is concentrated on motivational specialities like constancy and enthusiasm rather than emotion.

Also, the researches show that emotional and social skills support the development of the cognitive functions of the emotional and social skills. One of the kind of emotional intelligence keeping stress under control and directing emotions are also significant for success.

While emotional intelligence make decisions within life, it also includes the knowing and the usage of the emotions in terms of the individual. Emotional intelligence show itself as on the way to the individual's targets, controlling reactions, directing emotions under stress, and motivating himself towards positive and hopeful thinking. At the same time, emotional intelligence is a kind of social skills which forms the relations with the other individuals, directs the emotions in the relations, and serves basis for directing and perceiving emotions in relations (Oneil, 1996). Emotional intelligence is the emotional needs, drives, and true values of a person and guides all overt behavior. A person's interests tell you what a person likes to do. A person's mental and physical skills tell you what a person can do. However, a person's emotional intelligence determines what they do and will do (Simmons & Simmons, 1997). Emotional intelligence is a container term which encloses a series of skills one learns more or less intuitively (Merlevede; Bridoux & Vandamme, 2001).

This huge frame changes in individual differences and sex. The differences of emotional intelligence from IQ are that it can be teachable and learnable, also the skills that are apart from sole cognitive abilities and the abilities that just can complete it. Generally, cognitive abilities do not change after infancy period ends. While our emotional intelligence level is not genetically inherited, its development does not happen just at the first infancy periods (Goleman, 1999).

All the elements that form emotional intelligence have strengthening abilities for emotional intelligence with the others. They are lining up hierarchically and each step is bound to the other step. These four building stones are:

1. The ability to comprehending, commenting and identifying the emotion fully and precisely.
2. The ability to identify and produce the right emotion for the existing situation and to have the emotion control that will help to understand the emotions of himself and the others.
3. The ability to understand the emotions and the information that comes from the emotions.
4. The ability to arrange the emotions towards emotional and intellectual development as impulsive force (Weisinger, 1998).

As stated above emotional intelligence is explained with four dimensions:

The first dimension of the emotional intelligence starts with expressing and perceiving the emotions. Without this dimension, it is not possible to talk about emotional intelligence. Perception of the emotion concerns decoding, searching and recording the code of the emotional messages like facial expression and voice. The second dimension of the emotional intelligence is about the usage of emotions in cognitive activities. Emotions are the complex structures of psychological, experimental, cognitive and motivational substructures. Entering the emotions and both of the cognitive systems compose cognitive emotions. For instance, one thinks "I am sorry now." and this is a cognitive structure. The feeling of being sorry is the emotional side. This dimension focuses on how emotions effect cognitive system. Emotions are especially effective in problem solving, deciding, and creativity periods. Of course, cognitive structure can be interrupted by emotions, as it is in worry and fear. However, emotions may give priority to cognitive system to direct emotions to the important and also emotional state can be an incentive force to focus on the subject. Emotions change the cognitive structures. If the individual is happy s/he thinks positive, however if s/he is sad, s/he thinks negative. This changing power in cognitive system is because of different perspectives.

The third dimension is understanding emotions. At this level, the basic structure is to identify the emotion words and the relations among them. Individual emotional intelligence is the skill that identifies the terms which arranges emotion expression terms and groups. Results are gathered as a result of the relations of these terms. This is very significant. For example, if provocative stimulant is eliminated, some emotions like boredom and anger can manipulate us. The individual can get to know the emotions that directs him. He can get to know the meaning of the emotions, which of them come together, and their repeating periods. The capacity of understanding emotions is a significant part of human nature and interpersonal relations. Realizing his own feelings help the individual to perceive others' emotions in an emphatic way. Empathy is directing rather than imitating emotional bound and sharing belief and ideas .

The fourth dimension directing is used as arranging emotions from time to time. Though this fourth dimension is seen as a probable result of these four stages, it works as a director at the optimal level of emotion arrangement. Similarly, when another individual express his feelings or these feelings are perceived, though the others' feelings are in charge it adds little in arranging the feelings. The techniques of arranging other individuals' feelings have boundaries and these boundaries show individual differences. There is also an assumption that physical exercises are influential in arranging the relation between the individual's emotion state and and the others' emotion states.

Generally, a successful emotion arrangement method includes energy consumption which is because of active emotion situation manipulation that can make out a whole relief, stress manipulation, cognitive effort and bad mood. The centre of the individual's emotion arrangement is made up by the individual's direction and reflection of his own feelings and releasement of these feelings (Salovey et al., 2000). In emotional intelligence approaches, there are two models. The first model is the "ability model". It is based on the assumption that the emotions work as a determiner on relations. The model of Mayer and Salovey is an ability model. The second model is the Mix Model. This model includes intelligence definitions like social skills, personality specialities, and the abilities like behaviour. Goleman's Bar-on Model is a sample of Mix Model. At the same time, there are models similar to mix model and include the behaviour related to emotions, moreover there are models similar to intelligence-trait approach and emotional intelligence-ability models that include cognitive abilities related to intelligence. Though emotional intelligence models seem different, they have some similarities. For example; Salovey and Mayer's "reception of emotions" dimension is similar to Bar-on's "Emotional Awareness". The difference between Trait EI and Ability EI is their measurement. While Trait EI is related to behavioural tendencies and self perceived abilities, Ability EI is related to psychometric intelligence. In other words, Trait EI is handled with personality specialities, Ability EI is handled with cognitive abilities (Mayer; Roberts & Barsade, 2008).

Mayer and Salovey (1997) evaluated emotional intelligence model with four subheadings. These are: Perceiving and expressing the emotions, internalizing the emotions within thoughts, understanding and analyzing the emotions, ordering the emotions with thought. It focuses on emotional skills that can be developed through learning and experience (Lopes; Salovey&Straus, 2003). This conceptualization of Emotional Intelligence has been referred to as "Ability EI" (Warwick & Nettelbeck, 2004). Then, with Caruso (2004), they explained emotional intelligence with skill model which has four subheadings. First level is EQ skills, perception of emotions and evaluation. Second level is EQ skills, analysis of basic emotional expressions in mind. Third level is QE skills, understanding emotions, deducing from them and managing the emotions of others. Bar-on (2006) model is a mixed model which is the organization of personal, emotional, social, ability and skills. This model is divided into five subheadings as personal, interpersonal, adaptation, stress management, and general mood. The third approach to EI is often referred to as a Mixed Model approach because of the mixed qualities that such models target. Mixed model is a theoretical approach that equates diverse psychological traits, abilities, styles, and other characteristics to EI . Specific-Ability approaches to emotional intelligence is related to the individual's mental capacity and deals with the basic skills of emotional intelligence. E.g; how emotional information is used in thinking. These are considered; nonverbal perception, evaluation of emotions, labelling, managing language and emotions. What is meant by understanding emotions is how the individual defines his and the others' emotions. Managing the emotions is another skill that takes place in this approach. The integrative –model approaches focus on the universal and cohesive abilities of the individual. The specialities that take place within this approach happen within early childhood of the individual and this is a common point (Mayer; Roberts & Barsade, 2008).

Emotional intelligence is the basis of emotional abilities and these abilities are in relation with emotional intelligence. Yeşilyaprak (2001) states that emotional intelligence is the ability of the individual to use his feelings smartly, sensitively, beneficial and wisely. The concept emotional intelligence is identified under five headings.

1. Self-conscious: the ability to notice an emotion while it is being formed.
2. Controlling the emotions: the ability to control the emotions in an acceptable way.
3. Activating himself/herself: gathering the emotions around an aim, paying attention, activating himself or herself and controlling himself or herself.
4. Understanding others emotions: the ability of empathy in a general sense.
5. Continuing the relations: the ability to control others' emotions (Goleman, 1996).

The usage of emotion information is a helpful element in identifying an individual's intelligence. Nevertheless, the traditional school curriculum do not include neither intelligence researches nor systematic researches. As a result of these views, it is widely seen that emotional intelligence is a learnable and improvable type of intelligence. As a result, Thinking Skill of Emotional Intelligence Education Programme is developed and it is aimed to search the effect of this programme on the individuals' emotional intelligence levels.

There are scientific journals that inform about the education to improve individuals' emotional intelligence and its fruitful results. The skills concerning emotional intelligence are the skills that are related to realizing emotions, expressing emotions, directing emotions, motivating himself and controlling relations. Emotional intelligence skills can be acquired through living and through improving behaviour in learning process.

Thinking Skill of Emotional Intelligence Education Programme is a mixed model of intrapersonal and interpersonal skills. Intrapersonal skills are realizing one's his/her own feelings and the ability to express them. Interpersonal skills are realizing others' emotions and thoughts and using them for beneficial purposes. Educational model is made up of five dimensions. These five dimensions can be explained as;

1. Being aware of the emotions: It is the skill of understanding one's own feelings, being aware of the emotions, getting to know himself, getting to know the other individual and his feelings, expressing the emotions verbally and via body language, and linking the emotions and thoughts.
2. Directing the emotions: Realizing the emotion that underlies the emergent emotion, and the ability to show the appropriate feeling.
3. Motivating himself: Discovering the emotions that will motivate himself, not letting the emotions prevent himself and the ability to put up with stress.
4. Empathy: Understanding the others' emotions and thoughts, transferring the understood thoughts, and the ability to show the appropriate emotion.
5. Controlling the Relations: Realizing the relations of himself, and the emotional outcomes can effect his relationships, and the skill of evaluating the relationships.

2. The application of thinking skill of emotional intelligence

Education Model is prepared considering Philip Burnard's "Interpersonal Skills Training" book, Martin Orridge's "75 Ways to Liven Up Your Training", Debbie Pincus's"Manner Matter Activities to Teach Young People Social Skills", Seymour Epstein's "Constructive Thinking", Schilling and Palomores's "50 Activities for Teaching Emotional Intelligence", Mehmet E. Sarıdoğan's "The Effect of Florida Human Relations Skills Model on anxiety, loneliness, entreprising,opening himself, and empathic skills Level" and Seher Balcı's doctoral thesis "The Effect of Counselling Skills Education on University Students' Communication Skills Level". Thinking Skill of Emotional Intelligence Education Programme curricula, the rules to be obeyed, and the procedure are going to be presented.

Manner Matter is an activity book that offers students creative, imaginative ways to explore what manners are and are not, why they matter and how to use manners to get more from life. The book is divided into nine chapters such as getting to know one another, polite words and greetings, more mannerly ways. These parts are handled in a humorous way and at the end of each activity the attendants are asked open-ended questions about their ideas and insights, and the results are discussed. During the preparation of education programme, it is seen that the attendants can develop social awareness skills and they can also increase the number of sharings with the help of this book. "Interpersonal Skills Training" book is written as a sourcebook for participants to develop their interpersonal skills. The book has two parts. The first part of the book offers a theoretical context. It deals with issues such as: What are interpersonal skills?, What sort of training methods are available?. This part serves as a theoretical basis for the education programme. The second part of the book includes the activities. The education programme is inspired by the activities like "simple listening", "saying no". Doctoral thesis of Seher Balcı "The Effect of Counselling Skills Education on

University Students' Communication Skills Level" focuses on effective listening and effective responding. These skills are asking appropriate questions, summarizing, paraphrasing, responding with key words, defining the behaviour, words and emotions of the other person and reflecting them, controlling whether they have understood or not, and responding effectively. Mehmet E. Sarıdoğan's" The Effect of Florida Human Relations Skills Model on anxiety, loneliness, entreprising,opening himself, and empathic skills Level" study is designed to help the individuals to be succesful in human relations. This study, especially, adds much about identifying empathy expressions, showing empathy, understanding what opening oneself is, comprehending the positive results of opening oneself and expressing oneself. Martin Orridge's "75 Ways toLiven Up Your Training" and Schilling and Palomores's "50 Activities for Teaching Emotional Intelligence" include the activities concerning human relations and the ones related to emotional intelligence skills. These activities inspired the activities in the education programme.

The sources which were examined in order to determine the objectives of education and preparation of the programme have been influential in generating the activities that take place in educational curriculum. It is started to identify the gathered data, comprehend the data, in other words, each level of education is named. 1. The relationship of the individual with himself/herself 2.The relationship of the individual with the others 3. The activities that will make them like the parts number 1 and 2. First part is divided into subheadings as realizing the emotions, managing the emotions and motivating himself/herself, the relationship of the individual with the others is identified as empathy and controlling the relations. The references that are stated above are used in generating activities which aim the steps of these two objectives.

2.1 The aims of thinking skill of emotional intelligence education

The development of the emotional intelligence is bound to many conditions. This development is observed within the process step by step. There is no connection that not developed emotional intelligence skills cause problems in interpersonal relations. However, emotional intelligence skills have great role over realizing the individual's his/her own feelings, expressing his/her emotions, feeling empathy, and controlling relations. This means that; the sooner the awareness is settled, the more effective the risk of the interpersonal and intrapersonal problems can be prevented. Emotional intelligence skills education targets which are aimed to be acquired by individuals in education sessions and the activities that are going to be performed in these sessions are presented below.

1.   Being aware of the emotions

In order to help individuals to be aware of the emotions;

- Helping to be aware of the emotions;
- Helping to discover the emotions;
- Helping individuals to get to know themselves;
- Noticing the individual and being aware of the emotions about him/her;
- Expressing the emotions verbally and with body language;
- Viewing his/her own emotions;
- Relating the individuals' emotions and thoughts and help them to express;

- Helping the individuals to get to know their emotions about their bodies;
2.   Directing the Emotions

In order to fulfill this;

- Knowing the emotions;
- Reaching the be felt emotion, not the visible one;
- Reacting appropriately in appropriate situation;
3.   Motivating Himself

About the motivation of the individual himself;

- Helping them to discover the emotions that will help them to motivate themselves;
- Not letting emotions prevent their actions in any kind of situation;
- Confermenting themselves morally in any kind of situation:
4.   Empathy
- Improving the skills of listening the individual with sincerity and empathy;
- Thinking like the other individual;
- Understanding the feelings of the other individual;
- Re-delivering the understood emotions to the other individual;
5.   Controlling the Relations

About individuals' control over relations;

- All the relations need to be evaluated;
- The relations can be shaped with the evaluations;
- Comprehending that emotions and reactions control our relations.

2.2 The rules to be obeyed during session

The trainer informs the attendants about the requirements during the practition of the education programme process. These headings are emphasized:

1.   Thinking Skill of Emotional Intelligence Education will take 1 and half hour, be once a week and last 12 weeks;
2.   All the members should attend sessions properly;
3.   During the activities, all the members should attend carefully and actively;
4.   At the end of the activities, the members in education group should tell about their emotions and thoughts easily;
5.   After the activity process, members should listen to each other respectfully;
6.   At the end of the activities, all the members that attend will sit at the same level to see each other and this situation will be agreed.

Each education session is linked to the other session. Because of that it is important to continue the session. Also, the attendants benefit from the information transfer, development of the socializing techniques, learning within individuals by being active in the group. They see that they are not alone, and find the opportunity to share the emotions and ideas in common. There is an equality. With the help of this, the individual experiences the life, realizes, changes and make somebody change it. "Doing together" and "Feeling together" experience help the effectiveness of the education.

2.3 Procedure path

In Thinking Skill of Emotional Intelligence Education, the basis of emotional intelligence is considered. Some important points of this approach are stated below.

- Human nature cannot be understood by abstracting the power of emotions.
- Each emotion in our emotional repertoire has original role.
- Individuals have two kinds of intelligence, one thinks and the other feels. These two completely different comprehension style are in touch with each other to form our intellectual life.
- Emotion adds much to the processing of the rational intelligence, rational intelligence shapes the emotional data and sometimes refuses.
- Each emotion prepares us to act, each of them helps us to put of with the difficulties that are repeated in human life.
- The basis of the emotional intelligence is the individual's being aware of his/her own emotions. (Self-conscious)
- Emotional intelligence is identified as; activating himself/herself, going on in spite of obstacles, controlling the impulsions and delaying the satisfaction, arranging the mood, not letting boredom prevent thinking, showing empathy, and being hopeful.

The researcher , considering these scientific facts, can start applying the Thinking Skill of Emotional Intelligence Education.

First Session

In this session, informing grouping members and helping them get to know each other are planned.

Aim: Informing the group members about the process and and making the members in education group get to know each other.

Environment: The chairs are placed in circle to make the members see each other easily. Chairs do not touch each other and limit the individuals' movements. In order to use for information presentation there is a board.

Procedure: As mentioned in individual interviews beforehand, education group will meet at the same place, same hour and same sitting order, and if needed the activities in sessions can be recorded are expressed and the session starts. In the first session, the strategies that are going to be made use of are told to the individuals. This kind of information is very useful for the individuals that will attend a session for the first time At this stage, the aim of education, rules, the responsibilities and the utilization of the individuals are explained.

Second Session

In this session, Thinking Skill of Emotional Intelligence, there are activities to underline "Being Aware of the Emotions" and improving awareness.

Being aware of the Emotions

The ability to understand the emotions as soon as they come out is the basis of emotional intelligence. Feeling angry to someone and noticing that s/he is angry and saying "I am feeling angry now." are different things. Being aware of the emotions is a conscious state that serves base for improvement of another emotion conscious(Konrad&Hendl, 2001). Actually, all the emotions are impulse for us to move. The ability to be aware of the emotions is a must for psychological intuition and understanding own oneself. It is self-conscious that the individual is aware of what happens in his/her mental world. The mind which has consciousness towards itself, observes and investigates emotions and what has been lived. Self-conscious is not a type of attention mood that is vulnerable to be dispersed by an exaggerated reaction to the intensity of emotions and exaggerating what is perceived. Unlike, it is an objective situation even in hard emotions.

Aim: To discover being aware of the emotions.

Procedure: Group members sit in pairs by facing each other. Firstly, each member identifies two or three things as stated below."I notice that you are sitting opposite of me. I see your face and smile. That you have brown eyes and blonde hair but with brown waves attract my attention. You are sitting on a very old chair there are some pattern on the carpet underneath your chair…"

All the attendants do the same. The aim of this exercise is to notice as much as possible in five-minute time. After five minutes they change their roles and they do the same.

Finally, the attendants are encouraged to talk about their near future plans. Like holidays, weekend holidays, social events. The session is ended with encouraging the attendants to do this practice in their own lives.

Third Session

After talking about the observation of the previous session, the activities concerning the attitude and skills on "Expressing Emotions" take place.

Expressing Emotions

The people who are always in the mood of perceiving himself notice their own emotions as soon as they come out. This gives them the chance to act in the most appropriate way, controlling the emotions and use effectively. What do I feel now? Which emotions does this situation stimulate? the answers given to these questions are the determinant of how the emotions are expressed. When the emotions are told, they become owned. Individuals send emotional signals to the other people and these signals influence others(Goleman, 1996). Telling the emotions is the most significant part of satisfying the needs. The words that describes emotions like happy, excited, sad, worried, anxious, etc. is related to the emotions. The physiological identification of emotional state becomes a part of daily life vocabulary and this is very important in expressing how strong it is felt. Diagnosing the emotions and transmitting them is the most significant part of communication and a side of emotional control (Shapiro, 1997).

Aim: Expressing the individual's true emotions

Procedure: The group leader directs the session to talk about "Expressing Emotions". The individuals are encouraged to discuss these questions:

- Generally, which emotions can you express easily?
- What is the easiness of expressing these emotions to another person?

- Which emotions do you express hardly?

With the help of these, the discussion is directed from general to special and individual. Everybody joins the discussion. A relax and easy atmosphere is created. The reason for this is that if there is hard and emotional atmosphere, the individuals may think to stay away from discussion. Individuals investigate their emotions with discussion technique.

Fourth Session

After sharing ideas about the third session, "expressing ideas" is emphasized, in this session "manipulating the ideas" is presented.

Manipulating the Ideas

Keeping the the emotions under control can be viewed as a recipe of living comfortably in terms of emotion. Very powerful emotions can spoil the balance of the human. Also, just feeling one emotion is harmful,too. Good and bad moods, as long as they are in balance, are the most important elements of human life

Anger is the most outstanding emotion which is hardly manipulated. When people are angry, they have some extreme behaviour, and they become sorry for what they have done. Acting with emotions has three dimensions.

- Uncontrolling
- Extreme and powerful control
- Moderate control

In order to get along with other people, manipulating the emotions is very important. What is important is to find a beneficial and moderate control over the emotions. (Konrad&Hendl, 2001).

Aim: Expressing the emotions through manipulating.

Procedure: People hardly say no. throughout this activity, this problem is handled. The members in the group sit in pair facing each other. Then, one of the members become "yes" man and the other one becomes the "no" man. The pairs sit on yes and no chairs.

By keeping their quietness and by not keeping their quietness in a variety of situation, they make use of yes and no. It is aimed to discover which yes and no is hard to say.

This "yes" and "no" study takes approximately ten minutes during activity. Then, the process (what is felt while doing) and the content (what is talked about while doing) are discussed. This discussion is carried out with daily life examples.

Fifth Session

In the fourth session , the ideas about the previous session were presented and a similar study is planned to support the study on manipulating the emotions.

Aim: To help manipulating emotions animation study will be carried out.

Procedure: What is going to be acted is decided beforehand. Two volunteers are invited. One of the individuals is asked about the emotions when s/he could not manipulate his/he emotions. The told situation is acted in two parts. The other attendants make suggestions to the acting attendant on how to manipulate the emotions. In the second part, they act considering the suggestions of the other members. The ideas about the performance of the members are received. With this activity, the behaviour of telling and doing the things that they cannot do and tell in real life.

What is important for the researcher is to share in this session. Sharing has an important function. Sharing shows the universality of certain emotions, and sharing shows us that an event does not only happen in our own life. During sharing, some members talk about their personal life, there is a chance of catharsis and insight can be viewed (Dökmen, 1995).

Sixth Session

In this session, about the previous session are shared and an activity is planned about manipulating and a closely related item motivating "himself/herself".

Motivating Himself/Herself

The ones who motivate themselves have the desire to face and overcome the obstacles. Motivating himself is needed for gathering emotions for an aim, paying attention, controlling himself and creativity.

The control of stimulation, delaying satisfaction, arranging the emotion situation to help thinking but not preventing it, persevering, making effort, trying again when there is a problem or handling more effectively show the manipulating force of the emotion.

Aim: To observe the motivating of the attendants themselves while they are doing anything.

Procedure: The researcher requires the attendants to sit at a table or take an object with a smooth surface(e.g. a book)each attendant is given a matchstick and required to put them into an order on the table or the surface. The attendants are also required to form four equilateral triangle without breaking these six matchsticks. At the end, there should not be anything except for equilateral triangles. Time is thirty minutes.

At the end of thirty minutes the activity is discussed. During the activity, the individuals will get bored and leave and some of them will continue constantly.

Seventh Session

After discussing the ideas of the previous session, three skills are tried to be handled altogether. These are realizing the emotions, expressing the emotions and intrinsic motivation.

Aim: To enable the attendants to realize and express their own emotions fully and to develop intrinsic motivation.

Procedure: The researcher requires the attendants to develop an "emotion dictionary". Papers and pencils are given to the attendants. They are required to write emotion words they can find in ten-minute time. At the end of the given time, the attendants read the words they have written aloud and the papers are taken back. The common emotion words are eliminated, and the rest is listed on the board. Thus, an "emotion dictionary" is composed with the words that the attendants find.

The researcher tries to make the attendants imitate the words in the dictionary by facial expression, gesture, mimics, and behaviour. In this activity, the researcher tries to provide extrinsic motivation by saying " we can find more emotion words." Or "tell me the emotion word of this behaviour." It is aimed to keep the "we can find." idea alive and make the intrinsic motivation work.

Eighth Session

After discussing the views about the previous session, it is planned to inform about the significant part of the intelligence "empathy".

Empathy

Empathy is putting oneself in other people's shoes and understand his/her emotions and thoughts. The ones who have strong ability for empathy are less prone to aggression and more prone to social behaviour like helping, sharing.

Empathy is not an activity that is only beneficial to the one who is shown empathy. Empathy is also important for the one who shows empathy. The ones who have high empathic skills and aptitude and help people , are most likely to be loved by others (Dökmen, 1994).

Aim: To direct the attendants to put themselves in other people's shoes and think about the empathy skill.

Procedure: This activity is made up of two steps. In the first step, the group is informed about empathy. In the second step, the researcher delivers a piece of paper to each attendant and requires them to write an event as a title they have lived before. These papers are gathered and are put in a bag. The attendants choose papers of the event titles on which their names are not written. Each of them reads the paper and try to guess what s/he may have felt. After telling the ideas, whether the feedbacks are appropriate to the other attendant or not.

Showing empathy supports understanding and being understood emotions ideas are emphasized.

Ninth Session

Based on the empathy study in the eighth session, a similar study will be carried out to develop empathy skill in this session. Because empathy is a comprehensive skill and the thought that it cannot be acquired in two session time, it is aimed to direct the skill of empathic thinking.

Aim: To enable the attendants to realize one another's emotions and develop empathic thought.

Procedure: Group members sit in pairs facing each other. The researcher requires the pairs to talk silently, in order not to make the others hear what they say, with each other for the first six minutes of the ten-minute time. The other member tries to understand his emotions and show empathy. There will be no speech during the rest of the time and each attendant try to guess the emotions and thoughts of the other member. Then, the roles will be changed. At the end of the time, everything will be changed into group order and be discussed.

Firstly, the researcher asks what they have told each other and "what is felt?" thus the process is revised.

Tenth Session

After sharing the comments about the previous session, as it is needed to evaluate the relations of both daily life and the education programme, some activities are planned to develop the skills of controlling the relations for individuals, attendants.

Controlling the Relations

Reading the social and emotional signs, listening, resisting negative effects, viewing from other people's point of view, understanding which behaviour is acceptable in which situation are the abilities that have roles in interpersonal relations.

When the individual comprehends what s/he feels and starts to put up with emotions, it will be possible to understand others' emotions. Each person feels and thinks in a different way. For that reason, the messages that the other people send have great significance. Interpersonal relations are the basis of the society. Especially, the most of the problems of the individuals are the results of the emotions that are not expressed and misunderstanding of these emotions.

Communication is the criteria in interpersonal relations. By analyzing the individual relations, the relations with other people and their relations with him/her can be detected consciously (Jongeward&James, 1993).

Aim: to enable the attendants to say what s/he thinks about the other one at certain times directly and expression of the emotions is emphasized.

Procedure: The attendants sit in pairs facing each other. Each attendant tells his/her thoughts about the other attendant and his relations directly in five-minute time. Then, the roles are changed. The researcher gathers the attendants and requires them to tell what they have felt about their relations as a result of this activity.

Then the researcher invites all of the attendants to consider the relations in their real life.

Eleventh Session

After discussing the opinions about the previous session, a similar study is planned to evaluate relations based on the study of controlling relations.

Aim: To encourage the attendants to evaluate their group work experience.

Procedure: the attendants are required to wait silently and note their reactions within the group. After five minutes, they share their ideas with the group. Each attendants' relation with the group and whether they attend the study or not are discussed. The researcher has attended the study and shared his/her ideas. This activity is a need for a subjective evaluation process.

The attendants in the group evaluate what they feel for each other and for themselves.

Twelfth Session

After discussing the ideas about the previous sessions, an activity is planned to fulfill their desires about this education activity and to complete the missing items by concentrating on the acquired skills.

Evaluation

An evaluation of the education is done with the attendants in this session. "What did they hope?" and "What did they see?" and "what is missing and what are their suggestions?" questions are asked. With the questions similar to these, all the activities are shared that are done during these twelve sessions.

It is aimed to teach the techniques that they are going to use in the education period and improve their emotional intelligence levels of the individuals who attend the Thinking Skill of Emotional Intelligence Education. The techniques like noticing the individuals' own emotions, expressing their opinions, motivation themselves, evaluating the relations and empathy are in the centre of this frame programme.

Thinking Skill of Emotional Intelligence Education is carried out in two different thesis studies on mother and university students proved to be effective. In the first study performed by Yılmaz (2002) the influence on emotional intelligence thoughts is examined. A pretest, posttest model with a control group as study design was used and 10 individuals made up the study group and 10 individuals were in the control group. The mothers attending this study are the ones who have kids between the ages 0-5. The average age of the mother in the experimental group is 29.9 and their marriage periods are between 3-14 years. The average age of mothers in the control group is 30.3 and their marriage period is between 3-12 years. In the experimental group; 7 mothers have one child, 3 mothers have two children, whereas 5 mothers have one child, 4 mothers have 2, and 1 mother have 3 children in the control group. The mothers in each group were educated at high school and university level. Levels of emotional intelligence were assessed by the Emotional Intelligence Scale (Yılmaz & Ergin, 1999). In the data analysis, Mann-Whitney U Test, Wilcoxon Matched-Pairs Signed Ranks Test, and One-Way ANOVA for Repeated Measures were used. Results indicate that the level of emotional intelligence of those who attended the 12-session thinking skill emotional intelligence training program was lower than for those who did not attend this program ($p < .05$). A similar study is performed by Kurt (2007). In this research, Thinking Skill of Emotional Intelligence Education's influence over Guidance and Psychological Counseling Programme students' empathic skill levels. With 20 students control and experimental groups are made. 10 students who are in the experimental group received 1-1,5 hour education during 12 weeks. The attendants are the students of 1st, 2nd, 3rd, 4th grade in Samsun Ondokuz Mayıs University, Faculty of Education, Guidance and Psychological Counselling Department during the 2006-2007 educational term. 20 students who have mentioned that they could attend the sessions properly, are chosen for the study groups considering their scores they got from the test. Total 20 students; 10 for experimental and 10 for control group are chosen to make it appropriate for the group sharing and mutual effect. By the time, this situation is considered, 10 attendants are seen appropriate. In the experimental group; 6 students of 10 students are freshmen, three of them are 2nd graders, one of them is 3rd grader. In the control group; 8 of 10 students are freshmen, 2 of them are 2nd graders. In the experimental group, there are 8 female and 2 male students. In the control group, there are 6 female and 4 male students. Based on the evaluation of the empathic responds, EBÖB-B form is improved and in this form there are 6 problems and 12 empathic responds to these problems. Levels of empathic skill were assessed by the Empathic Skill Scale (B Form) (Dökmen, 1988). According to the statistical analysis, the level of empathic skill of those who attended the 12-session thinking skill emotional intelligence training program was higher than for those who did not attend this program ($p < .05$). The education increased the level of the students' empathic skill levels.

3. Conclusion

We all have different levels of emotional intelligence.the most importat feature of this concept is that it is improvable.however, we are not much aware of it. On the other hand, life and education experiences serve us many opportunuties to improve ourselves. It is an opportunity to think about our experiences and think about them. It is important to think about our experiences and be aware of the emotions that our thoughts have created. These experiences direct our lives. We decide, whether our direction will be positive or negative. Emotional Intelligence is made use of at this level. If we have the courage to improve our emotional intelligence, we know how our thoughts direct our emotions. As aresult of this, we use emotions while we are thinking, deciding, problemsolving, coping with stress and so on. What is important is to let ourselves to be improved. This permission is just letting ourselves to face some new emotion and thought while we are making use of the skills we have gained. This may be one of those enjoyable moments of life. Being open to be improved, learning, transferring what has been learned to life, needing to learn new things, learning more and more, thinking and feeling. In order to gather these experiences, many more education programmes are going to be needed.

Thinking skill of emotional intelligence education is a model that is developed in relation to different explanations of emotional intelligence. This programme which is based on skill education is thought to help the individuals who have difficulty in intrapersonal and interpersonal relations and with the help of teaching the information and the skills of emotional intelligence elements, the interpersonal relations are going to become more qualified. Adults can join this education programme. Being volunteer is compulsory for them to practise activities. Education groups are limited to 10-12 pupils in order for them to have effective communication. Education level of the attendants should be of same level. The discussions that are done in heterogeneous groups may not be effective. Education programme has been prepared in an order but the ones who practise this programme can be flexible and may add or extract items needed. Cultural and ethnical elements should be considered to understand the importance of emotional intelligence concept for further researches. The repetition of this education programme in different populations will make the model stronger. For that reason, the programmes that will develop the emotional intelligence dimensions will add much to their personal developments.

Emotional intelligence concept is a multi-dimensional approach that is suitable to some methods,concepts and educational practice. Educators who discovered emotional intelligence may think that it is just enough to explain this concept. However, experience cannot be underestimated concerning the behaviour change. Just understanding is not enough, but we need to practise. Of course, this education programme will always change. For this reason, I recommend the educators to practise each step of the programme on themselves. Doing this will help to understand the programme better. We can improve our emotional intelligence to have more meaningful relations in our interpersonal relations.

4. References

Ackerman, P. A. & Haggestad, E. D.,(1997) " Intelligence, Personality, and Interest: Evidence for Overlapping Traits", *Psychological Bulletin*, Vol:121, No:2, pp.219-245.

Balcı, S. (1996). "Danışma Becerileri Eğitiminin Üniversite Öğrencilerinin İletişim Beceri Düzeyine Etkisi" *Unpublished Doctorate Thesis, Ondokuz Mayıs University*, Samsun, Turkey.

Bar-On, R. (2006) "The Bar-On model of emotional-social intelligence (ESI)", *Psicothema*. Vol.18, supl., pp. 13-25. www.psicothema.com/pdf/3271.pdf

Brocket, S. & Braun, G., (2000) *Duygusal Zeka Testleri*, : trans: Nurettin Süleymangil, MNS Yayıncılık.

Burnard, P., (1992) *Interpersonal Skills training: Sourcebook of Activities for Trainers*, London, Kogan Page Limited.

Cherniss, C.,(2000) "Emotional Intelligence: What it is and Why it Matters", *Paper presented at the Annual Meeting of the Society for Industrial and Organizational Psychology*, New Orleans, LA, April.

Damasio, A. (1999) *Descartes'in Yanılgısı*, Trans: Bahar Atlamaz, Varlık Yayınları, Sayı:504, p.145

Dökmen, Ü. (1995) *Sosyometri ve Psikodrama*, Sistem Yayıncılık, İstanbul. pp: 165-166.

Dökmen, Ü. (1994) *İletişim Çatışmaları ve Empati*, Sistem Yayıncılık, İstanbul. pp: 137-138.

Ekman, P.&Davidson, R. J. (1994) *The Nature Of Emotion*, Newyork Oxford University Press, p. 16.

Epstein, S. (1998) *Constructive Thinking*, Prager Publishers, p.9.

Goleman, D. (1996) *Why It Can Matter More Than IQ*, Bloomsbury Publishing, p. 43.

Goleman, D. (1999) *Hayati Yalanlar Basit Gerçekler*, Trans: Betül Yanık, Arion, ISBN: 9789755710754, p.114. İstanbul.

Gürün, O.A. (1991) *Psikoloji Sözlüğü*, İnkılap Kitapevi, İstanbul, pp: 149-150,173.

Izard, C. (1989) *Human Emotions*, Plenum Press, Newyork, pp: 2-43.

Jongeward & James, (1993) *Kazanmak için doğarız*, Trans: Tülin Şenruh, İnkılap Kitapevi, 2nd Ed., p.69.

Konrad, S & Hendl, C. (2001) *Duygularla Güçlenmek*, Trans: Meral Taştan, Hayat Yayınları, İstanbul, pp:78-79.

Kurt, G. (2007) . Ondokuz Mayıs Üniversitesi Rehberlik ve Psikolojik Danışma Bölümü Öğrencilerine Verilen Duygusal Zeka Düşünme Becerileri Eğitiminin Empatik Beceri Düzeylerine Etkisi, *Unpublished master thesis, Ondokuz Mayıs University*, Samsun, Turkey.

Lopes, P.N.; Salovey, P & Straus, R. (2003) " Emotional intelligence, personality, and the perceived quality of social relationships", *Personality and Individual Differences*, 35, 641-658.

Mayer, J.D & Salovey, P., (1997) " What is Emotional Intelligence", *Emotional Intelligence: Key Readings on the Mayer and Salovey Model*, In Salovey, P., Brackett, M.A. & Mayer, J.D., (Eds.), (2004), *Emotional Intelligence: Key Reading on the Mayer and Salovey Model*, Newyork: Dude Publishing, pp: 29-59.

Mayer, J.D.; Salovey, P. & Caruso, D.R. (2000) "Emotional Intelligence as Zeitgeist, as Personality, and as a Mental Ability", The Handbook of Emotional Intelligence, Sanfrancisco: Jossey-Bass, a Wiley Company, pp: 92-117.

Mayer, J.D.; Salovey, P. & Caruso, D.R. (2004) "Emotional Intelligence: Theory, Findings, and Implications", *Psychological Inquiry*, Vol.15, No.3, 197-215.

Mayer, J.D.; Roberts, R.D. & Barsade, S.G. (2008) "Human Abilities: Emotional Intelligence", *Annu. Rev. Psychol.* 59: 507-536. http://psych.annualreviews.org

Merlevede, P.E.; Bridoux, D. & Vandamme, R. (2001) *7 Steps to Emotional Intelligence*. Crown House Publishing Limited. ISBN: 1899836500.

Oneil, J. (1996) "On Emotional Intelligence: A Conversation with Daniel Goleman", *Educational Leadership*, Vol:54, No:1, pp:6-11.

Orridge, M. (1998) *Eğitimlerinizi Canlandırmanın 75 Yolu*, Trans: Osman Akınhay, Sistem Yayıncılık.

Ortony, A.; Clore, G.L. & Collins, A. (1998) *The Cognitive Structure of Emotions*, Cambridge University Press, p.178.

Pincus, D. (1992) *Manners Matter Activities to Teach Young People Social Skills*, Carthage, IL: Good Apple.

Salovey, P. & Mayer, J.D., (1990) " Emotional Intelligence", *Imagination, Cognition, and Personality*, 9(3), pp: 185-211.

Salovey, P.; Mayer, J.D.& Caruso, D. (2000) The positive psychology of emotional intelligence. In *The Handbook of Positive Psychology*, C.R. Snyder & S. J. Lopez (Eds.) New York: Oxford University Press.

Salovey, P. & Sluyter, D. (1997) *Emotional Development And Emotional Intelligence: Educational Implications*. Basic Books.

Sardoğan, M.E. (1998) "Florida İnsan ilişkileri Becerileri Eğitimi Modelinin Grup Üyelerinin Kaygı, Yalnızlık, Atılganlık, Kendini Açma ve Empatik Beceri Düzeylerine Etkisi" *Unpublished Doctorate Thesis, Ondokuz Mayıs University*, Samsun, Turkey.

Schilling, D. & Palomares, S. (1996) *50 Activities for Teaching Emotional Intelligence*, Innerchoice Publication.

Shapiro, L. (1997). *Yüksek EQ'lu Bir Çocuk Yetiştirmek*, Trans: Ümran Kartal, Varlık Yayınları, İstanbul, pp:235-238.

Simmons, S. & Simmons, J.C. (1997). *Measuring Emotional Intelligence: The Groundbreaking Guide to Applying the Principles of Emotional Intelligence*. The Summit Publishing Group, Arlington, Texas.

Ülgen, G. (1995). *Eğitim Psikolojisi*, Bilim Yayınları, Ankara, pp:21-29.

Warwick, J. & Nettelbeck, T. (2004). " Emotional intelligence is…?", *Personality and Individual Differences*, 37, 1091-1100.

Weisinger, H. (1998). *İş Yaşamında Duygusal Zeka*, Trans:Nurettin Süleymangil, MNS Yayıncılık, p.13.

Yavuz, K.E. (2002) *7-12 Yaş Dönemi Çocuklarda Duygusal Zeka Gelişimi*, Özel Ceceli Okulları Eğitim Dizisi, No:4, p.13.

Yeşilyaprak, B. (2001) "Duygusal Zeka ve Eğitim Açısından Doğurguları" *Kuram ve Uygulamada Eğitim Yönetimi*, Yıl:7, Sayı: 25, pp:139-146.

Yılmaz, M. (2002) Duygusal Zeka Düşünme Becerileri Eğitiminin Annelerin Duygusal Zeka Düzeylerine Etkisi, *Unpublished Doctorate Thesis, Ondokuz Mayıs University*, Samsun, Turkey.

15

How to Influence the New Technologies in the Emotional Intelligence and Communication of Higher Education Student

Carmen Maria Salvador Ferrer
Unversity of Almería
Spain

1. Introduction

Throughout this chapter we will study how new technologies influence, used as basic tools in the university education system, in the emotional domain and communication skills of college students. To do this, we will, first, detailed analysis of two separate terms, to pass, expose the data in an empirical study conducted with a sample of university students. We hope that when the reader is immersed in the next chapter not only understand in detail the terms, but at the same time, find the content of that chapter of social relevance. Finally, the ultimate purpose is to invite readers to reflect on what happened in the new system of university education.

1.1 Emotional intelligence

In our view, emotional intelligence (ie), marks the way we relate to and understand the world (Salvador, 2010). This is a personal characteristic that takes into account the attitudes, feelings and, at the same time, includes skills like impulse control, self-awareness, self-motivation, confidence, enthusiasm and empathy, or ultimately feel sorry. From our humble view, one can consider the action necessary to provide, among other things, our largest professional services.

Emotional Intelligence, although it is present, it is in our view a clear precursor to the concept of Social Intelligence of a psychologist Edward Thorndike (1920), who defined it as the ability to understand and manage men and women, boys and girls, and act wisely in human relations. For Thorndike, in addition to social intelligence, there are two types of intelligence: the ability to handle abstract-ideas-and mechanical-ability to understand and manage objects.

This idea of a double intelligence Thorndike initially launched reflects the duality that is present in humans. Surely, the reader has ever tried has felt growing inside an emotion and at the same time, tried to reason so that does not dominate and take actions that make you regret later. However, this type of situation illustrates well the internal conflicts that we can feel when they are in control of emotions and reason. It is said, usually, that man is a reasonable, but we know that at the same time, sensitive and emotional. Sketching, we could say we have two brains, one emotional and one rational.

These two forms of intelligence seem to be related to two different mind styles. Thus, roughly as we might say that there are two types, a rational mind (works using approximations and assumptions, it is logical and pragmatic, perceive things and integrates them into a coherent and structured) and the other the emotional mind (fully irrational beliefs by taking their absolute truth and rejects everything that could otherwise). In general, a mind is responsible for thinking and feeling another. The rational mind is the way to understanding that we are typically conscious, more prominent in terms of reflective consciousness, able to analyze and meditate. But alongside this there is another system of knowledge, impulsive and powerful, although sometimes ideological: The emotional mind. These two minds fair operating in harmony, so the most part, interweaving different forms of knowledge to guide us in the world. Usually there is a balance between emotional and rational mind, which feeds and informs the emotion operations input power of emotions. However, the emotional mind and the rational mind are semi-independent powers and also reflect the operation of a separate circuit for interconnected in the brain.

As recorded by Salvador (2010), emotional intelligence could be described as emotional competence measures the ability to understand, process, control and express social and emotional aspects of our lives. In this sense, the degree to which we are capable of doing so is essential to productivity and life satisfaction. Furthermore, studies show that people find very productive workplace, and satisfied with life does not depend on the academic, emotional domain but with people (Goleman, 1995, Heath, 1991). Therefore, in our view, emotional competence is the ability to understand and express the emotional and social aspects of our lives. It is, therefore, conscious capacity, that is, thinking in one's mind, let´s think about the feelings, the more precise, we feel we feel. In this line, Salovey and Meyer (1990) define emotional intelligence as a set of skills used to assess fairly and express our own emotions and those of others and to use our feelings to motivate, plan and carried out full life. In this sense, the features that come to highlight these authors are (Salovey and Meyer, 1990):

1. *Knowing one's emotions*, it is self-consciousness, that is, recognizing a feeling as it occurs.
2. Improve emotions could be understood as controlling the feelings that are appropriate, which requires self-awareness.
3. *Control one's emotions*, understand and manage emotions in the service of a goal to pay attention to self-motivation and mastery, and at the same time for creativity.
4. *Recognizing emotions in others*. Empathy is the fundamental skill of the people. Individuals who display this predisposition are often more sensitive to social cues that indicate what others need.
5. *Manage emotions*, it is understood how to master the emotions of others.

One of the pioneers in the field of emotional intelligence testing has been Bar-On. Bar-On (1997) adds that emotional intelligence is an important factor in determining one's ability to succeed in life, to cope with everyday situations and get along with the world. In this regard, as noted by Bar-On (2006) the skills that comprise emotional intelligence and directly influence social welfare. Thus, Bar-On has developed a theoretical framework of social and emotional intelligence consists of five factors (intra-personal, interpersonal, adaptability, stress management and general mood) that constitute the EQ-i inventory.

Petrides and Furnham (2001), following the principles offered by Bar-On, conducted an investigation which shows that emotional intelligence should be understood as a set of skills and self-perceived characteristics. These results lead the authors to coin the term emotional self-efficacy. Of this work shows significant results for the scientific community in the first place, it is stated that there are few studies looking at emotional intelligence as an element related to personality traits and skills. For example, points out that the only study that meets these requirements is performed by Davies, Stankov y Roberts (1998). Second, Petrides and Furnham (2001) indicate that emotional intelligence should know the first to know the personality traits to pass, then the analysis of cognitive abilities. In this sense, these authors make the following taxonomy (adaptability, assertiveness, emotional assessment or perception of oneself and of others, emotional expression, emotional management of others, emotional regulation, low impulsivity, relationship skills, self esteem, motivation, social competence, stress management, empathy, trait, trait happiness, optimism, trait).

Goleman (2001), for its part, says that among the characteristics of emotional intelligence are some skills that allow us to motivate ourselves and to preserve the face of frustration, control our impulses and put ourselves in position to vary our sources of gratification; regulate our moods and acting, avoiding stress affects us. It's about being empathetic and to wait in life. According to Goleman (2001), the emotionally developed, ie the people who govern their emotions properly and also know how to interpret and interact effectively with the others emotion enjoy an advantage in all domains life. These people often feel more satisfied, are more effective and better able to master the mental habits that determine productivity. Customers, however, can't control his emotional life, are discussed in constant infighting that undermine their ability to work and prevents them from thinking clearly enough.
In summary, emotional intelligence is a learned skill that humans have that allows you to know and understand both their own emotions and those of others. This is without a doubt, an essential aspect of social-occupational adaptation of the person and at the same time, it is essential to the development and personal wellbeing.

As we have been saying, emotional intelligence is essential not only for the welfare of the individual but also to facilitate social integration. It is, in our view, a basic tool that significantly influenced even communication skills. We may consider that effective communication is related to emotional control. Roughly speaking, we could say that understanding and controlling our emotions during the speech communication, while understanding the emotions of the recipient is a key to the success of the message (Lillis and Tian, 2009).

1.2 Communication

Communication is a key event in our lives broadly speaking we could say that interpersonal communication is crucial to ensuring stability and individual survival (Mañas and Salvador, 2009). With it, we can get to know people, ie we find out what people think, feel and do. Personal dialogue is the most frequent way to exchange ideas, phrases and feelings, therefore, without it would be virtually impossible to achieve a deep knowledge about people. The media, as Mañas and Salvador (2009), can be defined as the exchange of information between sender and receiver and the interference (perceived) in meaning between them. The analysis of this exchange reveals that communication is a two way process elements linked in a row. In a generic sense, communication can be considered as one of the basic processes of any system of interaction. Following this line, the communication could be categorized as a dynamic process fundamental to the existence, growth, change and behavior of all systems of interaction, whether individual or collective-organized-(Thayer, 1975). In this vein, makes sense to argue that communication through people establish functional relationships that allow them to work together and achieve their intended goals. It therefore seems logical to assume that the communication process is not simple and, moreover, it involved a heterogeneous set of elements.

As pointed Mañas and Salvador (2009), effective communication can be altered by a number of factors that pose a barrier to the flow of communication. Undoubtedly, the most hinders the whole process is noise, which interferes with the accurate transmission and reception of the message. In addition, there are can highlight other barriers such as those of process, personal, physical and semantic (Munduate and Riquelme, 1994).

The obstacles to the transfer process can distort the meaning on all levels of the communication cycle mentioned above (for example, receive incorrect information, use a language not known, choose inappropriate means, etc.). For its part, the personal barriers are very heterogeneous, in which we would highlight: the ability to communicate effectively, how people process and interpret the information, the level of interpersonal trust between sender and receiver, skills communication, the natural tendency to evaluate or judge a message, and the ability to listen with understanding. As far as physical barriers are concerned, we would like to highlight the distance between sender and receiver because, as you can imagine, it is difficult to communicate with a person who is nine or ten feet away without using additional accessories to facilitate communication flow. Finally, semantic barriers shown in the form of encoding and decoding errors, since it is the communication phases that are transmitted and received symbols and words.

In summary, this communication process is becoming increasingly important in the existence and stability of the organization. In this sense, today, communication becomes a cornerstone for the survival of the institution, why then we will stop at a deeper analysis of it.

The application of new communication technologies is called electronic communication (Defever, 1991). Specifically, is defined as the discipline that deals with the use of electronic media in the activities of companies and organizations. Electronic communication allows more efficient communication and offers new possibilities for interaction, especially reducing the limitations of other forms of communication coming to alter the structure of the communication process by eliminating or reducing the limitations of spatial, temporal and social, connecting people in two different locations. The electronic media bring to the traditional media new opportunities to communicate, a more immediate contact, faster and richer returns (feedback) and increase the chances of interaction. Thus, the electronic media contribute to making the organization more available, providing new forms of relationships with stakeholders and interest groups.

In a sense, the Internet has disrupted many of the paradigms so far helped us to understand the processes of public communication media. In what follows, by way of summary, we highlight the ten paradigm shifts that lead to the e-communication, the new media landscape that emerges with Red (Orihuela, 2002): the user at the heart of the communication process, content vector media identity, universal multimedia, real-time requirement, the wealth management information, the disintermediation of communication processes, the emphasis on access to systems, the various dimensions of interactivity, hypertext as a grammar of the digital world and the appreciation of knowledge over information.

The new public communication scenarios posed by the Internet are to be interpreted as an opportunity to redefine the profile and professional requirements and the contents and procedures of their academic training. The media used are no longer the distinguishing factor of the profession, since all the carriers merge into the Red-and once again emerge as a differentiating factor content of identity and quality. However, it would make sense to consider how far this new road development affects personal communication, or whether the use of virtual communication impact in some way in basic skills for socio-professional integration of the individual.

1.3 New framework for teaching; European Higher Education area -EES-

The functions that the authors have proposed the possibilities that media vary considerably, ranging from those authors who limit their use to a few of them, even those who greatly expanded its field of action. For its part Aparici and Davis (1992) speak of four major functions and uses the media can play: a) use of media players such as transmitters, models, norms and stereotypes, from a technical perspective; b) critical use that uses the media to reflect on society and its environment; c) playful and creative use of media to children and acquire different codes and can be expressed with them, and finally, d) use more complete than unify the previous perspectives. In this line, Rowntree (1991), to analyze the functions that the media plays in self-instruction, the concrete in the following: a) To attract the interest of students; b) Make it easier to remember learning; c) Encourage new learning; d) Justify and provide learning; e) Get the student to actively address; f) Providing rapid and specific feedback to their responses; g) To encourage the practice and review; and h) To assist students in their own progress.

For his part, Martinez (1995), points between the functions of the media: a) serve as a resource to improve and maintain the motivation of learning; b) function carries information or content; c) methodological guide the learning process; d) be a means of expression of the pupil. In another angle, as indicated by Cebrian (1992), raising the curriculum integration is to recognize the possibilities that have the means to act in the curriculum as: a) academic content structure; b) solidified the curriculum in practice; c) interpreter and signifiers of the curriculum; d) of professional development facilitators; e) Cause and effect for educational innovation; f) Representatives of legitimate content; g) drivers of the curriculum established and h) exemplifies teaching models and learning.

As Toffler (1985), complex organizations, such as universities, change significantly when three conditions are met: significant external pressure, people who are members dissatisfied with the existing order and presented in a coherent alternative plan, model or vision. So, like any organization that seeks quality, the university, to carry out real change and real innovation processes should provide, first, attention to environment and messages. The changes are affecting higher education institutions can´t be understood without reference to the context of changes that occur in different orders and that constitute the external pressure:

1. The changes in the way of organizing the university fostered by the European Higher Education, the teaching approaches in relation to powers, ECTS, etc.
2. The changes brought by ICT.
3. Changes in knowledge (in the generation, management and distribution of it).
4. The changes in the student, in the city, in what may be a person trained today, and so on.

As noted by Salinas (2004), the innovation processes concerning the use of ICT in university teaching often start with, most of the time, the availability and existing technology solutions. However, a balanced view of the phenomenon should lead to the integration of technological innovations in the context of the tradition of our institutions, institutions that do not forget, have an important educational function. We consider the idiosyncrasies of each of the institutions to integrate information and knowledge technologies (ICT) in higher education processes, too, that the dynamics of society can leave the sidelines.

In summary, we could understand that new technologies bring to education with a triple function, namely, informative, motivating and informative. It is, therefore, three basic pillars of development and human training, in our view, must be in the same proportion, ie, computer media should not only be motivating, but they should also contribute to the formation students. It is therefore imperative that academic institutions should be relaxed and develop ways of integrating information technology and communication in the formation processes (Salinas, 2004).

1.4 Objectives

From our humble view, we consider that college students succeed in their training cycle, in particular, and in your work setting, more broadly, it is essential to have excellent communication skills and optimal emotional domain. However, the new higher education system is part of the use of technologies there is little empirical evidence to demonstrate how this new way of teaching impact in individual variables (communication and emotional control).

In this sense, the fundamental objective of this work is an empirical approach to study new technologies in the context of higher education. In particular, interested in knowing to what extent the use of new technologies affect the communication process and the emotional domain. Thus, we propose the following *hypothesis*:

1. New technologies applied to the framework of Higher Education have basic effects on the emotional domain and communication.
2. We hope that the use of new technologies present a negative impact on the knowledge of others' emotions and emotional control.
3. We believe that the use of new technologies in the context of Higher Education had a negative impact on communication styles.

1.5 Method

1.5.1 Participants

This research presents a descriptive and cross, consisting of a total of 92 first-year university students (52% men and 48% female), aged 18-25 years (mean 20 and standard deviation of 4). For the most part, use new media technology such as mobile phone, chat, video games, among others. In addition, the average time used in these items is more than 20 hours per week, in regard to video games, 30 hours a week to chat, etc. All indications, then, that our university students are immersed in the culture of new technologies. However, as noted earlier, this new dynamic of interaction has been transferred to the classroom. This implies that the dynamics of classes using a computer platform (Web-Ct) to facilitate teacher-student interaction and at the same time, student-student. This is a computer system where, in addition to link tasks, assessment tasks, there are windows of interaction of the type chat, forum, e-mail. The number of weekly hours that students spend on this platform is 20 hours per week.

1.5.2 Instrument

The instruments used were previously adapted to Spanish, through a process of expert validation. The following table shows the characteristics of the scales and the most relevant psychometric properties of instruments used:

Emotional intelligence. This instrument includes all the items used to assess emotional intelligence, from the two traditional tools, as in Castilian (Salvador, 2008). In this sense, the total number of questions on this scale amounts to 53 which assesses the degree of agreement on a Likert scale of 5 points, indicating the value 1 "complete disagreement" and the value 5 to the contrary. The reliability coefficient in this case was .90.

Communication. The scale used was Communicative Competence Scale (Rubin, Palmgren and Sypher, 1994), which measures the ability to choose among the available communication behaviors to achieve their own interpersonal goals during an encounter, keeping your face and the line of interactants colleagues within the constraints of the situation. The analysis yielded a Cronbach alpha score of .93.

1.5.3 Procedure

The questionnaire was filled in anonymously and voluntarily. One researcher was responsible for overseeing the procedure, to ensure that there were no problems. After finishing the procedure of collection of data will be passed to the analysis of the data. This was done in SPSS 18 for Windows.

1.6 Results

We explored the correlation matrix of Pearson, noting the relationship in the direction indicated by the hypotheses, being most significant (see Table 1). After analysis of the correlation matrix provides preliminary support the proposed hypotheses. Thus, intra-dimensional analysis of the dimensions that make up emotional intelligence, it should be noted that the relationship shows a higher score is the one between IE i.e. self-knowledge and management (r =. 687, significance =. 001), followed by IE i.e. self-management and self-knowledge (r =. 588, significance =. 001). Similarly, it would make sense to highlight the lack of relationship between self-management and IE knowledge.

	Communication	I.E. Self-Knowledge	I.E. Self-Management	I.E. Knowledge	I.E Management
Communication	--				
I.E. *Self-Knowledge*	-.27(**)	--			
I.E. Self-Management	.94(**)	.55(**)	--		
I.E. Knowledge	-.89(**)	.30(**)	-.00	--	
I.E Management	-.34(**)	.69(**)	-.20(**)	.39(**)	--

P=.001(**); p=.05(*)

Table 1. Correlation matrix of the study (N = 92)

Finally, when analyzing the relationship between communication and integrate the different dimensions of emotional intelligence (self-knowledge, self-management, knowledge management), we found that all relationships are statistically significant. However, this section would be pointless to note that in most cases the relationships that emerge have a negative sign. In particular, the positive relationship is the couple that emerges from self-management, communication (r=.935, significance=.001). With respect to the negative relationship, we find that the communication is related to IE knowledge management and self- knowledge IE (r=-.886, r=-.344, r=-.265, significance =.001; respectively). In short, these data indicate that our youth are characterized by deficits in communication and poor emotional skills.

2. Discussion and conclusions

The main objective of this study was to determine whether college students are immersed in the culture of new technologies have emotional control and communication skills. The results show that, in general terms, the objective has been covered. In more detail, we could say that the first scenario, where we predicted that new technologies used in the context of Higher Education have crucial effects on emotional control and communication, is fulfilled. Even more broadly appreciated that all college students have certain weaknesses in communication and at the same time, some deficits in the emotional domain, especially in understanding the feelings of others. Regarding the second scenario, where we hoped that the use of new technologies present a negative impact on the knowledge of others' emotions and emotional control, it is confirmed. Specifically, the data show no correlation between knowledge of the emotions of others and self-management.

Finally, the third hypothesis, we estimated that the use of new technologies in the context of higher education had a negative impact on communication styles, is also confirmed. Specifically, the findings show that college students have poor communication skills.

Thus, in view of the findings, we note also that the greater emotional self-management, interpersonal communication. Similarly, it should be noted that the higher the self-knowledge, the lower the communication. In another angle, the findings appear to indicate that the greater understanding of the emotions of other, lower communication and, finally, the higher is the domain of the emotions of others, the lower the communication. In conclusion, it is interesting to note two additional results.

On the one hand, they seem to have predictive power of new technologies on communication skills and emotional intelligence. On the other hand, the great impact that the efforts and fate of emotional control. This indicates that if we train students in mastering their emotions and their communication skills should take into account new technologies. In summary, the results show that the use of virtual systems streamlines education, although this innovative teaching-learning method has some negative consequences for students. Thus, broadly speaking, the data from our research shows that students learn computer skills, but lack other skills. Specifically, the paper presents certain shortcomings and also the emotional domain. Being a bit more precise, the weakness in the emotional control is achieved in understanding the feelings of others.

In a sense, these results would demonstrate that ICTs are not a panacea and not a "silver bullet" in the education system. Yet this is not to deny the relevance of showing the same, but on the contrary, we come to say that ICTs are a way more in the process of teaching and, contrary to popular belief, are not the only way of teaching.

We, too, emphasized the integral role of education, therefore we believe that ICTs can help the education system. As they tell (Cabero, Castaño, Cebreiro, Gisbert, Martinez, Morales, Prendergast, Romero and Salinas, 2003) education can't be excluded from the development of new information technologies, arguing several reasons. On the one hand, new media form a new society that the education system will serve. And, moreover, the system always uses the media used in social communication, and now this happens, among other things, the use of telecommunication networks. It would, therefore, to understand ICT as a challenge in the education system.

However, given its exploratory nature, the results of this study should be interpreted with caution because our work is not without limitations. We might note that probably the most important is inherent to the study, brought about mainly by the sample size. Another disadvantage is the time to carry out the collection of data, exactly what we mean is that the results were obtained in a single moment in time which could interfere with the relationships found between variables. Therefore, we emphasize the need to continue working in this line, with the main purpose of deepening the concept of emotional intelligence, focusing our attention at the traits of personality and cognitive abilities.

So, it is important in *future research* that this find be replicated with more comprehensive constructs. To our knowledge, and following the arguments of Perez, Petrides and Furnham (2007), it is necessary to progress in research, breaking with the belief still exists that emotional intelligence is a unitary construct. Another relevant question refers to the elements of emotional intelligence. Similarly, as demonstrated in this paper, need to further deepen the relationship IE and new technologies, with the main purpose of achieving personal well-being and socio-cultural integration.

3. References

Aparicio, R. and Davis, B. (1992). Education in the media. In VARIOUS: *European conference about information technology in education: A critical insight.* Barcelona: TIE Congress, 546-556.

Bar-On, R. (1997). *The emotional inventory (EQ-I): Technical manual.* Toronto: Multi-health Systems.

Bar-On, R. (2006). The Bar-On model of emotional-social intelligence. *Psicothema,* 18, 13-25.

Cabrero, J. Castaño, C. Cebreiro, B., Gisbert, M., Martínez, F., Morales, J. Prendergast, M.P., Romero, R. and Salinas, J. (2003). New technologies in university activities. *Pixel-Bit. Media and Education Magazine,* 20, 81-100.

Cebrian, M. (1992). *Television: Believe to see. The credibility of children for television.* Málaga: Anydamar.

Davies, M., Stankov, L. y Roberts, R.D. (1998). Emotional intelligence: in search an elusive construct. *Journal of Personality and Social Psychology,* 75, 989-1015.

Goleman, D. (1995). *Emotional intelligence.* Barcelona: Kairos.

Goleman, D. (2001). An EI-Based theory of performance. In Cherniss, C. and Goleman, D. (Eds). *The Emotionally Intelligent Workplace: How to select for, measure, and Improve Emotional Intelligence in Individuals, groups, and Organizations.* San Francisco, CA: Jossey-Bass, págs.27-44.

Heath, D.H. (1991). *Fulfilling Lives: Paths to maturity and success.* San Francisco: Jossey-Bass.

Lillis, M. and Tian, R.G. (2009). Cross-cultural communication and emotional intelligence. Inference from case studies of gender diverse groups. *Marketing Intelligence & Planning,* 27, 3, 428-438.

Mañas, M.A. and Salvador, C. (2009). Communication in organizations. In Rodriguez, A. (Ed.), *Psychology of groups and organizations.* Madrid: Piramide.

Martínez, F. (1995): Culture, media and education. In Ballesta, J. (Cood), *Teaching with the media.* Barcelona: PPU Diego Marín, 11-30.

Munduate, L. and Riquelme, J.M. (1994). *Conflict and negotiation.* Madrid: Piramide.

Pérez-González, J.C., Petrides, K.V., and Furnham, A. (2007). La medida de la inteligencia emocional rasgo. En J. M. Mestre y P. Fernández-Berrocal, *Manual de Inteligencia Emocional* (pp. 81-97). Madrid: Pirámide.

Petrides, K.V. y Furnham, A. (2001). Trait emotional intelligence: Psychometric investigation with reference to established trait taxonomies. *European Journal of Personality,* 15, 425-448.

Rowntree, D. (1991): *Teaching Through Self-instruction,* London: Kogan Page.

Rubin, R. B., Palmgren, P., & Sypher, H. E. (1994*). Communication research measures: A sourcebook.* New York: Guilford Press.

Salinas, J. (2004). Educational innovation and the use of ICT in university education. *Journal of University and Knowledge Society,* 1, 1.

Salovey, P. and Mayer, J. D. (1990). *Emotional intelligence. Imagination, cognition and personality.* New York, vol. 9, No. 3, pp. 185-211.

Salvador, C. (2010). *Transcultural analysis of emotional intelligence.* University of Almería: Publishing Service.

Thayer, L. (1975). *Communication and communication systems.* Barcelona: Ediciones Peninsula.

Thorndike, E. L. (1920). *Intelligence and Its uses. Harper's Magazine.* New York, Jan., No. 140, pp. 227-35.

Toffler, A. (1985). *The Adaptive Corporation.* New York: McGraw Hill.

Permissions

The contributors of this book come from diverse backgrounds, making this book a truly international effort. This book will bring forth new frontiers with its revolutionizing research information and detailed analysis of the nascent developments around the world.

We would like to thank Dr. Annamaria Di Fabio, for lending her expertise to make the book truly unique. She has played a crucial role in the development of this book. Without her invaluable contribution this book wouldn't have been possible. She has made vital efforts to compile up to date information on the varied aspects of this subject to make this book a valuable addition to the collection of many professionals and students.

This book was conceptualized with the vision of imparting up-to-date information and advanced data in this field. To ensure the same, a matchless editorial board was set up. Every individual on the board went through rigorous rounds of assessment to prove their worth. After which they invested a large part of their time researching and compiling the most relevant data for our readers. Conferences and sessions were held from time to time between the editorial board and the contributing authors to present the data in the most comprehensible form. The editorial team has worked tirelessly to provide valuable and valid information to help people across the globe.

Every chapter published in this book has been scrutinized by our experts. Their significance has been extensively debated. The topics covered herein carry significant findings which will fuel the growth of the discipline. They may even be implemented as practical applications or may be referred to as a beginning point for another development. Chapters in this book were first published by InTech; hereby published with permission under the Creative Commons Attribution License or equivalent.

The editorial board has been involved in producing this book since its inception. They have spent rigorous hours researching and exploring the diverse topics which have resulted in the successful publishing of this book. They have passed on their knowledge of decades through this book. To expedite this challenging task, the publisher supported the team at every step. A small team of assistant editors was also appointed to further simplify the editing procedure and attain best results for the readers.

Our editorial team has been hand-picked from every corner of the world. Their multi-ethnicity adds dynamic inputs to the discussions which result in innovative outcomes. These outcomes are then further discussed with the researchers and contributors who give their valuable feedback and opinion regarding the same. The feedback is then collaborated with the researches and they are edited in a comprehensive manner to aid the understanding of the subject.

Apart from the editorial board, the designing team has also invested a significant amount of their time in understanding the subject and creating the most relevant covers. They scrutinized every image to scout for the most suitable representation of the subject and create an appropriate cover for the book.

The publishing team has been involved in this book since its early stages. They were actively engaged in every process, be it collecting the data, connecting with the contributors or procuring relevant information. The team has been an ardent support to the editorial, designing and production team. Their endless efforts to recruit the best for this project, has resulted in the accomplishment of this book. They are a veteran in the field of academics and their pool of knowledge is as vast as their experience in printing. Their expertise and guidance has proved useful at every step. Their uncompromising quality standards have made this book an exceptional effort. Their encouragement from time to time has been an inspiration for everyone.

The publisher and the editorial board hope that this book will prove to be a valuable piece of knowledge for researchers, students, practitioners and scholars across the globe.

List of Contributors

Adrian Furnham
Research Department of Clinical, Educational and Health Psychology, University College London, UK

Annamaria Di Fabio
Department of Psychology, University of Florence, Italy

Reuven Bar-On
University of Texas Medical Branch, USA

Michel Hansenne
University of Liège, Department of Psychology, Belgium

Hui-Wen Vivian Tang
Department of Applied English, Ming Chuan University, Taoyuan, Taiwan

Mu-Shang Yin
Department of Travel Management, Hsing Wu Institute of Technology, Taipei, Taiwan

Reza Gharoie Ahangar
Department of Management and Economics, Science and Research Branch, Islamic Azad University, Iran

Laban Peter Ayiro and James K. Sang
Department of Educational Management and Policy Studies, Moi University, Eldoret, Kenya

Antti Syväjärvi and Marko Kesti
University of Lapland, Rovaniemi, Finland

Ilkay Ulutas and Esra Omeroglu
Department of Early Childhood, Development and Education, Gazi University, Ankara, Turkey

Barbara B. Meyer, Susan E. Cashin and William V. Massey
University of Wisconsin, Milwaukee, USA

Roisin P. Corcoran and Roland Tormey
Yale University, USA
École Polytechnique Fédérale de Lausanne, Switzerland

Gladys Shuk-fong Li, Wei Ting Li and Hsiu Hua Wang
Department of Athletic Sports, National Chung Cheng University, Taiwan

Claudia S. P. Fernandez, Herbert B. Peterson and AnnaMarie Connolly
The University of North Carolina at Chapel Hill, USA

Shelly W. Holmström
The University of South Florida, USA

Müge Yılmaz
Ondokuzmayıs University, Turkey

Carmen Maria Salvador Ferrer
Unversity of Almería, Spain

Printed in the USA
CPSIA information can be obtained
at www.ICGtesting.com
JSHW011501221024
72173JS00005B/1166